Nurse's
Clinical
Guide

W9-BSJ-961

HEALTH
ASSESSMENT

SECOND EDITION

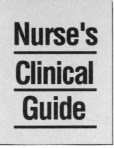

HEALTH
ASSESSMENT

SECOND EDITION

Patricia Gonce Morton, RN, PhD
Associate Professor
Graduate Program in Trauma and Critical Care Nursing
University of Maryland, Baltimore

Springhouse Corporation
Springhouse, Pennsylvania

STAFF

Executive Director, Editorial
Stanley Loeb

Senior Publisher, Trade and Textbooks
Minnie B. Rose, RN, BSN, MEd

Art Director
John Hubbard

Editor
Nancy Priff (senior editor), Mary Hohenhaus Hardy

Clinical Consultant
Patricia Dillon, RN, MSN

Associate Acquisitions Editor
Betsy K. Snyder

Copy Editor
Debra Davis

Editorial Assistant
Louise Quinn

Designers
Stephanie Peters (associate art director), Elaine Ezrow, Laurie Mirijanian

Typography
Diane Paluba (manager), Elizabeth Bergman, Joyce Rossi Biletz, Phyllis Marron, Robin Mayer, Valerie L. Rosenberger

Manufacturing
Deborah Meiris (director), Anna Brindisi, Kate Davis, T.A. Landis

Printed in the United States of America.
ISBN 0-874340-704-1
CGHA2E-011094

A member of the Reed Elsevier plc group

Library of Congress Cataloging-in-Publication Data

Nurse's clinical guide to health assessment / [edited by] Patricia Gonce Morton. – 2nd ed.
   p. cm.
   Rev. ed. of: Nurse's clinical guide – health assessment / Patricia Gonce Morton. c1990.
   Includes bibliographical references and index.
   1. Nursing assessment. 2. Physical diagnosis.
I. Morton, Patricia Gonce, 1952- Nurse's clinical guide – health assessment. II. Title: Health assessment.
   [DNLM: 1. Nursing Assessment – handbooks. 2. Physical Examination – nurses' instruction. 3. Physical Examination – handbooks. WY 39 N97347 1994]
RT48.M68 1995
616.07′5 – dc20
DNLM/DLC   94-28318
ISBN 0-87434-704-1   CIP

TABLE OF CONTENTS

GUIDE TO ILLUSTRATIONS

ADVISORY BOARD

CONTRIBUTORS

Linda S. Baas, RN, PhD, CCRN
Assistant Professor, College of Nursing
and Health, University of Cincinnati

Marie Scott Brown, RN, PhD, PNP
Professor of Family Nursing, School of
Nursing, Oregon Health Sciences
University, Portland

Karen E. Burgess, RN, MSN
Research Assistant, University of
California, Los Angeles

Kathryn J. Conrad, RN, MSN, OCN
Clinical Director, Cancer Education
Resources and Services, Pittsburgh Cancer
Institute

Joan Corder-Mabe, RN,C, MS, OGNP
Nurse Practitioner, Kaiser Permanente,
Springfield, Va.

Patricia Dillon, RN, MSN
Assistant Professor, Gwynedd Mercy
College, Gwynedd Valley, Pa.

Linda L. Grabbe, RN, PhD
Health Policy Analyst, ABT Associates,
Cambridge, Mass.

Linda Brune Haas, RN, MN, CDE
Endocrinology Clinical Nurse Specialist,
Department of Veterans Affairs Medical
Center, Seattle

Marcia Jo Hill, RN, MSN
Nursing Manager, The Methodist
Hospital, Houston; Assistant Clinical
Professor, Department of Dermatology,
Baylor College of Medicine, Houston

Roxana Huebscher, RN, PhD, FNP-C
Assistant Professor, University of
Wisconsin College of Nursing, Oshkosh

JoAnn Hungelmann, RN, DNSc
Community Volunteer Project with Older
Adults, Milwaukee

Karen A. Landis, RN, MS, CCRN
Pulmonary Clinical Nurse Specialist,
Lehigh Valley Hospital, Allentown, Pa.

Margaret Massoni, RN,CS MSN
Assistant Professor, The College of Staten
Island, City University of New York

Elizabeth D. Metzgar, RN,C, MPH, FNP
Assistant Professor, Community Health
Nursing, College of Nursing, Montana
State University, Missoula

Patricia Gonce Morton, RN, PhD
Associate Professor, Graduate Program in
Trauma and Critical Care Nursing,
University of Maryland, Baltimore

Catherine Paradiso, RN,CS, MS, CCRN
Instructor, Hunter-Bellevue College of
Nursing, Brookdale Health Science
Center, New York

Ann E. Rogers, RN, PhD, ACP
Assistant Professor, School of Nursing,
University of Michigan, Ann Arbor

Regina Shannon-Bodnar, RN, MS, MSN, OCN
Clinical Manager, Oncology, Greater
Baltimore Medical Center

Julia L. Swager, RN, MSN
Medical-Surgical Clinical Nurse
Specialist, Memorial Hospitals
Association, Modesto, Calif.

Susan Heidenwolf Weaver, RN, MSN,
CCRN, CNA
Assistant Director of Nursing, St. Clares-
Riverside Medical Center, Denville, N.J.

Ellis Quinn Youngkin, RN,C, PhD, OGNP
Associate Professor, School of Nursing,
Medical College of Virginia, Virginia
Commonwealth University, Richmond

FOREWORD

The nurse who practices in this era of health care reform must be able to perform efficient, knowledgeable, and accurate assessments in any setting. Because of budget constraints in hospitals and other acute care settings, the nurse must be able to assess clients quickly, yet competently. In home health care and similar settings, the nurse must be prepared to evaluate clients who are sicker than in the past because of earlier discharge from hospitals. And in settings that focus on health and wellness, the nurse is becoming more of a primary care provider, making assessment skills more critical than ever. Consequently, an in-depth knowledge of assessment procedures — and the rationales behind them — now is expected of all practicing nurses.

For these reasons, *Nurse's Clinical Guide to Health Assessment, Second Edition,* puts all the assessment information a practitioner will need in one convenient book. This comprehensive, yet portable, guide is perfectly suited to today's practical nursing needs and busy clinical settings. Easy to carry, hold, and consult, it also presents information clearly and directly.

In keeping with its comprehensiveness, this guide takes a holistic approach to nursing assessment, showing how to evaluate physiologic systems as well as aspects of life that affect physiologic function, such as activities of daily living, sleep and eating patterns, cultural heritage, and developmental status.

Among its many features are:
• a brief, illustrated review of pertinent anatomy to help focus assessment on appropriate body systems or structures
• health history questions and rationales specific to the client's reason for seeking care
• detailed physical assessment guidelines, including many step-by-step illustrated procedures and checklists of helpful assessment reminders
• a summary of common laboratory studies and their normal values
• clear descriptions of common normal and abnormal assessment findings

• special assessment considerations that accommodate the client's cultural heritage or physical and emotional development
• sample documentation of assessment findings using the SOAPIE format.

This Second Edition is longer than its predecessor and offers several new and easy-to-use features: a guide to illustrations; updated suggested readings; the North American Nursing Diagnosis Association's latest taxonomy; a comprehensive listing of common laboratory tests, including abnormal results and possible causes; and a glossary of terms.

Used as a practical clinical reference or as a source for learning and practicing assessment skills, *Nurse's Clinical Guide to Health Assessment, Second Edition,* will function as one of the clinician's most valuable tools. It provides everything needed for competent, caring assessment of clients in any setting.

Marie Scott Brown, RN, PhD
Professor of Family Nursing
School of Nursing
Oregon Health Sciences University
Portland

PREFACE

Every nurse – whether neophyte or expert practitioner – needs top-notch assessment skills, because assessment forms the basis for all the other nursing process steps and ultimately helps determine all client care.

To help its reader obtain or refine these vital assessment skills, *Nurse's Clinical Guide to Health Assessment, Second Edition,* describes how to conduct informative health history interviews, perform effective physical assessments, and interpret laboratory studies accurately. Written by and for nurses, this expanded edition also explains how to analyze assessment data, formulate nursing diagnoses, and document all findings appropriately. Perhaps of greatest appeal to today's nurse is having a handy, pocket-sized, highly readable, extensively illustrated, and extremely well-organized assessment guide.

Throughout its four units, *Nurse's Clinical Guide to Health Assessment, Second Edition,* takes a holistic health-oriented approach to assessment. Unit One reviews basic assessment skills. Chapter 1, which tells how to interview clients and gather health history data, highlights psychosocial and cultural influences on health. Chapter 2 describes how to use equipment and perform basic physical assessment techniques.

In Unit Two, Chapter 3 explores assessment of activities of daily living and sleep patterns, and Chapter 4 explains how to evaluate nutritional status.

Unit Three details assessment of specific body systems and structures, including the urinary, immune, and endocrine systems – a particular strength of this guide. For each aspect of the assessment, chapters describe normal – and abnormal – findings. When appropriate, they also present cultural and developmental considerations.

In Unit Three, each chapter begins with an illustrated overview of anatomy. Then it presents all three sections of the health history: health and illness patterns, health promotion and protection patterns, and

role and relationship patterns. It continues with physical assessment, including a list of applicable equipment and assessment techniques, descriptions of specific assessment procedures, and illustrations of various steps and techniques. Each chapter also describes common laboratory studies and, when appropriate, advanced assessment skills. It concludes with an example of SOAPIE documentation.

Three recurring features help focus the reader's attention in these chapters:
• *Assessment checklist* prepares the nurse to perform the physical assessment by asking for answers to several important questions.
• *Common laboratory studies* identifies commonly ordered laboratory tests and their normal values.
• *Selected nursing diagnosis categories* supplies the most recent NANDA nursing diagnosis categories typically used for each body system assessment.

Unit Four details these special assessments:
• comprehensive head-to-toe assessment, which may be performed when a new client seeks care or when a known client requests an annual checkup.
• partial assessment, which is used when time is limited or when the client does not need or cannot tolerate a complete assessment
• perinatal and neonatal assessments, which usually are performed in family planning, maternity, neonatal, and other settings.

New for this edition, a guide to illustrations helps the nurse locate specific illustrations more quickly than ever. A list of updated suggested readings ends every chapter. Also, two new appendices and a master glossary enhance this edition and make it easier to use.

Users of this current, accurate, and quick reference will have in hand all that they need to assess clients with skill and confidence.

Patricia Gonce Morton, RN, PhD

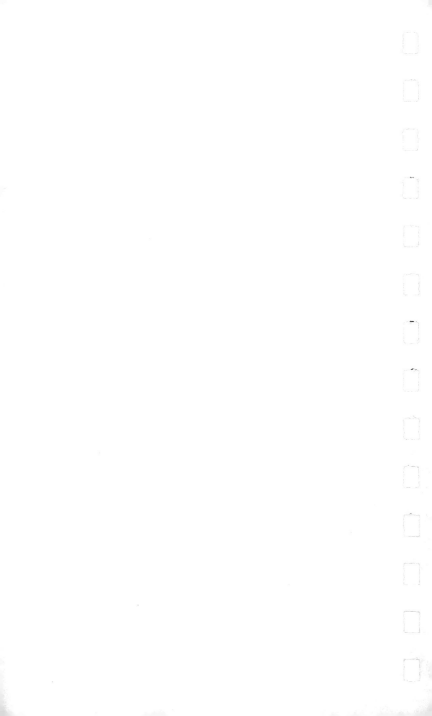

UNIT ONE

Reviewing Assessment Skills

1

The Health History ∎

The health history, the major subjective data source about a client's health status, provides insights into actual or potential health problems. A guide to subsequent physical assessment, the health history organizes pertinent physiologic, psychological, cultural, and psychosocial information; relates to the client's current health status; and accounts for such factors as life-style, family relationships, and cultural influences.

DEVELOPING INTERVIEWING SKILLS

To obtain an accurate health history, the nurse needs a basic knowledge of pathophysiology and psychosocial principles, of interpersonal and communication skills, and of the "therapeutic use of self." The following paragraphs provide guidelines for a successful interview.

Nurse-client communication

Effective health interviews require good communication and interpersonal skills. The interview is a nurse-client dialogue, not a simple question-and-answer session. The nurse can overcome common barriers to effective communication, including emotional or cultural biases, by developing self-awareness and acceptance of different life-styles. Self-awareness—recognizing and accepting one's feelings, beliefs, and values, including personal biases, strengths, and weaknesses—allows the nurse to communicate more effectively with others, which is important in obtaining accurate, unbiased information.

The nurse's personal health and experiences can influence the therapeutic effectiveness of the nurse-client relationship.

Effective interview skills rely on nonverbal as well as verbal communication. Be aware of such nonverbal communications as eye movements, facial expressions, body gestures, and posture. Disparities between the client's words and actions may provide important insights.

Therapeutic use of self

Using personal skills in a healing way to help the client is "therapeutic use of self." Central to this concept is self-awareness, which permits approaching a client with empathy and acceptance, and establishes the open, nonthreatening environment needed to obtain a more accurate health history. Three important techniques enhance a nurse's therapeutic use of self: exhibiting empathy, demonstrating acceptance, and giving recognition.

Empathy, the capacity for understanding another's feelings, helps establish a trust-based relationship and encourages the client to share personal information. To show empathy, use phrases that address the client's feelings; for example, "That must have upset you."

Accepting the client's verbal and nonverbal communication is crucial to a successful interview. Acceptance does not signify

The nursing health history

The nursing health history provides subjective data about the client as a person. The list below includes all the components of a comprehensive nursing health history.

1. BIOGRAPHICAL DATA

Name; address; telephone number; contact person; sex; age and birth date; birthplace; Social Security number; race, nationality and cultural background; marital status and names of persons living with the client; education; religion; occupation.

2. HEALTH AND ILLNESS PATTERNS

- Reason for seeking health care
- Current health status
- Past health status
- Family health status
- Status of physiologic systems
- Developmental considerations

3. HEALTH PROMOTION AND PROTECTION PATTERNS

- Health beliefs
- Personal habits
- Sleep and wake patterns
- Exercise and activity patterns
- Recreational patterns
- Nutritional patterns
- Stress and coping patterns
- Socioeconomic patterns
- Environmental health patterns
- Occupational health patterns

4. ROLE AND RELATIONSHIP PATTERNS

- Self-concept
- Cultural and religious influences
- Family role and relationship patterns
- Sexuality and reproductive patterns
- Social support patterns
- Other psychosocial considerations

5. SUMMARY OF HEALTH HISTORY DATA

agreement or disagreement with the client; rather, it demonstrates an effort to remain neutral and nonjudgmental. Neutral statements ("I hear what you are saying," "I see") show acceptance. Nonverbal behaviors, such as nodding or making momentary eye contact, also provide encouragement without indicating agreement or disagreement. However, the "right" words may be useless if nonverbal communication, such as rigid posture or an uninterested look, reveal different feelings.

Put the client at ease during the interview by recognizing the client's communication efforts. To give recognition, listen actively to what the client says, occasionally providing verbal or nonverbal acknowledgment to encourage the client to continue speaking.

Client's expectations

Personal values and previous experiences with the health care system can affect the client's health history expectations.

Help the client clarify expectations, concerns, and questions. If possible, provide answers that rectify client misconceptions appropriately. A client may be uncomfortable providing personal information; reassure the client that the information is confidential and accessible only to authorized health care professionals. Affirm that, legally, no information can be released to any person or organization without the client's written consent.

Behavioral considerations

Encounters with a hostile or angry client occur occasionally. To maintain control of the interview, do not waste time or energy arguing or feeling insulted. Rather, listen without showing disapproval. Try to relax. Speak in a firm, quiet voice and use short sentences. Avoid abstract ideas or detailed explanations. A composed, unobtrusive, and nonthreatening manner usually soothes the client. However, if this technique fails, postpone the interview and call for assistance, if needed.

Cultural and ethnic considerations

A client's cultural and ethnic background can have a subtle and complex effect on the health history interview. Culture refers to an integrated system of learned behavior patterns that are characteristic of members of a society and are not biologically inherited. Ethnicity is an affiliation with a group of people classified according to a common racial, national, religious, linguistic, or cultural origin or background.

A person's culture and ethnicity affect beliefs, values, attitudes, and customs. They also help shape educational, occupational, and familial opportunities and expectations. Culture also affects the way a person experiences health and illness. The degree of these effects depends on whether the client has undergone acculturation (modification caused by contact with another culture) or assimilation (loss of cultural identity when an individual becomes part of a different, dominant culture).

Avoid stereotyping a client based on cultural background. Although a client may share certain characteristics with others of the same culture, the client will also exhibit individual differences. You should respect cultural factors and individual differences that influence the client's habits, beliefs, and attitudes about health care. Concentrate on developing the client's trust in and rapport with you.

Effective interviewing techniques

To obtain the most benefit from a health history interview, the nurse should try to make the client feel comfortable, respected, and trusting. The nurse should use effective interviewing techniques to help the client identify resources and improve problem-solving abilities. Remember, however, that successful techniques in one situation may not be effective in another, depending on your attitude and the client's interpretation of your questions. Examples of effective interviewing techniques follow.

Offering general leads. General questions give the client an opportunity to speak freely. Such questions as "What brought you here today?" or "Are you concerned about any other things?" direct the client to discuss the most significant concerns.

Restating. To help clarify what the client means, restate the essence of a client's comments.

Reflection. This technique gives the client an opportunity to reconsider a response and add information.

Verbalizing the implied. Stating what is implied or unspoken sometimes helps interpret a client's statement accurately or yields additional insight into a client's symptoms or concerns.

Focusing the discussion. To help the client identify significant health concerns, focus on important discussion points.

Sequencing the problem. To identify a problem, determine its course, and draw a conclusion, define the time limits and other factors associated with the problem by asking, "What events led to this?" or "Did this happen before or after (another event)?"

Encouraging client participation. This technique affirms the client's individual value by encouraging the expression of opinions, concerns, or doubts.

Encouraging client evaluation. Promote the client's cooperation in developing a health care action plan by actively encouraging comments on implementation strategies. This technique ensures greater client compliance, leading to a desired outcome.

Clarification. Because many variables affect the interview and because interpretations of health behaviors or symptoms vary, you may have to clarify meanings. Admitting, for example, "I'm not sure what you mean," or clarifying a particular symptom or concern prevents misunderstandings.

Presenting reality. When a client makes unrealistic statements or exaggerates, presenting reality usually encourages the client to reevaluate and modify statements.

Making observations. Observing the client helps you interpret and validate nonverbal behavior. Observations may increase the client's situational awareness and suggest possible alternatives, or open new areas for discussion.

Giving information. Share information and facts with a client to encourage direct involvement in health care decisions.

Using silence. Silence sometimes lets the client reorganize thoughts and consider what to say next, while allowing you an opportunity to observe. Although long silences can be awkward, avoid saying something just to reduce anxiety. Using silence effectively is a crucial skill; it can even convey empathy.

Summarizing. To help clarify information and ease the transition between health history sections, provide a brief summary after each major health history component.

Interviewing techniques to avoid

The following interviewing techniques may create communication problems between nurse and client, and thus should be avoided.

Asking how or why. A question that begins with *why* or *how* may be perceived as a threat or a challenge because it forces the client to justify feelings and thoughts. Some clients feel they should invent an answer if they do not have one. "Why" questions may also be difficult for clients who lack specific knowledge or are unaware of a crucial fact.

Using probing, persistent questioning. This style of questioning usually increases client discomfort, creates defensive feelings, and makes the client feel manipulated. One or two attempts to elicit information about a particular topic are sufficient.

Using inappropriate language. Do not block communication by using technical jargon or abstract terms that are inappropriate for the client's developmental level, education, or background. Clients may perceive this as an unwillingness to share information or an attempt to hide something from them.

Be sure to phrase questions appropriately, based on the client's age, education, and background.

Giving advice. Sharing personal experiences or opinions and giving advice imply that you know what is best for the client— the opposite of collaborating with and encouraging the client to participate in health care decisions. Frequently, a client who asks for advice has already made a decision and wants a sounding board for ideas.

Giving false assurances. Glib statements and false reassurances, such as "Everything will be fine," devalue a client's feelings and communicate a lack of sensitivity. Avoid offering false reassurance to relieve your anxiety if you are unable to help the client.

Changing the subject or interrupting. These techniques prevent the client from completing a thought and shifts the conversation's focus. Such behavior indicates a lack of empathy. Also, by interrupting the client's idea flow, you may confuse the client. Wait until the client completes a thought before clarifying a relevant point.

Using clichés. Avoid using phrases such as, "You'll feel better in the morning," or "Where there's life there's hope." These phrases may make the client feel uncomfortable or disappointed, and they may discourage the client from expressing genuine feelings.

Giving excessive approval. Telling the client that a response is particularly good implies that an opposing response is bad. Similarly, excessive agreement may make the client feel that modifying information is wrong. Also, excessive approval or agreement may be perceived as phoniness, or it may set narrow limits on other client responses by encouraging answers that will gain approval. Of course, the nurse can approve of or agree with a client's statements or thoughts. However, the agreement or approval should be appropriate—not excessive.

Jumping to conclusions. Premature interpretations and hasty conclusions invite inadequate or inaccurate information.

Using defensive responses. A client may express anger and frustration about a treatment program or health care facility with a verbal attack. Realize that a defensive response from you will imply that the client has no right to express such feelings or opinions, which may increase the client's anger.

Making too many literal responses. A client who cannot state feelings directly may use figurative language with hidden meanings. If you respond literally to such statements, you will lose an opportunity to explore a client's real feelings. To avoid misunderstandings, always base your responses on the client's affect and the conversational context.

Asking leading questions. By its phrasing, a leading question suggests the "right" answer. This type of question may force the client to supply a socially acceptable response rather than an honest one. For example, the question "You've never had a venereal disease, have you?" may force the client to answer "No."

CONDUCTING THE INTERVIEW

During the interview, the physical surroundings can directly affect the client's comfort and willingness to provide accurate information. A private room with a door helps ensure freedom from interruptions. An arrangement of comfortable chairs facing but slightly offset from each other creates a friendly feeling. Position the chairs 1 to 4 feet apart to facilitate eye contact and hearing. However, if the client seems to feel this is uncomfortably close, increase the distance.

The interview structure

Ideally, the interview includes an introductory phase, a working phase, and a termination phase. Each requires a different communication style to establish the proper tone and provide transition to the next phase.

In the *introductory phase*, use nonprobing, client-centered questions and comments to put the client at ease and to explain the health history purpose and desired outcome. Begin by introducing yourself. Show the client where to sit, establish an interview time frame, and ask if the client has any questions about the interview procedure. Spend a few minutes chatting informally before starting the working phase.

Obtain detailed health history information in the *working phase* of the interview. Temper the natural impulse to take interview notes by recognizing that lengthy note-taking may distract the client, who may wonder if you are listening. If you must take notes, tell the client before the interview starts. Experience will show how to compile pertinent information immediately after the interview and organize the final form later.

The health history ends with the *termination phase*. Provide a smooth closing by summarizing salient interview points, informing the client about the interview results, explaining how the physical assessment will be conducted, and discussing follow-up plans.

OBTAINING HEALTH HISTORY DATA

Modify the health history structure to meet the client's current health status. For example, if the client is moderately or acutely ill, collect pertinent medical information first. Do the less-structured, more-time-consuming interview parts last, or postpone them until the client feels better.

Major health history components include biographic data, health and illness patterns, health promotion and protection patterns, role and relationship patterns, and a summary of health history data.

Biographical data

The first information gathered in a complete health history, biographic data identify the client and provide important sociocultural information. Record the following information:

- client's full name
- current address

Symptom analysis

When assessing a client with a symptom or health concern, the nurse uses a symptom analysis to help the client describe the problem fully. (A condition the client perceives subjectively is a *symptom;* a condition the examiner perceives objectively is a *sign.*) A method for obtaining a systematic and thorough assessment, the symptom analysis is easy to remember with the mnemonic device PQRST. The following questions serve as a guide to effective symptom analysis.

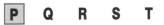

PROVOCATIVE OR PALLIATIVE
What causes the symptom? What makes it better or worse?
• First occurrence. What were you doing when you first experienced or noticed the symptom? What seems to trigger it: stress? position? certain activities? arguments? (For a physical symptom such as a discharge: What seems to cause it or make it worse? For a psychological symptom: Does the depression occur when you feel rejected?) What relieves the symptom: changing diet? changing position? taking medication? being active?
• Aggravation. What makes the symptom worse?

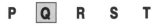

QUALITY OR QUANTITY
How does the symptom feel, look, or sound? How much of it are you experiencing now?
• Quality. How would you describe the symptom—how it feels, looks, or sounds?
• Quantity. How much are you experiencing now? Is it so much that it prevents you from performing any activities? Is it more or less than you experienced at any other time?

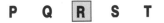

REGION OR RADIATION
Where is the symptom located? Does it spread?
• Region. Where does the symptom occur?
• Radiation. In the case of pain, does it travel down your back or arms, up your neck, or down your legs?

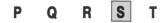

SEVERITY SCALE
How does the symptom rate on a severity scale of 1 to 10, with 10 being the most extreme?
• Severity. How bad is the symptom at its worst? Does it force you to lie down, sit down, or slow down?
• Course. Does the symptom seem to be getting better, getting worse, or staying about the same?

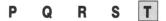

TIMING
When did the symptom begin? How often does it occur? Is it sudden or gradual?
• Onset. On what date did the symptom first occur? What time did it begin?
• Type of onset. How did the symptom start: suddenly? gradually?
• Frequency. How often do you experience the symptom: hourly? daily? weekly? monthly? When do you usually experience it: during the day? at night? in the early morning? Does it awaken you? Does it occur before, during, or after meals? Does it occur seasonally?
• Duration. How long does an episode of the symptom last?

- telephone number
- contact person
- sex
- age and birth date
- Social Security number
- place of birth
- race, nationality, and cultural background
- marital status and names of any persons living with the client
- education
- religion
- occupation.

Health and illness patterns

This section of the comprehensive health history includes the client's reason for seeking health care; current, past, and family health history; status of physiologic systems; and developmental considerations.

Health promotion and protection patterns

What a client does (or does not do) to stay healthy is affected by such factors as health beliefs, personal habits, sleep and wake patterns, exercise and activity, recreation, nutrition, stress and coping, socioeconomic status, environmental health patterns, and occupational health patterns. Although data will overlap, be sure to assess all (or most) elements, depending on the client.

Role and relationship patterns

A client's role and relationship patterns reflect the client's psychosocial health (psychological, emotional, social, spiritual, and sexual development). To assess role and relationship patterns, investigate the client's self-concept, cultural influences, religious influences, family role and relationship patterns, sexuality and reproductive patterns, social support patterns, and other psychosocial considerations.

Summary of health history data

Conclude the health history by summarizing all findings. For the well client, list the client's health promotion strengths and resources along with defined health education needs. If the interview points out a significant health problem, tell the client what it is and what to do about it.

Occasionally, the client's health history indicates an immediate need for referral to a physician or psychotherapist. Inform the client about any concerns and the reason for them based on the health history. Then make plans with the client about the referral. Offering to set up the appointment for the client increases the likelihood of compliance. Always conclude the interview by giving the client an opportunity to have the last word: "Should we talk about anything else?" or "Do you have any information you want to add or questions you want to ask?"

Assessing the family

Assessment of how and to what extent the client's family has fulfilled and does fulfill its functions is an important part of the health history. The nurse should assess the family into which the client was born (family of origin) and, if different, the current family.

Use these guidelines to assess how the client perceives family functions. Because the questions target a nuclear family—that is, mother, father, and children—they may need modification for single-parent families, families that include grandparents, elderly clients who live alone, or unrelated individuals who live as a family.

Affective function

Assessing how family members feel about, and get along with, each other provides important information. In some families, one person performs the "sick role," and the other family members support the illness and keep the member sick. For example, a child whose parents have marital problems may be sick to get attention. The parents may allow the child to be sick so they can focus their attention on the child and avoid dealing with their problems.

To assess affective function, ask the following questions:
- Do family members regard each other positively?
- How do the members of your family treat each other?
- How do the members of your family regard each other's needs and wants?

(Text continues on page 12.)

Assessing physiologic systems

When assessing a client's health and illness patterns, the nurse asks selected questions about the function of each body system. Use the phrases below as guidelines for the questions, and perform a symptom analysis on any reported symptoms.

GENERAL HEALTH STATUS

☐ Unusual symptoms or problems
☐ Excessive fatigue
☐ Inability to tolerate exercise
☐ Number of colds or other minor illnesses per year

☐ Unexplained episodes of fever, weakness, or night sweats
☐ Impaired ability to carry out activities of daily living (ADLs)

SKIN, HAIR, AND NAILS

☐ Known skin disease, such as psoriasis
☐ Itching
☐ Skin reaction to hot or cold weather
☐ Presence and location of scars, sores, ulcers
☐ Presence and location of skin growths, such as warts, moles, tumors, or masses
☐ Color changes noted in any of the above lesions

☐ Changes in amount, texture, or character of hair
☐ Presence or development of baldness
☐ Hair care practices, including frequency of shampooing, permanent, or hair coloring
☐ Changes in nail color or texture
☐ Excessive nail splitting, cracking, or breaking

HEAD AND NECK

☐ Lumps, bumps, or scars from old injuries
☐ Headaches (Perform a symptom analysis.)
☐ Recent head trauma, injury, or surgery
☐ Concussion or unconsciousness from head injury
☐ Dizzy spells or fainting

☐ Interference with normal range of motion
☐ Pain or stiffness (Perform a symptom analysis.)
☐ Swelling or masses
☐ Enlarged lymph nodes or "glands"

NOSE AND SINUSES

☐ History of frequent nosebleeds
☐ History of allergies
☐ Postnasal drip
☐ Frequent sneezing
☐ Frequent nasal drainage (Note color, frequency, and amount.)

☐ Impaired ability to smell
☐ Pain over the sinuses
☐ History of nasal trauma or fracture
☐ Difficulty breathing through nostrils
☐ History of sinus infection and treatment received

MOUTH AND THROAT

☐ History of frequent sore throats—especially streptococcal (Perform a symptom analysis.)
☐ Current or past mouth lesions, such as abscesses, ulcers, or sores
☐ History of oral herpes infections
☐ Date and results of last dental examination
☐ Overall description of dental health

☐ Use of proper dental hygiene, including fluoride toothpaste, where applicable
☐ Use of dentures or bridges
☐ Bleeding gums
☐ History of hoarseness
☐ Changes in voice quality
☐ Difficulty chewing or swallowing
☐ Changes in ability to taste

continued

Assessing physiologic systems continued

EYES

- ☐ Date and results of last vision examination
- ☐ Date and results of last check for glaucoma (for clients over age 40 or with a family history of glaucoma)
- ☐ History of eye infections or eye trauma
- ☐ Use of corrective lenses
- ☐ Itching, tearing, or discharge (Note color, amount, and time of occurrence as well as treatment received.)
- ☐ Eye pain; spots or floaters in visual field
- ☐ History of glaucoma or cataracts
- ☐ Blurred or double vision
- ☐ Unusual sensations, such as twitching
- ☐ Light sensitivity
- ☐ Swelling around eyes or eyelids
- ☐ Visual disturbances, such as rainbows around lights, blind spots, or flashing lights
- ☐ History of retinal detachment
- ☐ History of strabismus or amblyopia

EARS

- ☐ Date and results of last hearing evaluation
- ☐ Abnormal sensitivity to noise
- ☐ Ear pain
- ☐ Ringing or crackling in the ears
- ☐ Recent changes in hearing ability
- ☐ Use of hearing aids
- ☐ History of ear infection
- ☐ History of vertigo
- ☐ Feeling of fullness in the ear
- ☐ Ear care habits, including use of cotton-tipped swabs for ear wax removal
- ☐ Ear wax characteristics
- ☐ Number of ear infections per year for pediatric clients

RESPIRATORY SYSTEM

- ☐ History of asthma or other breathing problem (Perform a symptom analysis.)
- ☐ Chronic cough (Perform a symptom analysis.)
- ☐ History of coughing up blood
- ☐ Breathing problems after physical exertion
- ☐ Sputum production (Note color, odor, and amount.)
- ☐ Wheezing or noisy respirations
- ☐ History of pneumonia or bronchitis

CARDIOVASCULAR SYSTEM

- ☐ History of chest pain
- ☐ History of palpitations
- ☐ History of heart murmur
- ☐ History of irregular pulses
- ☐ Hypertension
- ☐ Need to sit up to breathe, especially at night
- ☐ Coldness or numbness in extremities
- ☐ Color changes in fingers or toes
- ☐ Swelling or edema in extremities
- ☐ Leg pain when walking; relieved by rest
- ☐ Hair loss on legs

BREASTS

- ☐ Date and results of last breast examination (including baseline mammography for women between ages 35 and 40)
- ☐ Pattern of breast self-examination
- ☐ Breast pain, tenderness, or swelling (Perform a symptom analysis.)
- ☐ History of nipple changes or nipple discharge (Note color, odor, amount, and frequency.)
- ☐ History of breast-feeding

Assessing physiologic systems continued

GASTROINTESTINAL SYSTEM

☐ Indigestion or pain associated with eating (Perform a symptom analysis.)
☐ History of ulcers
☐ History of vomiting blood
☐ Burning sensation in windpipe
☐ Frequent nausea and vomiting (Perform a symptom analysis.)
☐ History of liver disease, jaundice

☐ History of gallbladder disease
☐ Abdominal swelling or ascites
☐ Changes in bowel elimination pattern
☐ History of diarrhea or constipation
☐ History of hemorrhoids
☐ Use of digestive aids or laxatives
☐ Date and results of last Hemoccult exam (for clients over age 40)

URINARY SYSTEM

☐ Painful urination
☐ Characteristics of urine and pattern of urination
☐ Hesitancy in starting urine stream
☐ Changes in urine stream
☐ History of kidney stones
☐ History of flank pain
☐ Blood in urine

☐ History of decreased or excessive urine output
☐ Dribbling, incontinence, or stress incontinence
☐ Frequent urination at night
☐ History of bladder, kidney, or urinary tract infections

FEMALE REPRODUCTIVE SYSTEM

☐ Menstrual history, including age of onset, duration, and amount of flow
☐ Date of last menstrual period
☐ Painful menstruation
☐ History of excessive menstrual bleeding
☐ History of missed periods
☐ History of bleeding between periods
☐ Date and results of last Pap smear
☐ Obstetrical history (for women of childbearing age), including number of pregnancies, miscarriages, abortions, live births, and stillbirths
☐ Satisfaction with sexual performance
☐ History of painful intercourse
☐ Contraceptive practices
☐ History of sexually transmitted disease
☐ Knowledge of how to prevent sexually transmitted disease, including acquired immunodeficiency syndrome (AIDS)
☐ Problems with infertility

MALE REPRODUCTIVE SYSTEM

☐ Presence of penile or scrotal lesions
☐ Prostate problems
☐ Pattern of testicular self-examination
☐ Satisfaction with sexual performance
☐ History of venereal disease

☐ Contraceptive practices
☐ Knowledge of how to prevent sexually transmitted disease, including AIDS
☐ Concern about impotence or sterility

NERVOUS SYSTEM

☐ History of fainting or loss of consciousness
☐ History of seizures or other nervous system problems; use of medication for seizure control
☐ History of cognitive disturbances, including recent or remote memory loss, hallucinations, disorientation, speech and language dysfunction

☐ History of sensory disturbances, including tingling, numbness, sensory loss
☐ History of motor problems, including problems with gait, balance, coordination, tremor, spasm, or paralysis
☐ Interference by cognitive, sensory, or motor symptoms with ADLs

continued

Assessing physiologic systems continued

MUSCULOSKELETAL SYSTEM

☐ General health status
☐ History of fractures
☐ Muscle cramping, twitching, pain, or weakness (Perform a symptom analysis.)
☐ Limitations on walking, running, or participating in sports
☐ Joint swelling, redness, or pain
☐ Joint deformity

☐ Joint stiffness, including time and duration
☐ Noise with joint movement
☐ Spinal deformity
☐ Chronic back pain (Perform a symptom analysis.)
☐ Musculoskeletal-related interference with ADLs

IMMUNE SYSTEM AND BLOOD

☐ History of anemia
☐ History of bleeding tendencies
☐ History of easy bruising
☐ History of low platelet count
☐ History of becoming easily fatigued
☐ History of blood transfusion
☐ History of allergies, including eczema, hives, and itching
☐ Chronic clear nasal discharge

☐ Frequent sneezing
☐ Conjunctivitis
☐ Interference of allergies with ADLs
☐ Usual method for treating allergic symptoms
☐ History of frequent unexplained systemic infections
☐ Unexplained gland swelling

ENDOCRINE SYSTEM

☐ History of endocrine disease, such as thyroid problems, adrenal problems, or diabetes
☐ Unexplained changes in height or weight
☐ Increased thirst
☐ Increased urinary output

☐ Increased food intake
☐ Heat or cold intolerance
☐ History of goiter
☐ Unexplained weakness
☐ Previous hormone therapy
☐ Changes in hair distribution
☐ Changes in skin pigmentation

• How are feelings expressed in your family?
• Can family members safely express both positive and negative feelings?
• What happens in the family when members disagree?
• Do family members deal with conflict in a constructive manner?

Socialization and social placement

These questions provide information about the flexibility of family responsibilities, which is helpful for planning a client's discharge. For example, a mother of small children who has just had major surgery may need household help when she goes home, if the husband is not expected to help or does not want to.

To assess socialization and social placement, ask the following questions:
• As a couple, are you satisfied with your role and your spouse's role as a spouse and a parent?
• Do you and your spouse agree about how to bring up the children? If not, how do you work out differences?
• Who is responsible for taking care of the children?
• How well do you feel your children are growing up?
• Are family roles negotiable within the limits of age and ability?

• Do you share cultural values and beliefs with the children?

Health care function

This assesssment will uncover many cultural beliefs. Identify the family caregiver and then use that information when planning care. For example, if the client is the caregiver, then the client may need household help when discharged.

To assess health care function, ask the following questions:

• Who takes care of family members when they are sick? Who makes doctor appointments?

• Are your children learning skills, such as personal hygiene, healthful eating habits, and the importance of sleep and rest?

• Can your family adjust to your being ill and unable to care for them?

Family and social structures

The client's view of the family and of other social structures affects health care. For example, if the client needing home health care belongs to an ethnic group with a strong sense of family responsibility, then the family probably will care for the client.

To assess the importance of family and social structures, ask the following questions:

• How important is your family to you?

• Do you have any friends that you consider family?

• Does anyone other than your immediate family (for example, grandparents) live with you?

• Are you involved in community affairs? Do you enjoy these activities?

Economic function

Financial problems frequently cause family conflict. Ask these questions to explore money issues and how they relate to power roles within the family:

• Does your family income meet the family's basic needs?

• Does money allocation consider family needs before individual needs?

• Who makes decisions about family money allocation?

DOCUMENTING THE HEALTH HISTORY

The system used to document the health history and other parts of the assessment varies with each health care facility. Some facilities use computerized records that provide standardized formats for documentation. Others use source-oriented records, in which each professional group documents separate data on each client. For example, one part of the record contains physician orders, another contains laboratory data, and another contains nursing data. In a source-oriented record, health care professionals usually document data in narrative (paragraph) form.

Still other health care facilities use problem-oriented records (POR), also known as problem-oriented medical records (POMR). Unlike the source-oriented record system, the POR system focuses on the client's problems. With the POR system, data are documented according to the SOAPIE format, which closely follows the nursing process steps.

The SOAPIE format consists of:

• **S**ubjective (history) data—what the client reports

• **O**bjective (physical) data—what the nurse observes, inspects, palpates, percusses, and auscultates

• **A**ssessment—nursing diagnosis and a statement of the client's progress or lack of progress

• **P**lan—plan of client care

• **I**mplementation—nursing interventions that carry out the plan

• **E**valuation—review of the results of the implemented plan.

However, regardless of the system used to document the health history, data must be documented according to the following legal guidelines:

• Use the appropriate form and document in ink.

• Be sure the client's name and identification number are on each page.

• Record the date and time of each entry.

• Use standard accepted abbreviations only.

• Document symptoms in the client's own words.

Pediatric health history

Although the pediatric health history varies somewhat from the one used for adults, it still covers the five basic health history components. Each component includes specific areas the nurse needs to assess for a pediatric client, as shown in the list below. To gain even more information, observe the parent-child interaction and behavior during the interview.

1. BIOGRAPHICAL DATA

Child's name; parent's name; contact person; address; telephone number; sex; age; birth date; place of birth; race, nationality, and cultural background; religious affiliation

2. HEALTH AND ILLNESS PATTERNS

- Current health status
- Prenatal and birth history
- Past health status
- Immunization and screening test history
- Family health status
- Status of physiologic systems
- Developmental milestones and considerations

3. HEALTH PROMOTION AND PROTECTION PATTERNS

- Child's or parent's health beliefs
- Personal habits (for adolescents)
- Sleep and wake patterns
- Temperamental assessment
- Behavior and discipline assessment
- Infant and child safety patterns
- Nutritional assessment
- Stress and coping patterns
- Family economic patterns
- Environmental health patterns
- School performance patterns
- Description of a typical day

4. ROLE AND RELATIONSHIP PATTERNS

- Child's self-concept
- Child's or parent's description of cognitive ability
- Role socialization patterns
- Cultural, spiritual, and religious influences on child's role socialization
- Child's communication patterns
- Sibling relationships
- Child's role in the family
- Child's knowledge of sexuality and reproduction
- Sexuality and sexual relationships (for adolescents)
- Child's peer relationships
- Emotional health status

5. SUMMARY OF HEALTH HISTORY DATA

- Be specific; avoid generalizations and vague expressions.
- Write on every line. Do not leave blank spaces.
- If a certain space does not apply to the client, write NA (not applicable) in the space.
- Do not backdate or squeeze writing into a previously documented entry.
- Document only work done personally; never document for someone else.

- Do not document value judgments and opinions.
- Sign every entry with your first and last name and title.

The client's record is used by other health care professionals to determine subsequent health needs. Before recording the health history, analyze notes and recollections to formulate a careful assessment of the client-supplied subjective data. Follow the guidelines discussed below when documenting the health history.

Write the history clearly and concisely, omitting information or opinions that might bias the reader. Avoid specific descriptions that label a finding as normal. Normal can be interpreted in many ways. If a particular section of the health history has no significant data, note that fact. This is called recording pertinent negatives; for example, "Client denies family history of diabetes, heart disease, or cancer."

The written history need not contain full sentences, except where the client's own words are revealing. Use only standardized abbreviations for medical terms. Because the recorded history is a legal document, be sure to date and sign it. Include a written summary of significant health history data at the end. The summary is particularly important as a source for the nursing diagnoses derived from subjective data.

SUGGESTED READINGS

Braverman, B. (1990). Eliciting assessment data from the patient who is difficult to interview. *Nursing Clinics of North America* 25(4), 743-750.

Clevenger, F. (1990). Interviewing the elderly client. *Advancing Clinical Care,* 5(6), 26-27.

Gehring, P. (1991). Physical assessment begins with a history. *RN,* 54(11), 26-32.

Gilliss, C., and Kulkin, I. (1991). Monitoring nursing interventions and data collection in a randomized clinical trial. *Western Journal of Nursing Research,* 13(3), 416-422.

Rosenbaum, J. (1991). A cultural assessment guide: Learning cultural sensitivity. *Canadian Nurse,* 87(4), 32-33.

2

Physical Assessment Skills

Assessment begins with subjective findings, including the health history and review of systems. Then the nurse moves to the physical assessment to obtain objective data about a client.

The physical assessment has four main parts:

• general survey (the nurse's initial observations of the client's general appearance and behavior)

• vital sign measurements (assessment of temperature, pulse and respiration rates, and blood pressure)

• assessment of height and weight

• physical examination (assessment of all structures, organs, and body systems).

An accurate physical assessment requires use of all of the nurse's senses and an intelligent, systematic approach. The nurse must develop expertise in using special equipment and in performing the four basic assessment techniques: inspection (observing), palpation (feeling body surfaces with the fingers), percussion (striking the fingers against body surfaces), and auscultation (listening to body sounds).

In a complete physical assessment, the nurse uses these techniques to evaluate each body structure, organ, or system in detail. The information obtained completes the client's health picture, substantiating or dispelling the nurse's or client's health concerns and possibly providing new information. Physical assessment findings and the client's history data help the nurse develop nursing diagnoses.

ASSESSMENT EQUIPMENT

For much of the physical assessment, the nurse relies directly on the senses—sight, hearing, smell, and touch—using the eyes, ears, nose, and hands as basic tools. To complete certain assessment steps, however, the nurse must use special equipment.

Basic assessment equipment

Usually, the physical assessment requires a thermometer, stethoscope, sphygmomanometer, visual acuity chart, penlight or flashlight, measuring tape and pocket ruler, marking pencil, and a scale.

Other basic assessment equipment

A complete collection of basic physical assessment equipment includes these additional items:

• a wooden tongue depressor to help assess the gag reflex and reveal the pharynx

• safety pins to test how well a client differentiates between dull and sharp pain

• cotton balls to check fine-touch sensitivity

• test tubes filled with hot and cold water to assess temperature sensitivity

• common, easily identified substances, such as ground coffee and vanilla extract, to evaluate smell and taste sensations

• a water-soluble lubricant and disposable latex gloves for rectal and vaginal assessment. (*Note:* The nurse must wear gloves when handling body fluids or touching open lesions or wounds.)

Advanced assessment equipment

Certain steps in the physical assessment may require specialized equipment – ophthalmoscope, nasal illuminator, otoscope, and tuning fork. Although these devices usually are reserved for nurses with special training and expanded roles, all nurses should be familiar with them and their applications. Other equipment sometimes used in advanced assessment includes the reflex hammer, skin calipers, vaginal speculum, goniometer, and transilluminator.

Ophthalmoscope

The nurse uses an ophthalmoscope (a light source and a system of lenses and mirrors) to assess internal eye structures (collectively called the fundus). Light intensity is adjustable, but the nurse should protect the client's comfort by using the lowest intensity possible.

Switching the aperture (ophthalmoscope opening) changes the color or size of the light beam. The large, round aperture proves suitable for most clients; the small, round aperture (sometimes a half circle), for clients with small pupils. To localize and measure fundal lesions, the nurse can use the grid or target aperture; to assess lesion elevation and examine the anterior eye, the slit beam; to assess specific fundal details, the green filter. To identify these apertures, shine the light onto a white piece of paper.

To use the ophthalmoscope, the nurse follows this procedure: hold it in the palm of your hand and place your index finger on the lens selection disk. This disk – a rotating dial on the instrument head – allows you to change the lens to compensate for the client's or your own myopia (nearsightedness) or hyperopia (farsightedness). Lens power is measured in diopters, marked by numbers that appear in an illuminated window as you turn the dial. Diopter values range from about -25 to $+40$. Positive diopters, numbered in black, show closer structures or compensate for a short, hyperopic eyeball. Negative diopters, numbered in red, help compensate for a longer, myopic eyeball. For positive diopters, turn the dial clockwise; for negative diopters, turn it counterclockwise.

Some ophthalmoscopes must be recharged periodically. To do this, disassemble the handle and plug it into a wall outlet. Also, change batteries and light bulbs as needed. (For details on ophthalmoscope use, see Chapter 7, Eyes and Ears.)

Nasal illuminator

The nurse uses a nasal illuminator to assess the nasal interior. The simplest type of nasal illuminator, the nasal speculum, is a double-bladed metal instrument used with a penlight to assess the lower and middle nasal turbinates and nasal mucosa. Alternatively, assess nasal structures by attaching to the ophthalmoscope handle a short, wide speculum designed especially for the nostrils (nares). The third type of nasal illuminator has a handle similar to an ophthalmoscope handle and a short, narrow head containing a light source. Any of these devices can cause the client discomfort if the nurse is not skilled.

Otoscope

The nurse uses an otoscope to assess the external auditory canal and tympanic membrane. The otoscope head, fixed to the same handle used for the ophthalmoscope, attaches and turns on just as the ophthalmoscope does; it provides light and magnification. Various funnel-like specula, ranging from $\frac{1}{8}''$ to $\frac{3}{8}''$ (0.32 to 1 cm) in diameter, fit onto the otoscope head. (For details on using the otoscope, see Chapter 7, Eyes and Ears.)

Tuning fork

The nurse uses a tuning fork to test sound conduction during the auditory assessment and vibratory sensation during the neurologic assessment. Vibrating a specific number of times per second, the tuning fork creates a characteristic sound known as its frequency. Different tuning forks have different frequencies, measured in cycles per second (CPS) or hertz (Hz). A high-frequency (500-Hz to 1,000-Hz) fork helps assess auditory function; a low-frequency (100-Hz to 400-Hz) fork helps assess vibratory sensation.

To use a tuning fork, the nurse follows this procedure: strike it lightly against a firm object, such as a desk top, or against your knee, to activate the vibrations. If the fork tines have knobs, pluck these to activate the vibrations. Then, depending on whether the assessment is for touch or hearing, place the base of the fork on a bony prominence or hold the fork near the client's ear. Do not touch the tines while they vibrate; this dampens the vibrations and interferes with accurate assessment. (For more information on using a tuning fork, see Chapter 7, Eyes and Ears, and Chapter 15, Nervous System.)

PHYSICAL ASSESSMENT TECHNIQUES

To perform the physical assessment, the nurse uses four basic techniques: inspection, palpation, percussion, and auscultation.

Inspection

Critical observation or inspection is the most frequently used assessment technique. Performed correctly, it also reveals more than the other techniques. However, an incomplete or hasty inspection may neglect important details or even yield false or misleading findings. To ensure accurate, useful information, the nurse should approach inspection in a careful, unhurried manner, pay close attention to details, and try to draw logical conclusions from the findings.

Unlike palpation, percussion, and auscultation, inspection is not a single, self-contained assessment step. Instead, it begins on first contact with the client and continues throughout the health history interview, general survey, vital sign measurement, and detailed body systems assessment. With each of these assessment phases, inspection findings enhance and refine the knowledge base.

Inspection can be direct or indirect. During direct inspection, rely totally on sight, hearing, and smell. During indirect inspection, use equipment, such as a nasal or vaginal speculum or an ophthalmoscope, to expose internal tissues or to enhance the view of a specific body area.

To inspect a specific body area, first make sure the area is sufficiently exposed and adequately lit. Then, survey the entire area, noting key landmarks and checking the overall condition. Next, focus on specifics—color, shape, texture, size, and movement.

While inspecting the client, always maintain objectivity; do not be misled by preconceived ideas and expectations. Stay alert for unusual and unexpected findings as well as for predictable ones.

Palpation

During palpation, the nurse touches the body to feel pulsations and vibrations, to locate body structures (particularly in the abdomen), and to assess such characteristics as size, texture, warmth, mobility, and tenderness. Palpation allows detection of a pulse, muscle rigidity, enlarged lymph nodes, skin or hair dryness, organ tenderness or breast lumps, and measurement of the chest rising and falling with each respiration. (See *Using the hands in palpation* for more information.)

Usually, palpation follows inspection as the second technique in physical assessment. For example, if a rash is present on

Using the hands in palpation

To enhance palpation technique, the nurse can take advantage of the tactile sensitivity specific to each hand region. The tips and pads of the fingers can best distinguish texture and shape. The back, or dorsal surface, of the hand can best feel for warmth. The ulnar surface, or ball, of the hand (at the base of the fingers on the palmar side) can best feel thrills (fine vibrations over the precordium) and fremitus (tremulous vibrations over the chest wall) as well as vocal vibrations through the chest wall. The thumb and index finger can best assess hair texture, grasp tissues, and feel for lymph node enlargement. The flattened finger pads can best palpate tender tissues, feel for crepitus (crackling) at joints, and lightly probe the abdomen. A single finger or nail tip can best stroke the skin when attempting to elicit the cremasteric (testicular retraction) or abdominal reflexes in the neurologic examination. The whole hand can best test handgrip strength.

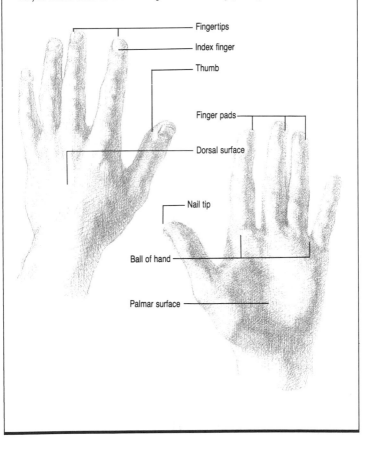

Fingertips

Index finger

Thumb

Finger pads

Dorsal surface

Nail tip

Ball of hand

Palmar surface

inspection, the nurse determines through palpation if the rash has a raised surface or feels tender or warm. However, during an abdominal or urinary system assessment, palpation should come at the end of the examination to avoid causing client discomfort and stimulating peristalsis (smooth muscle contractions that force food through the GI tract, bile through the bile duct, and urine through the ureters).

To perform thorough assessments, the nurse needs to master the several palpation techniques described here. Light palpation involves using the tips and pads of the fingers to apply light pressure to the skin surface. Ballottement, a light palpation variation, involves gentle, repetitive bouncing of tissues against the hand (think of bouncing a small ball gently) to assess free-floating or partially attached structures. Deep palpation requires use of both hands and heavier pressure.

Light palpation
To perform light palpation, press gently on the skin, indenting it ½″ to ¾″ (1 to 2 cm). Use the lightest touch possible; too much pressure blunts your sensitivity. Close your eyes to concentrate on what your fingers are feeling.

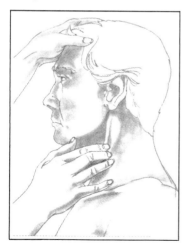

Deep palpation
To perform deep palpation, increase your fingertip pressure, indenting the skin about 1½″ (4 cm). Place your other hand on top of the palpating hand to control and guide your movements. To perform a variation of deep palpation that allows pinpointing an inflamed area, press firmly with one hand, then lift your hand away quickly. If the client complains of increased pain as you release the pressure, you have identified rebound tenderness. (Suspect peritonitis if you elicit rebound tenderness when examining the abdomen.)

Use both hands (bimanual palpation) to trap a deep, underlying, hard-to-palpate organ (such as the kidney or spleen) or to fix or stabilize an organ (such as the uterus) with one hand and palpate it with the other.

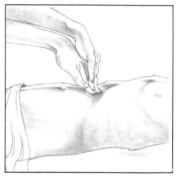

Light ballottement
To perform light ballottement, apply light, rapid pressure from quadrant to quadrant of the client's abdomen. Keep your hand on the skin surface to detect any tissue rebound.

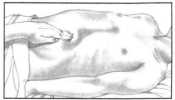

Deep ballottement
To perform deep ballottement, apply abrupt, deep pressure; then release the pressure, but maintain fingertip contact with the skin.

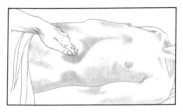

Percussion
During percussion, the nurse uses quick, sharp tapping of the fingers or hands against body surfaces (usually the chest and abdomen) to produce sounds, elicit (detect) tenderness, or assess reflexes. Percussing for sound—the most common percussion goal—helps locate organ borders, identify organ shape and position, and determine if an organ is solid or filled with fluid or gas.

Percussing for sound requires a skilled touch and an ear trained to detect slight sound variations. Organs and tissues produce sounds of varying loudness, pitch, and duration, depending upon their density. For instance, air-filled cavities, such as the lungs, produce markedly different sounds from those produced by the liver and other dense tissues.

To assess the client completely, the nurse needs to be able to perform these three percussion techniques: indirect, direct, and blunt percussion.

Indirect percussion
To perform indirect percussion, use the middle finger of your nondominant hand as the pleximeter (the mediating device used to receive the taps) and the middle finger of your dominant hand as the plexor (the device used to tap the pleximeter). Place the pleximeter finger firmly against a body surface, such as the upper back. With your wrist flexed loosely, use the tip of your plexor finger to deliver a crisp blow just beneath the distal joint of the pleximeter. Be sure to hold the plexor perpendicular to the pleximeter. Tap lightly and quickly, removing the plexor as soon as you have delivered each blow.

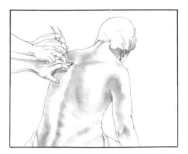

Direct percussion
To perform direct percussion, tap your hand or fingertip directly against the body surface. This method helps assess an adult's sinuses for tenderness or elicit sounds in a child's thorax.

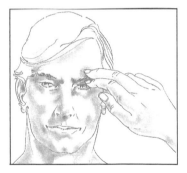

Blunt percussion
To perform blunt percussion, strike the ulnar surface of your fist against the body surface. Alternatively, you may use both hands by placing the palm of one hand over the area to be percussed, then making a fist with the other hand and using it to strike the back of the first hand. (See illustration on page 22.) Both techniques aim to elicit tenderness—not to create a sound—over such organs as the kidneys, gallbladder, or liver. (Another blunt percussion method, used in the neurologic examination, involves tapping a rubber-tipped reflex hammer against a tendon to create a reflexive muscle contraction.)

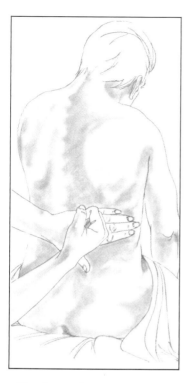

Normal percussion sounds over the chest and abdomen include:

• resonance—the long, low, hollow sound heard over an intercostal space lying above healthy lung tissue

• tympany—the loud, high-pitched, drum-like sound heard over a gastric air bubble or gas-filled bowel

• dullness—the soft, high-pitched, thudding sound normally heard over more solid organs, such as the liver and heart. (*Note:* Dullness heard in a normally resonant or tympanic area warrants further investigation.)

Abnormal percussion sounds may be heard over body organs. Consider hyperresonance – a long, loud, low-pitched sound – a classic sign of lung hyperinflation, as in emphysema. Flatness – similar to dullness but shorter in duration and softer in intensity – may also be heard over pleural fluid accumulation or pleural thickening. (For a summary, see *Percussion sounds.*)

When percussing, the nurse moves from resonant areas to dull areas to accentuate any sound differences, as in these examples: to identify the lower border of liver dullness, begin percussing over the tympanic abdominal regions, then move up toward the dull liver area. To identify the upper border of liver dullness, begin over the lungs and percuss downward. Compare from side to side, tapping a few times in each area. Except for areas over such organs as the liver, gallbladder, and spleen, percussion findings should be symmetrical.

Auscultation

During auscultation, the nurse listens to body sounds – particularly those produced by the heart, lungs, vessels, stomach, and intestines. Most auscultated sounds result from air or fluid movement – for example, the rush of air through respiratory pathways, the turbulent flow of blood through vessels, and the movement of gas (agitated by peristalsis) through the bowels.

Usually, the nurse performs auscultation after the other assessment techniques. When examining the abdomen, however, auscultate after inspecting, but before percussing and palpating. That way, bowel sounds are heard before palpation disrupts them.

The nurse can hear body sounds, such as the voice, loud wheezing, or stomach growls, fairly easily, but will need a stethoscope to hear softer ones. An appropriate procedure is this one: Use a high-quality, properly fitting stethoscope with a diaphragm and bell. (The diaphragm, when applied firmly, is best for detecting high-pitched sounds; the bell, when applied lightly, is best for detecting low-pitched sounds.) Provide a quiet environment and make sure that the body area to be auscultated is sufficiently exposed. Remember that a gown or bed linens can interfere with sound transmission. Instruct the client to remain quiet and still. Before starting, warm the stethoscope head (diaphragm and bell) in your hand; otherwise, the cold metal may make the client shiver, possibly producing unwanted sounds. Place the diaphragm or bell over the appropriate area. Closing your eyes to help focus your attention, listen intently to individual sounds and try to iden-

Percussion sounds

Percussion produces sounds that vary according to the tissue being percussed. This chart shows important percussion sounds along with their characteristics and typical locations.

SOUND	INTENSITY	PITCH	DURATION	QUALITY	SOURCE
Resonance	Moderate to loud	Low	Long	Hollow	Normal lung
Tympany	Loud	High	Moderate	Drumlike	Gastric air bubble; intestinal air
Dullness	Soft to moderate	High	Moderate	Thudlike	Liver; full bladder; pregnant uterus
Hyperresonance	Very loud	Very low	Long	Booming	Hyperinflated lung (as in emphysema)
Flatness	Soft	High	Short	Flat	Muscle

tify their characteristics. Determine the intensity, pitch, and duration of each sound and check the frequency of recurring sounds.

APPROACH TO ASSESSMENT

The physical assessment may take various forms. A complete physical assessment—appropriate for periodic health checks—includes a general survey, vital sign measurements, height and weight measurements, and assessment of all organs and body systems.

However, in the hospital and many other settings, the nurse rarely has the opportunity to perform a complete assessment. In such cases, the nurse may conduct a modified assessment, using knowledge of the client's history and complaints. For example, if the client has peripheral vascular disease, include skin and peripheral pulse examination in the assessment; if the client has a herniated lumbar disk, test motor function and sensation in the legs and feet.

No matter which type of assessment is performed or where—hospital, clinic, or home—the nurse should keep in mind that the procedure can cause anxiety or fear. The client may worry that the assessment will confirm a suspected illness or uncover an unexpected problem, or may even consider the assessment an invasion of privacy because the nurse must observe and touch sensitive, private, and perhaps painful body areas.

Using the following guidelines can help ensure the correct approach to physical assessment, thereby enhancing the client's and the nurse's comfort. Some guidelines for the nurse serve at all times; others help with a specific type of assessment.
• Begin by introducing yourself. Give your full name. If you wish, explain that you may take longer than a more experienced examiner to complete the assessment. (In many cases, the client appreciates the extra attention.)
• Make sure your grooming, dress, and behavior reflect a professional attitude. This enhances the client's sense of dignity and promotes respect for you. For example, ad-

dress an adult client by title and last name (such as Mr. Murphy, Mrs. Harper, Rev. Smith, Dr. Jones) unless asked to do otherwise.

• Before starting the assessment, briefly explain what you will do and why; include any position changes that you will ask the client to make. (For more information, see *Client positioning and draping guidelines*.) As you proceed with the assessment, explain each step in detail. By reassuring the client that the assessment will hold no surprises or unexpected discomfort, you promote trust and cooperation.

• Have all necessary equipment on hand and in working order. Leaving the room to search for equipment could interrupt your concentration and make the client doubt your competence.

• Make sure the examination room is well lighted with natural lighting (preferable) or adequate artificial light.

• To help ensure accurate findings and promote client comfort, ask the client to void before you begin the assessment.

• Respect the client's privacy and modesty. Ask family members and other visitors to leave, then close the door and pull drapes, as appropriate. Let the client undress in privacy, if possible, and provide a gown or sheet to cover up. Drape the client so that you can easily expose body areas for examination. (Allow a modest client to wait until absolutely necessary before removing undergarments.)

• Make the client as comfortable as possible by offering a pillow and making sure that the room and assessment equipment are warm.

• Always warn the client before performing a procedure that may cause discomfort. If posssible, avoid touching tender or painful areas until the end of the assessment.

• Use the same communication skills you applied in the interview. Politely ask the client to follow your instructions. Answer any questions and express thanks for cooperation—but do not let conversation interfere with your concentration. Avoid inappropriate jokes and disparaging comments.

• Be sensitive, unhurried, and reassuring—especially with an elderly client, who may move slowly. If the client seems to be tiring, provide a rest period. Concerned, caring behavior markedly enhances the client's comfort and builds confidence in you.

• Wash your hands before and after the assessment, in the client's presence. Using good hand-washing technique in the client's presence shows that you care for the safety of this client, other clients, and yourself.

• Dress comfortably and minimize position changes during the assessment. When assessing a bedridden client, raise the bed to a level comfortable for you.

• Always use the same systematic approach to assessment, varying it only to accommodate the client's particular needs. This reduces the risk of overlooking a significant finding. For example, develop the habit of working from the same side for all clients so that you assess body regions in the same way each time.

• Avoid negative reactions, such as grimaces or exclamations, to abnormal or unexpected findings and unpleasant odors or sights. Even a seriously ill client may notice your reaction and become anxious, embarrassed, or angry.

Special considerations for pediatric clients

The nurse may perform a pediatric assessment for various purposes, including well-baby visits; routine screenings for eyesight, hearing, and growth and development; and follow-up visits after an illness. Whatever the purpose, use a gentle, patient approach and be sure to assess how well the child has achieved developmental milestones. If possible, also evaluate the parent-child relationship.

Tailor your assessment to the child's age and developmental level. Infants (up to age 1) usually respond and cooperate readily, and rarely mind being undressed and examined naked. To help the infant relax, coo and smile during the examination. As appropriate, allow the parent to hold the infant. With an infant who breast-feeds during the assessment, assess feeding technique.

A child ages 1 to 2 may be more fearful and harder to examine. You may need to calm or distract an upset or uncooperative child with a toy or another diversion, such

Client positioning and draping guidelines

Requirements for client positioning and draping vary with the body system or region being assessed. These illustrations show the primary positioning and draping arrangements that the nurse uses during a routine assessment.

To examine the head, neck, and anterior and posterior thorax, have the client sit on the edge of the examination table.

To perform some portions of the neurologic and musculoskeletal examinations, have the client stand (when feasible) or sit.

To begin examining the female client's breasts, place her in a seated position. For the second part of the examination, ask her to lie down. When she does, place a small pillow or folded towel beneath her shoulder on the side being examined. To spread her breast more evenly over the chest, ask her to place her arm (on the side being examined) over her head.

To examine the abdomen and cardiovascular system, place the client supine and stand on the right. For a female client, ensure privacy during abdominal assessment by placing a towel over her breasts and upper thorax. Pull the sheet down as far as her symphysis pubis, but do not expose this area.

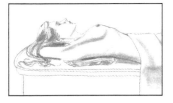

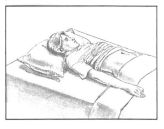

To perform a rectal examination on a male client, have him lean across the examination table. If he cannot stand upright, have him lie on his left side, with his right hip and knee slightly flexed and his buttocks close to the edge of the table.

To examine the female client's reproductive system, place her in the lithotomy position. Drape a sheet diagonally over her chest and knees and between her legs. Her buttocks should be at or just past the edge of the table and her feet in the stirrups. The rectal examination may be done in this position, also.

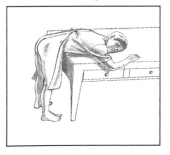

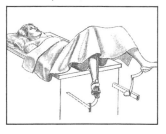

as funny noises or a game of peek-a-boo. Keep in mind that young children typically find eye, ear, and mouth assessment more distressing than assessment of other body areas. For this reason, examine the head last instead of following the standard head-to-toe format. Hip abduction evaluation also can cause distress, so delay this until late in the examination. Also delay assessment of a crying child, if possible. Crying tenses the muscles, preventing accurate musculoskeletal and neurologic assessment. When accompanied by sobs, crying also can interfere with auscultation of heart sounds.

A child ages 2 to 3 may be the most difficult to assess. This child may dislike being undressed and touched and may cling to the parent. To improve the assessment, develop a supportive relationship with the parent and take the time to gain the trust of both parent and child. Encourage the parent to participate, and let the child sit on the parent's lap. Explain each examination instrument and demonstrate its use on the parent. If appropriate, let the child touch the equipment and help with the assessment, such as by holding the stethoscope in place on the chest. When possible, integrate play into the assessment. For example, let the child pretend to listen to your heart or to a doll's heart. These creative touches improve cooperation by developing trust and teaching the child about the body.

By age 4 or 5, a child typically becomes more cooperative and less fearful of the assessment. This child responds especially well when play is incorporated into the assessment, as appropriate.

Compared to a young child, an older child or adolescent proves easier to engage in conversation, follows instructions more willingly, and has a better understanding of the goal of assessment. More independent, this client may ask not to have a parent present during the assessment; if so, respect this request. Also, be sensitive to the client's increased sense of modesty. Provide adequate privacy and let the client keep undergarments on until the last minute. Let the adolescent know that you will answer any questions about physical changes related to emerging sexuality—a topic of particular concern at this age.

Special considerations for pregnant clients

Assessment of a pregnant client has a dual focus—the client and her developing fetus. While assessing the maternal and fetal parameters that mark the normal course of pregnancy—fundal height, nutritional status, weight gain, pelvic size, fetal growth, and the changing appearance of the breasts and vagina—the nurse also checks for evidence of pregnancy-related complications. (For detailed assessment steps, see Chapter 20, Perinatal and Neonatal Assessment.)

To help assess a pregnant client properly, the nurse follows these guidelines:

• Be prepared to perform a comprehensive assessment—pregnancy affects a woman's entire body.

• Provide a chair that offers adequate support. A pregnant client in the third trimester usually has trouble getting into and rising from a soft, low chair. Help the client onto the examination table and into position, and drape her appropriately.

• Allow ample time for the assessment so that the client does not feel rushed. Also keep in mind that normal hormonal swings during pregnancy may make the client feel impatient, then embarrassed by her impatience.

Special considerations for elderly clients

When assessing an elderly client, the nurse should be aware that aging normally causes physiologic changes and impairs the body's response to stress, illness, and injury. Specific aging-related changes may include reduced muscle strength and range of motion, vital sign changes, slowed reflexes, impaired sensory perception, and slowed or impaired thought processes. These changes may contribute to the elderly client's increased risk for interrelated and chronic health problems—most notably, cardiovascular and cerebrovascular disease, cancer, dementia, cataracts, diabetes, and lung disease. To complicate matters, an elderly client may take many medications, possibly leading to adverse reactions or unexpected drug interactions that can interfere with interpretation of assessment findings.

During the assessment, address the client respectfully, using the title and last name unless the client requests otherwise. Keep in mind that this client may prefer more formal social conventions than those widely used today and may find an overly casual manner offensive.

Be sure to phrase your instructions simply and slowly, addressing one point at a time. Give the client plenty of time to respond. Because an elderly client may tire easily and have trouble changing positions, allow extra time for each assessment step. However, do not assume that all elderly clients are frail, move slowly, or are hard of hearing. Such preconceptions can interfere with accurate assessment.

Special considerations for disabled clients

The nurse may assess a disabled client during a routine health screening or for a special reason, such as determining eligibility for rehabilitation or setting vocational goals. Whatever the purpose, focus on the client's functional ability and mental capacity. Tailor your assessment to the client's specific needs, assets, and limitations. For example, provide detailed verbal instructions to a blind client; simplify instructions for a developmentally disabled (mentally retarded) client.

A disabled client may reveal beforehand whether the disability limits participation in the assessment. Take the time to learn as much as possible about the client's abilities and impairments before starting the assessment. The client will appreciate this step and may respond with increased cooperation. As with other clients, avoid stereotyping the disabled client; show sensitivity and consideration at all times.

THE GENERAL SURVEY

As the first step in the physical assessment, the general survey provides vital information about the client's behavior and health status. During this step, the nurse documents initial impressions of the client in a one-paragraph statement—a summary that provides an overall picture guiding subsequent assessment.

The general survey requires skilled, focused observation and a confident, professional approach. The inexperienced nurse may feel self-conscious and may worry about the client's impressions. However, to detect subtle clues from behavior and appearance and derive an accurate client profile, learn to focus all your attention on the client—a skill that comes with practice and experience.

During the first contact with the client, be prepared to receive a steady stream of impressions, mostly visual. The client's sex, race, and approximate age will be obvious. Because some health concerns may relate to these factors, be sure to note them. Also note less obvious factors that may contribute to your overall impression, including signs of distress; facial characteristics; body type, posture, and movements; speech; dress, grooming, and personal hygiene; and psychological state.

Signs of distress

First check for obvious signs of physical or emotional distress. Dyspnea (shortness of breath)—probably the most common sign of distress—suggests a cardiac or respiratory problem. Note any restlessness or wheezing, which may accompany asthma, or shallow, labored respirations, which may signal pneumonia. Determine if dyspnea occurs only with a particular position, such as recumbency; this may indicate cardiac involvement.

Pain, another clue to distress, typically shows in a client's facial expression, body movements, and posture. Check for halting, limited movements and an overly rigid or otherwise odd posture. If the client grimaces, writhes, clutches the abdomen, or shows other obvious signs of pain, stop the assessment and notify a physician.

Be aware that clients express emotional distress in varying ways. One client, for instance, may show distress through jerking hand movements or rapid speech; another may withdraw or sit with the head bowed and arms crossed over the chest.

Facial characteristics

A client's face provides valuable clues to physical, emotional, and psychological well-being. Observe the face for expression, contour, and symmetry. Obvious tension, staring, trembling, a downcast or shifting gaze, or constant blinking suggests a neurologic or psychological problem. Facial trembling, for example, may result from anxiety or a facial nerve problem. A flat expression with no affect (outward manifestation of feelings) commonly accompanies Parkinson's disease (a progressive, degenerative neurologic disorder) and myasthenia gravis (a neuromuscular disorder causing muscle weakness). In some cases, facial trembling may indicate a psychological disturbance.

Abnormal features, such as an enlarged nose and lips, a protruding jaw, and a prominent supraorbital ridge, suggest acromegaly (a chronic metabolic disorder characterized by growth hormone overproduction). Facial asymmetry, with incomplete eye closure and one-sided mouth drooping, may result from the facial nerve paralysis typical of Bell's palsy.

Also, determine whether facial characteristics suggest the client's stated age. Chronic illness can cause dull, sagging, wrinkled skin and other signs of premature aging.

Body type, posture, and movements

Assess the client's general body type, classifying the build as stocky, average, or slender. Check for cachexia (extreme thinness) or obesity. With an obese client, assess for abnormal fat distribution, as in Cushing's syndrome (characterized by truncal obesity and thin limbs). Note any unusual physical features; a rounded (barrel) chest, for example, may signal chronic lung disease.

While observing the client's overall body structure, pay especially close attention to the hands. Observe the fingers for clubbing (enlargement) or edema (swelling), which may indicate a cardiovascular problem; also check for contractures (abnormally stiff joint positions), suggesting arthritis.

Observe gait and other movements for symmetry, coordination, and smoothness. Note any obvious involuntary movements or deformities—for instance, an amputated limb. Gait problems, such as shuffling, may accompany Parkinson's disease. Limping may stem from previous injury; spasticity, from cerebral palsy. Note any use of assistive devices, such as a cane, walker, brace, or prosthesis (noting this also helps determine whether the client needs assistance with walking). In the hospital, your observations of body movement may take a different focus. For instance, note whether a bedridden client can sit up, turn, and reposition.

Also observe the client's posture—a clue to energy level, psychological status, and skeletal structure. If the client slumps, look for other signs of possible fatigue or depression. A hunched-over posture may mean merely that the client is cold; however, it could reflect guarding (a tense, protective reaction to abdominal pain) or a pulmonary problem. In the classic posture of chronic obstructive lung disease, the client hunches over a bedside table in an attempt to ease breathing.

Speech

Assess the client's speech for tone, clarity, vocal strength, vocabulary, sentence structure, and pace. Hoarseness or softness may indicate laryngitis or cranial nerve paralysis. Inappropriate loudness suggests nervousness. A monotone may reflect depression. Fast, garbled speech may accompany a mental disorder; slow, garbled speech, a cerebrovascular accident (stroke). Note the client's vocabulary and word usage pattern—possible clues to educational level. (This information may help later when you plan the client's care and teaching sessions.)

Listen carefully to the speech pattern. A client with expressive aphasia (a neurologic condition impairing the ability to form words) may speak hesitantly and deliberately. Note whether the client constantly searches for words, repeats your words, or uses rhyming words—possible clues to a psychological disorder. Also identify other obvious speech characteristics, such as stuttering, lisping, or a foreign accent.

Dress, grooming, and personal hygiene

A client's dress, grooming, and personal hygiene may reflect physical and psychological health status. Look for signs of apparent indifference to appearance or inability to perform self-care. Note whether the client's hair looks clean and neat, and evaluate facial and oral hygiene.

Closely observe the client's clothing, and note its appropriateness for the season and situation. Observe how well garments fit and match, and assess their cleanliness and general condition. Clashing colors, for example, could signal mental dysfunction or a visual deficit. However, avoid drawing final conclusions from these observations: although loose hems, holes, or incorrectly buttoned clothing may indicate failing vision or a psychological problem, it could also reflect financial problems.

Note any frank odors, such as alcohol, which may indicate alcoholism; urine, suggesting incontinence or poor hygiene; or excessive perfume or cologne, which may reflect an attempt to mask body odor. However, always consider these findings in context. Not all clients who smell of alcohol are alcoholics; also, certain sociocultural customs may account for specific body odors.

Psychological state

Besides facial expression and posture, other behavioral components can supply important clues to the client's psychological status. For instance, note whether the client cooperates and understands and follows simple instructions, such as "Please sit down." Assess the client's level of awareness, attentiveness, and attention span. Assess the client's orientation to time, place, and person. Note lethargy, drowsiness, or other signs of decreased level of consciousness. (For an explanation of assessing mental status and level of consciousness, See Chapter 15, Nervous System.)

Also note whether the client appears relaxed and comfortable or nervous and fidgety. Extreme anxiety may cause rigidity, trembling, and restlessness; the client may experience abdominal pain and hold the arms against the stomach for relief.

Observe for any bizarre or repeated mannerisms or movements, such as involuntary, spasmodic movements. Check hand position and movement and use of gestures. A client who clasps the hands tightly, uses wildly flailing gestures, or experiences hand trembling may be psychologically disturbed.

If you shake hands, notice whether the client has a firm, steady grasp or a weak one; the latter may signal a neurologic problem or reflect aging-related changes. Also note whether the palm is dry; damp with sweat, as from anxiety; or cold and clammy, as from shock. Watch to see if the client bites the fingernails or constantly plays with an object, such as a tie or purse strap.

Special considerations for pediatric clients

When conducting a general survey of an infant or child, expect certain behaviors to vary according to the child's age. A newborn usually lies quietly in the parent's arms or cries softly when uncomfortable or disturbed. A child ages 6 months to 2 years usually clings to the parent and may be scared or uncooperative. Expect a preschooler to show more confidence and curiosity and, after initial shyness, to cooperate with the assessment. A school-age child typically has a longer attention span and follows instructions better.

Evaluate the same details as for an adult, focusing on signs of distress, facial characteristics, posture, activity level, motor coordination, language function, maturity level, and ability to understand and cooperate with the assessment.

Keep in mind that a child may be more spontaneous and restless than an adult, may stare with frank curiosity, and may express emotion readily. Look for signs of anxiety, including thumb sucking, nail biting, and rocking. If a parent is present, observe how the parent and child interact. Note the amount and quality of physical contact and verbal communication, and assess how well the parent responds to the child's needs and copes with any crying or uncooperative behavior.

Special considerations for elderly clients

The general survey of an elderly client resembles that of any adult, but focuses more intensely on certain areas. For example, when observing the client's skin, gait, and posture, expect the normal physiologic changes of aging—loose, wrinkled, dry skin; a stiff, slow gait resulting from bone mineral loss; and a bent, stooped posture and knee flexion from kyphosis (increased thoracic spine curvature). Stay alert for clues to reduced self-care capacity, such as missing buttons or a misbuttoned shirt. Learn to identify key signs of aging-related disorders, such as the flat affect and shuffling gait of Parkinson's disease.

Although many elderly clients remain alert, independent, and active, some are at risk for special problems, including chronic disease, depression, and confusion. Most have endured numerous losses and have grieved for these losses in a healthy manner. However, some react with prolonged depression, anxiety, or other maladaptive responses. Early signs of depression include a short attention span, emotional lability (instability), and inattention to personal dress or hygiene.

Confusion, another finding in some elderly clients, can result from adverse drug reactions or interactions, dehydration, infection, nutritional problems, organic brain changes, and other factors. Unfamiliar surroundings and routines, such as during hospitalization or a stay in an extended-care facility, can contribute to confusion.

While assessing the elderly client, be aware that your attitudes toward aging and elderly persons can color your interpretation of the client's appearance and functional ability. For instance, if you respect the experience and wisdom that come with advanced age, you are more likely to assess a client's abilities in a positive light. If, on the other hand, you view most elderly persons as impaired or helpless, you may diminish the client's abilities.

Special considerations for disabled clients

When assessing the client with a disability, deficit, or deformity that impairs functioning, be sure to address special areas of client concern. Note any obvious signs of disability, such as use of a wheelchair or seeing-eye dog. Assess the client's functional ability, independence level, and attitude toward the disability and the assessment. As always, avoid stereotyping the client, and take a caring, sensitive approach.

Cultural and ethnic considerations

Caring for clients of diverse cultural and ethnic backgrounds is commonplace for the nurse. A client's life-style, values, beliefs, and cultural and ethnic customs can play a key role in appearance, behavior, and attitude toward health and illness. Be aware that your values and beliefs may distort your assessment of a client whose background differs from yours. To obtain the most accurate and useful general survey findings, remain as objective as possible and avoid imposing your values on the client.

During the general survey, attempt to assess the client's values and health beliefs accurately. Take care not to mistake cultural preferences in dress, manner, and physical appearance for abnormal behavior or signs of a physical or psychological disorder. For example, what you may consider poor hygiene might be considered normal in certain cultures. Likewise, behavior that may strike you as apathetic, seductive, or hostile might be a standard response to stress in clients from a particular family background.

Avoid stereotyping a client on the basis of ethnic or cultural background. Doing so tends to limit your appreciation of the client's uniqueness.

Documenting the general survey

The nurse documents general survey findings in a short, concise paragraph. Include only the information that you consider essential to communicating your overall impression of the client. Do not comment on everything you observe—only the most important points. For example, mention that the client has a facial rash, but do not describe the rash in detail until later, when documenting the complete physical assessment findings.

VITAL SIGNS

Assessment of vital signs—temperature, pulse, respirations, and blood pressure—is a basic nursing responsibility and an important method for measuring and monitoring vital body functions. Vital signs give insight into the function of specific organs—especially the heart and lungs—as well as entire body systems. The nurse obtains vital signs to establish baseline measurements, observe for trends, identify physiologic problems, and monitor a client's response to therapy.

During a complete physical assessment, the nurse will take all vital signs at once, or will integrate vital signs into different assessment steps. Because an abnormal finding can alert you to possible problems to investigate further as you proceed, you may prefer to take all vital signs at the beginning.

An ill client requires frequent vital sign assessment, with frequency depending on the nature and severity of the disorder. Expect to assess vital signs every 4 to 6 hours in a hospitalized client. In an acute situation, however, you may assess vital signs every 1 to 2 hours. After certain types of surgery and other procedures, a client may need extremely frequent monitoring—perhaps every 15 minutes. With any client, do not hesitate to obtain vital signs as often as you think appropriate.

When assessing vital signs, keep in mind that a single measurement usually proves far less clinically valuable than a series of measurements, which can substantiate a trend. In most cases, look for a change—from the normal range, from the client's normal measurement, or from previous measurements.

If you obtain an unusual measurement or if you doubt a finding, repeat the measurement or, if possible, have another nurse repeat it. If you still feel uncertain, check your equipment and, if necessary, replace it and take another measurement.

If you obtain an abnormal vital sign finding, maintain a calm, professional demeanor; an anxious expression or exclamation could upset the client. If the client expresses concern over repeated measurements, calmly explain that you obtained a slightly high or low measurement and you just want to check it again.

Consider how vital sign findings relate to each other and to other physical assessment findings. Because vital signs reflect basic body functions, any significant change warrants further investigation.

HEIGHT AND WEIGHT MEASUREMENTS

With every client—in any setting—the nurse should record height and weight (anthropometric measurements) as part of the basic assessment profile. Although the general survey gives an overall impression of body size and type, height and weight measurements provide more specific information about a client's general health and nutritional status. In routine physical assessment, these measurements should be taken periodically throughout the client's life to help evaluate normal growth and development and to identify abnormal patterns of weight gain or loss—frequently an early sign of acute or chronic illness. (For information on determining optimal body weights as well as other anthropometric measurements, such as midarm circumference and triceps skinfold thickness, see Chapter 4, Nutritional Status.)

Accurate height and weight measurements also serve other important purposes. In children, they guide dosage calculations for various drugs; in adults, they help guide cancer chemotherapy and anesthesia administration, and they help evaluate the response to I.V. fluids, drugs, or nutritional therapy.

SUGGESTED READINGS

Brown, M. (1991). How do you spell assessment?...Simple mnemonic device to organize your work. *American Journal of Nursing*, 91(9), 55-56.

Kain, C., et al. (1990). The older adult: A comparative assessment. *Nursing Clinics of North America*, 25(4), 833-848.

McConnell, W. (1990). Orderly assessment. *Emergency*, 22(10), 34-38.

Nettina, S., and Gregonis, S. (1990). Triage: Assigning priorities. *Nursing90*, 20(11), 86.

Reed, J., and Bond, S. (1991). Nurses' assessment of elderly patients in hospital. *International Journal of Nursing Studies*, 28(1), 55-64.

Sony, S. (1992). Baccalaureate nurse graduates' perception of barriers to the use of physical assessment skills in the clinical setting. *Journal of Continuing Education in Nursing*, 23(2), 83-87.

UNIT TWO

Assessing Activity, Sleep, and Nutrition

3

ADLs and Sleep Patterns

Maintaining a constant balance between activities of daily living (ADLs) and sleep is vital to the promotion and maintenance of physiologic and psychosocial health. Daily activity affects a person's ability to sleep soundly, and in turn the quality of sleep affects a person's ability to carry out daily activities. Therefore, the nurse must carefully assess the client's ability to perform ADLs, the client's ability to achieve and maintain restful sleep patterns, and the balance between the two. Alterations in ADLs or disturbances in sleep patterns can signal actual or potential health problems.

ASSESSING ADLs

A thorough assessment ascertains a client's functional status and identifies actual and potential health problems related to ADLs. It also suggests interventions to help promote the client's independent function at home and in the community and provides a method for measuring progress.

The nurse uses the interview and observation to gather information on ADLs. During the interview, gather data from the client and the family. Focus on their perceptions of the client's ability to perform ADLs, and identify the client's and family's goals for functioning. Determine whether the client and the family have realistic views, have developed attainable goals, and have similar perspectives. Observe the client performing ADLs whenever possible.

The following sample interview questions provide a guide to assessing a client's ability to perform ADLs.

Personal care activities

Do you have any difficulty standing, walking, or climbing stairs? Can you get in and out of a chair? Can you get in and out of bed? What assistive devices do you use to aid in mobility? If the client uses a wheelchair, ask, *Can you propel the chair yourself?*
(RATIONALE: An alteration in mobility may hinder a client's ability to engage in other ADLs.)

Can you open packages and containers? Can you use utensils for eating? Can you cut your food? Do you have any other problems feeding yourself? What times do you usually eat? Who prepares your meals? Where do you eat your meals? With whom do you eat?
(RATIONALE: These questions help investigate the client's ability to prepare meals and to eat independently. The ability to feed oneself is an important personal care activity. Besides providing nourishment, meals may provide a time for socializing.)

Can you use the toilet alone, or do you require assistance? Do you have any problems with bowel or bladder control? If so, how do you manage these problems? Do you use any assistive devices for elimination, such as a catheter or colostomy bag? If so, can you care for these devices? How have elimination problems affected your other activities?

(RATIONALE: An elimination problem can interfere with work, school, recreational, and socialization activities. These questions give the client an opportunity to discuss problems, fears, and anxieties regarding elimination, and give the nurse an opportunity to teach the client ways to manage these problems. Keep in mind that elimination activities are private matters to adults; the client or family may hesitate to discuss them because of embarrassment. Ask questions in a matter-of-fact way and try to put the client at ease.)

What are your usual bathing habits? Do you have any problems with personal hygiene and bathing? Can you get in and out of a tub or shower? Can you shave? Can you care for your teeth, hair, fingernails, and toenails? Can you care for your dentures, hearing aids, or any other prostheses?

(RATIONALE: For many clients, an inability to manage personal hygiene activities can reduce self-esteem and alter self-concept. These questions help investigate the client's ability to perform these activities. Remember that most clients consider personal hygiene activities to be private; they may hesitate to discuss problems. Also, some clients may have experienced a gradual, unnoticed decline in their ability to perform personal hygiene.)

Do you have any difficulties with dressing and grooming? If so, are these problems more pronounced on the left side, the right side, the upper part, or the lower part of your body? Can you work buttons, snaps, and zippers? Is dressing easier with certain types of clothing? If so, which kinds?

(RATIONALE: Musculoskeletal or neuromuscular abnormalities can disrupt fine or gross motor coordination, making dressing and grooming—activities that most adults perform independently—difficult for the client.

To help prevent frustration with these normal ADLs, suggest different types of clothing or assistive devices.)

Family responsibility activities

What are your living arrangements? Does your home need structural changes so that you can fulfill your family responsibilities and perform activities of daily living? Do you have any problems with food management, such as shopping or food preparation? Can you do your own laundry? What type of cleaning can you do? If you have a yard, can you care for it? Are you having any difficulties managing your money, such as getting to a bank? What arrangements have you made for child care? Does your family responsibility include caring for any sick or disabled persons in the home? If so, do you have any difficulties with this role? Do you care for a pet in your home?

(RATIONALE: These questions help investigate the structure and composition of the client's family, the client's developmental status, and the responsibilities the client has assumed in the family. A client who cannot perform usual family responsibility activities may develop role and relationship problems and may benefit from a referral to a social agency for help with such responsibilities as food management or child care.)

Work and school activities

What does your typical day involve? Do you work outside the home? Where and what type of work do you do? How many hours per week do you work? What is your work schedule like? Do you have any conflicts between your work schedule and other responsibilities or activities of daily living? What is your job like? Is work mainly a source of satisfaction or frustration? Do you participate in any volunteer work?

(RATIONALE: These questions help investigate the type of work the client participates in and the role of work in the client's life. A client with a heavy, stressful work schedule may feel that he or she is neglecting family and self, causing guilt feelings that add to the stress. Suggest stress-reduction techniques for such a client.)

What do you see yourself doing in the future? How do you feel about retirement? What plans have you made for retirement? (RATIONALE: These questions help investigate the client's view of retirement, including alterations in ADLs caused by retirement.)

Are you going to school? If so, where and for what purpose? What do you like most about school? What do you like least about school? Do you have any difficulties balancing school activities with other life responsibilities? (RATIONALE: These questions help investigate the nature and demands of any schoolwork in which the client participates, and help assess the effects of school on other activities. A client whose school activities interfere with personal care activities, family responsibilities, or work activities may benefit from counseling.)

Recreational activities

What do you do when you're not working or in school? How do your days off differ from your work or school days? How much recreational time do you have in a day and in a week? Are you satisfied with the amount of your recreational time and what you can do during that time? With whom do you share your recreational time? How often do you get physical exercise? Do you participate in any special exercise program? If so, what kind and for how long? How do you feel after you exercise? Has your physician ever restricted your activity or exercise? If so, why? What benefits have you gained from exercise? (RATIONALE: These questions help investigate the type, amount, timing, purpose, and benefits of the client's recreational and physical exercise activities. A decrease in usual activity levels may result from a physical disorder, and may lead to an emotional problem, such as depression.)

Are you retired? If so, how would you describe your day? What recreational and exercise activities do you participate in now that you are retired?

(RATIONALE: These questions help discover the type of activities enjoyed by a retired client, who may have more time for recreation than a younger adult. For a retired client, recreation and exercise activities may take the place of work activities, providing stimulation, satisfaction, and interpersonal relationships.)

Socialization activities

What kinds of things do you do when you are alone? Can you use a phone, write clearly, and see well enough to enjoy reading or watching television? Do you have many close friends? Who would you confide in if you had a problem? Do you depend on your family for help? How often do you get together with family members? Can you travel outside the home? Which activities are you involved in outside your home? Do you belong to any social groups, such as clubs or church groups? Do you drive your own car or use public transportation? (RATIONALE: These questions help investigate the client's role in society, the structure of the client's social network, and any barriers to socialization the client may have. Illness, relocation, or the loss or change of a job can disrupt the client's usual social network, leading to social isolation, loneliness, and depression. Help such a client adjust by suggesting social activities that are available in the community.)

Developmental considerations

The nurse must devise special questions to assess a child's ADLs. Sample questions follow.

Does your child eat independently? Does your child use utensils or fingers to eat? Does your child eat with other members of the family? (RATIONALE: The ability to feed oneself is an important personal care activity and, for a child, an important developmental step. A child who eats with other family members not only receives nourishment but also develops social skills.)

Is your child toilet trained? If so, when did this occur? Does your child have problems with incontinence during the day or bedwet-

ting at night? How does your child communicate the need to eliminate? Does your child need any type of assistance with toileting?
(RATIONALE: These questions assess elimination activities, which are important milestones for children. They uncover any special needs the child may have so that these needs can be met during hospitalization, if necessary.)

Can your child get dressed alone? Does your child have any difficulties when dressing?
(RATIONALE: Children gradually assume responsibility for dressing and grooming—two important components of personal care activities. Slowness to assume these responsibilities may indicate a developmental lag.)

Where does your child go to school? In which grade is your child? What does your child enjoy most and least in school? Has your child's school performance changed recently? If so, in what way?
(RATIONALE: For most older children, school activities are their work activities. Questions such as these evaluate a child's involvement in, and feelings about, school.)

What is your child's daily schedule? Does your child prefer to play alone, with peers, or with adults? What are your child's favorite activities and toys? Does your child participate in sports? How much time each day does your child have for play? What type of physical exercise does your child perform as a part of normal play?
(RATIONALE: These questions evaluate the type of play the child enjoys and the factors affecting it. Play provides the child with a sense of control, a means of self-expression, and a way to learn about the world. Play also encourages sensorimotor and intellectual development.)

ASSESSING SLEEP PATTERNS

A person's age, exercise level, personal habits, diet, environment, and mood all affect the quality and duration of sleep. Altering one or more of these factors, with the ob-

vious exception of age, often can improve sleep. The first steps in assessing a client's sleep patterns are identifying the factors affecting sleep, distinguishing between normal and abnormal sleep patterns, and knowing when to refer a client to a sleep disorder center for specialized diagnostic procedures and treatment. Then, after collecting appropriate data, the nurse can formulate a specific nursing diagnosis and plan interventions. (For more information, see *Sleep pattern assessment* on page 38.) Sample interview questions related to sleep patterns follow.

Sleep-wake patterns
How old are you?
((RATIONALE: Age and developmental status affect the amount, timing, and quality of sleep.)

What do you do for a living? What are your normal working hours?
(RATIONALE: Certain occupations require shift work, which can disrupt sleep.)

What time do you usually go to bed? What time do you usually wake up in the morning?
(RATIONALE: The usual times for retiring and arising provide accurate information about the duration of sleep.)

Do you fall asleep easily? Do you usually sleep all night without waking up? If awakened, do you fall asleep again quickly?
(RATIONALE: Difficulty falling asleep or staying asleep at night may indicate a sleep disorder. If so, this would indicate the need for a more detailed sleep assessment.)

Does anything help you sleep? Does anything make it more difficult to sleep?
(RATIONALE: The answers to these questions provide information about the use of sleeping pills and the client's bedtime rituals.)

Do you feel rested when you awaken in the morning?
(RATIONALE: A complaint of feeling tired upon awakening suggests insufficient sleep or a lack of restful sleep because of mood changes, medical problems, or a sleep dis-

Sleep pattern assessment

When a client reports a sleep problem or is at risk for sleep disruption, assess the severity of the problem by following these basic steps. Obtain more detailed information, as needed, based on the client's responses to your questions.

1. Ask if the client has difficulty initiating and maintaining sleep. If so, carefully assess the duration of the problem as well as the client's habits, mood, stress level, snoring, and use of medications. Also, observe and document nighttime sleep.

2. Find out if the client is excessively sleepy during the day. If so, ask about the onset and duration of symptoms, type of problems encountered, presence of other symptoms, snoring, and character of nocturnal sleep. Also, observe and document the client's sleep patterns.

3. Determine if the client sleeps normally, but at an inappropriate time of day. Ask if the client must work evenings, nights, or rotating shifts. If so, assess how long difficulties have been present, and how the client has tried to resolve them.

4. Ask if the client sleepwalks, experiences night terrors or enuresis, or makes unexplained movements or noises at night. If so, check for a family history of these activities and a history of seizures. Also note the client's age and any stressors.

5. If no abnormal sleep patterns are present, no further assessment is needed. Provide preventive information, if appropriate. However, if abnormal sleep patterns are present, perform a detailed sleep assessment.

6. After the detailed sleep assessment, expect the physician to refer the client to a sleep disorder center if the client has symptoms of chronic insomnia, sleep apnea, narcolepsy, sleep-wake cycle disturbances, or nocturnal seizures. If no referral is needed, plan interventions with the client to normalize sleep patterns.

order. In this instance, perform a more detailed assessment of the client's sleep patterns.)

Do you take naps during the day? Can you stay awake when driving, at work, and around the house?
(RATIONALE: Although daytime naps are common for children and elderly clients, most adults can remain awake and alert during the day. If the client has difficulty remaining awake when carrying out ADLs, perform a more detailed assessment.)

How is your health? Do you have any acute or chronic illnesses? What prescription and nonprescription medications do you take? Do you use alcohol or recreational drugs?
(RATIONALE: Certain medications, such as diet pills, and some illnesses, such as emphysema, can interfere with sleep.)

Are you satisfied with your sleep? If not, what bothers you about it?
(RATIONALE: The answer to this question uncovers the client's perception of sleep. If the client has concerns, perform a further assessment or, if indicated, educate the client about normal sleep patterns.)

Excessive daytime sleepiness
When did you first notice that you had difficulty staying awake during the day? Could you stay awake in high school or in college? Could you stay awake during your 20s or 30s?
(RATIONALE: The answers to these questions help pinpoint the onset of the symptoms. Also question the client's spouse, friends, or family members about the client's ability to stay awake during the day.)

Does your sleepiness cause you any difficulties? Can you stay awake while driving?

Have you had any accidents because of sleepiness? Do you fall asleep at work, when talking, or while watching TV or reading? Do you fall asleep at unusual times and places?
(RATIONALE: Brief attacks of sleep during activity and rest may indicate narcolepsy or sleep apnea.)

Do you take naps? How long are the naps? Do you feel refreshed after a nap?
(RATIONALE: These questions obtain information about whether the client can resist naps and about the duration of naps. Naps usually refresh clients with disorders of excessive daytime sleepiness, but only briefly.)

Does anything improve your alertness or make you especially sleepy?
(RATIONALE: This question provides information about ways the client has tried to increase alertness and conditions that provoke sleepiness.)

Does anything unusual happen—such as a feeling of weakness or feeling that you will fall down—when you laugh, become angry, or feel startled or surprised?
(RATIONALE: Positive answers to these questions indicate cataplexy. If the symptoms exist, ask when they first began and what circumstances trigger them. Refer a client with these symptoms to a sleep disorder center for definitive diagnosis and treatment.)

Have you ever felt momentarily paralyzed just before falling asleep or upon awakening?
(RATIONALE: If the client has experienced sleep paralysis, ask about onset and frequency. Sleep paralysis can be normal and does not by itself suggest a sleep disorder.)

Have you ever had dreams more frightening than nightmares, and so vivid that they seemed real? If so, when did these dreams occur? Did they occur while you were falling asleep, on awakening, or during the night?
(RATIONALE: These symptoms suggest hypnagogic hallucinations, which are vivid and realistic and usually occur while falling asleep or on awakening.)

Assessment checklist

The nurse should ask herself or himself these questions before beginning the assessment:
☐ Does the client require any special assistance, such as a cane or walker? If so, have I provided for it?
☐ Have I reviewed the appropriate ADLs for this client? Have I reviewed the appropriate hours of sleep?
☐ How might the client's culture influence ADLs and sleep patterns?
☐ Have I observed and evaluated the client's home environment, where practical?
☐ Have I reviewed relevant laboratory data?

Have you ever been told that you snore? If so, how loudly? Can people in the next room hear you? How about several rooms away? When did you start snoring? Has it recently become louder or more frequent?
(RATIONALE: Snoring often accompanies sleep apnea. The loudness of the snoring provides a rough index of the problem's severity. The client's bed partner is an excellent source for this information.)

Have you ever been told that you stop breathing at night, that you make grunting or snorting noises, or that you are a restless sleeper? If so, when did these things first happen? Have they recently increased in frequency?
(RATIONALE: Breathing difficulties and restless sleep commonly occur in a client with obstructive sleep apnea. The client's bed partner, and not the client, usually notices these signs and symptoms.)

Have you recently gained weight? Do you weigh more now than you did 5 years ago, 10 years ago, or 15 years ago? Has your collar size increased in recent years?
(RATIONALE: Weight gain often triggers the onset of obstructive sleep apnea.)

Do you drink alcohol? If so, how much?
(RATIONALE: Alcohol exacerbates sleep apnea.)

Do you have headaches in the morning? How is your memory? Is it worse than it used to be? Have you been told that you are more irritable than you used to be?
(RATIONALE: Clients with sleep apnea frequently experience morning headaches, memory loss, and irritability. The client's spouse or family members are often the first to notice memory and personality changes.)

Does anyone else in your family have similar problems with sleep?
(RATIONALE: Approximately half of the clients with narcolepsy have family members who suffer from excessive sleepiness.)

Insomnia
When did you first notice that you had difficulty sleeping at night? What was going on in your life at that time? Were you ill, stressed, or having family problems?
(RATIONALE: These questions establish the approximate date of symptom onset and help identify the precipitating circumstances.)

Has the problem worsened, improved, or remained the same? Do you have problems every night or only once in a while?
(RATIONALE: Besides describing the severity of the complaint, the answers to these questions help assess for factors affecting the client's ability to sleep.)

What do you do when you can't sleep? Do you worry about not being able to sleep? Do you stare at the clock, get up and do something else, or take a sleeping pill?
(RATIONALE: Besides identifying the use of sleeping pills, these questions help identify behaviors that might increase sleeplessness.)

After a sleepless night, how do you feel the next day? Do you have difficulty staying awake? Do you take a nap?
(RATIONALE: Napping, particularly in the evening, may disrupt nocturnal sleep.)

Do you exercise regularly? If so, what time of day do you usually exercise?
(RATIONALE: Regular exercise, especially in the late afternoon, may facilitate sleep for some individuals. Irregular exercise or exercise just before retiring may inhibit sleep.)

Do you smoke cigarettes?
(RATIONALE: A smoker may have more difficulty falling asleep than a nonsmoker.)

Is your bedroom noisy or uncomfortably hot or cold? Does your bed partner snore or disrupt your sleep?
(RATIONALE: Noise [including snoring], a restless bed partner, or an uncomfortable room temperature can disrupt sleep.)

How would you describe your recent moods? Are you depressed or under stress?
(RATIONALE: Most insomnia results from anxiety or psychological problems.)

Do you have any other concerns about your sleep that you would like to discuss?
(RATIONALE: This open-ended question provides an opportunity to discuss concerns and reassure the client that the body obtains all the sleep it needs and that sleep loss rarely leads to illness or other problems.)

Developmental considerations
Pose the following types of questions to a child's parent or guardian.
What is your child's usual bedtime and naptime? How long does your child sleep at night?
(RATIONALE: Evaluate the child's sleep patterns according to the child's age. Teach the parents about the normal changes that occur with age. For example, many 5 year olds stop taking naps.)

What is your child's usual bedtime routine? Does it include such activities as eating a snack, listening to a story, or brushing teeth?
(RATIONALE: Toddlers commonly have elaborate bedtime routines. Use this information to continue the child's usual bedtime routine during hospitalization. Also, if the child has difficulty falling asleep at night, assess the child's activities just before bedtime.)

Does your child have any particular security objects, such as a toy or a night-light? Does your child have any security behaviors, such as thumb sucking?

(RATIONALE: Use this information to continue the child's usual routine during hospitalization. Also, reassure parents that many children need security objects and behaviors, and will relinquish them with maturity.)

Does your child have any sleep difficulties? Does your child have difficulty falling asleep? Does your child awaken during the night (if not appropriate for the child's developmental age)? Does your child have nightmares or night terrors? If so, please describe. Does your child wet the bed, snore, or breathe loudly?

(RATIONALE: Many difficulties associated with bedtime and awakening at night occur because of inconsistent routines, a lack of parental limit-setting, and the parent's response to the child awakening at night. For example, feeding and holding the child whenever the child awakens at night positively reinforces nighttime awakenings. Reassure the parents that children commonly have night terrors and nightmares between ages 2 and 4. Provide information about enuresis, if appropriate. Also, loud, noisy breathing or snoring suggests sleep apnea, which requires referral to a sleep disorder center for evaluation and treatment.)

Do you have any other concerns about your child's sleep patterns that you would like to discuss?
(RATIONALE: This open-ended question gives the parents the opportunity to discuss any additional concerns.)

DOCUMENTATION

The SOAPIE method of documentation includes the following components: subjective (history) data, objective (physical) data, assessment, planning, implementation, and evaluation. The following example shows how to document nursing care for a client with sleeping difficulty.

Case history

Mrs. Jones, 72 years old, has a history of hypertension. Three weeks ago, she moved with her husband of 44 years from their single-family home into a senior citizen

Selected nursing diagnosis categories

The nurse can use these diagnosis categories to formulate nursing diagnoses for a client with modified ADLs or with sleep disorders.

- Activity intolerance
- Altered role performance
- Bathing or hygiene self-care deficit
- Body image disturbance
- Bowel incontinence
- Constipation
- Diarrhea
- Diversional activity deficit
- Dressing or grooming self-care deficit
- Feeding self-care deficit
- High risk for injury
- Impaired adjustment
- Impaired home maintenance management
- Impaired physical mobility
- Ineffective family coping: Compromised
- Ineffective individual coping
- Self-esteem disturbance
- Sleep pattern disturbance
- Toileting self-care deficit

apartment complex. While the visiting nurse checks her blood pressure, Mrs. Jones complains of having difficulty sleeping at night and of feeling tired and sluggish during the day.

S   O   A   P   I   E

Client states, "I am having trouble falling asleep and wake up several times during the night. My husband and I just moved to a new apartment, and I'm having trouble sleeping in a different place. I'm tired and have difficulty doing my usual activities during the day. I often have to take a nap, which is not my usual routine."

S   **O**   A   P   I   E

Temperature 98.4° F., pulse 78 and regular, respirations 18 and regular, blood pressure 136/84. Skin pale, dark circles under the eyes. Eyelids appear puffy. Client yawned frequently during the interview.

S   O   **A**   P   I   E

Sleep pattern disturbance related to changes in home environment.

S   O   A   **P**   I   E

Identify factors interfering with client's
sleep. Develop strategies to eliminate or reduce environmental disturbances. Discuss
foods and medications that may interfere
with restful sleep. Teach client additional
measures to promote restful sleep.

S   O   A   P   **I**   E

Discussed with client noise, temperature,
light, and newness of surroundings as possible factors interfering with sleep. Taught
strategies to reduce environmental disturbances, such as closing door and curtains.
Discussed why reliance on sleeping medications is not advised and pointed out the
effect of caffeine and alcohol consumption
on sleep. Instructed client in relaxation techniques, such as a warm bath and reading at
bedtime.

S   O   A   P   I   **E**

Client identified factors that interfere with
sleep and strategies to eliminate them. Client
described the role of medications and food
in the promotion of restful sleep. Client
identified relaxation methods she will employ to promote sleep.

SUGGESTED READINGS

Dorociak, Y. (1991). Aspects of sleep.
Nursing Times, 86(51), 38-40.

Fisher, A. (1992). Functional measures:
What is function, what should we measure, and how should we measure it? Part
1. *American Journal of Occupational
Therapy, 46*(2), 183-185.

Fisher, A., et al. (1992). Cross-cultural assessment of process skills. *American
Journal of Occupational Therapy, 46*(10),
876-885.

Hodgson, L. (1991). Why do we need sleep?
Relating theory to nursing practice. *Journal of Advanced Nursing, 16*(12), 1503-
1510.

Weiler, K. (1991). Functional assessment
in the determination of the need for a
substitute decision maker. *Journal of
Professional Nursing, 7*(6), 328.

4

Nutritional Status

From birth, the quality of a client's life is affected by the quality and quantity of nutrients consumed and used. The body's nutritional status—the balance between nutrient intake and energy expenditure or need—reflects the degree to which the physiologic need for nutrients is being met. Proper nutrition promotes growth, maintains health, and helps the body resist infection and recover from disease or surgery. Malnutrition impedes these natural processes.

HEALTH HISTORY

The nutritional health history includes a dietary history, intake record, and psychosocial assessment. It can confirm good nutrition or detect an altered nutritional status and the need for more in-depth assessment and follow-up; it also identifies potential nutrition-related health problems, detects the need for education, and permits realistic planning for short- and long-term goals.

Three groups of sample questions follow. Those on *health and illness patterns* help the nurse identify actual or potential nutrition-related health problems; those on *health promotion and protection patterns* help the nurse determine what the client does to maintain adequate nutrition; and those on *role and relationship patterns* help the nurse determine the client's body image and relationships with others.

Health and illness patterns

Have you had any recent change in diet? If so, can you describe the duration and specific changes? To what degree has your caloric intake increased or decreased?
(RATIONALE: A decreased intake contributes to weight loss and may lead to nutritional deficiency. An increased intake may lead to weight gain, but does not rule out nutritional deficiency.)

Have you experienced any significant weight gain or loss, or a change in appetite, bowel habits, mobility, physical exercise, or lifestyle?
(RATIONALE: Significant changes may indicate an underlying disease. For example, weight gain may indicate an endocrine imbalance, such as Cushing's syndrome or hypothyroidism; weight loss may be related to cancer, GI disorders, diabetes mellitus, or hyperthyroidism.)

Do you take any prescription or over-the-counter medications, especially vitamin or mineral supplements or appetite suppressants? If so, what is the purpose, starting date, dose, and frequency of each? Do you use any "natural" or "health" foods? If so, which ones and how much of each do you use, and why?
(RATIONALE: The client's response to these questions may indicate a nutritional deficiency requiring supplementation, or that the client perceives a nutritional deficiency

and self-prescribes. In other cases, the response may reveal routine drug use that can cause nutritional deficiencies or related problems.)

Do you drink alcoholic beverages? If so, how much per day or week and what kind? How long have you been drinking alcohol? (RATIONALE: Alcohol intake provides calories, but no essential nutrients. Chronic alcohol abuse may lead to malnutrition.)

How much per day do you consume of the following beverages: coffee, tea, cola, cocoa? (RATIONALE: These beverages contain caffeine, a habit-forming stimulant that increases heart rate, respiration rate, blood pressure, and secretion of stress hormones. In moderate amounts of 50 to 200 mg/day, caffeine is relatively harmless. Intake of greater amounts can cause sensations of nervousness and intestinal discomfort. Clients who drink 8 or more cups of coffee may complain of insomnia, restlessness, agitation, palpitations, and recurring headaches. Sudden abstinence after long periods of even moderate daily intake can cause withdrawal symptoms, usually headache.)

Do you have any food allergies? If so, please describe them. (RATIONALE: Food allergies may have caused the client to eliminate certain foods, thus increasing the hazard of nutritional deficiencies. The nurse can use information about food allergies to help the client plan safe, balanced meals or to prevent the hospitalized client from being served food that can cause an allergic reaction.)

Have you ever had (or been told that you have) an eating disorder, such as anorexia nervosa or bulimia, or a problem with substance abuse? (RATIONALE: These conditions compromise nutritional status.)

Have you followed a planned weight-loss or weight-gain program within the past 6 months? If so, please describe the program. (RATIONALE: Because fad dieting can lead to altered nutritional status, evaluate the client's eating program.)

Do you have a family history of any of the following disorders: cardiovascular disease, Crohn's disease, diabetes mellitus, cancer, GI tract disorders, sickle-cell anemia, allergies, food intolerance (for example, lactose intolerance), or obesity? (RATIONALE: These genetic or familial disorders may affect digestion or metabolism of food and can alter the client's nutritional status.)

Developmental considerations
Use the following sample questions as a guide to assessing nutritional status in a pediatric, pregnant, lactating, or elderly client.

Infant
If the infant is breast-fed, how often and how long does he or she nurse at each breast? How much water does the infant drink, and how often? Do you use relief bottles? If so, what type of bottle or nipple do you use? What type of formula do you use, and how much and how often do you give it? Do you give the infant supplementary food or cereal? If so, how much? (RATIONALE: During the 1st year of life, energy needs are high in relation to body size. The normal full-term neonate needs 110 to 120 calories per kg of body weight per 24 hours. Human milk and properly prepared formula supply adequate fluid intake under normal circumstances. A "rule-of-thumb" gauge for the fluid requirement for normal infants is approximately 100 ml of fluid per kilogram of body weight in a 24-hour period. Neither whole cow's milk nor skim milk is suitable for use in formula during the 1st year of life. Solid food is usually not introduced until the 4th to 6th month for formula-fed infants and the 6th month for breast-fed infants. Cereal is usually the first solid food added to the infant's diet. Strained fruits and vegetables may be introduced gradually at about the 6th month.)

Toddler
How much fluid does your child drink in a typical 24-hour period? How much of it is milk (specify kind), juice, or carbonated drinks? Does the child drink from a cup? Does the child feed himself? How often and

what kind of snacks are eaten? Is the child allergic to any foods? Does the child particularly like or dislike any food(s)?
(RATIONALE: Growth rate slows during this time, but muscle mass development and bone mineralization increase. At the beginning of the toddler period [age 1], the child needs approximately 1,000 Kcal/day; the amount increases to 1,300 to 1,500 Kcal by the end of the toddler period [age 3]. In developing autonomy, a toddler may refuse food at times.)

School-age child
What does the child eat for breakfast? Does the child take lunch to school or eat the school lunch? Is the child involved in sports or other physical activities at school?
(RATIONALE: Body changes continue gradually during these years. Girls usually advance at a faster rate than boys. Breakfast is a particularly important meal during this time, preparing the child for learning and school activities. Food likes and dislikes continue in the established pattern, and may be affected by television viewing. Nutrition information usually is included in the curriculum. School-related activities may conflict with family mealtimes.)

Adolescent
What do you eat in a typical day (24 hours)? What snacks and fluids do you consume? Do you use any alcohol, drugs, tobacco, caffeine (coffee, tea, cola, or cocoa), salt, or vitamin supplements? If so, what effects do they produce? Do you follow any special diets? Have you gained or lost weight recently?
(RATIONALE: Adolescence is a time of rapid growth, with the onset of puberty increasing nutritional requirements. The growth rate varies widely among individuals, and includes sex-related differences. The growth rate of boys is usually slower than that of girls; however, boys' total weight and height gains are usually greater than girls'.)

Pregnant client
How have your eating patterns changed since you have become pregnant?
(RATIONALE: The nutritional status of the mother during pregnancy contributes to the future health of the child. An increase in protein and other nutrients—particularly calcium, iron, and folic acid—is needed during pregnancy. The daily requirement of folic acid is doubled during pregnancy, from 0.4 mg to 0.8 mg, because of increased fetal needs. Some pregnant women have pica [a craving for nonfood substances, such as starch or clay].)

Are you taking any nutritional supplements, such as vitamins?
(RATIONALE: Physicians usually prescribe supplements that contain all of the needed additional nutrients for pregnant clients. If the pregnant client is a teenager, the need for nutrients is greater from demands of the developing fetus added to the growth and development of the mother.)

How has your weight changed since you have become pregnant?
(RATIONALE: Caloric intake should be increased by about 1,000 Kcal/day. Sometimes, however, a woman may overeat, believing she must eat for two. The weight gain should be at the rate of 0.5 to 1 pound per week, with approximately 4 pounds in the 1st trimester, 10 to 12 pounds in the 2nd trimester, and 8 to 10 pounds in the 3rd trimester.)

Are you currently breast-feeding another baby?
(RATIONALE: Breast-feeding is contraindicated during pregnancy because both processes increase nutritional requirements and compete for available nutrients.)

Breast-feeding client
Do you have any questions regarding breast-feeding, or any personal concerns or problems? Have you noticed any changes or problems in your breasts? Is breast-feeding pleasurable?
(RATIONALE: A change in the mother's physical or emotional health can alter breast milk supply.)

Elderly client
Do you wear dentures? If so, do they interfere with your eating patterns in any way?

(RATIONALE: Poorly fitted dentures can decrease nutritional intake and limit variety in diet, predisposing the client to certain nutritional deficiencies.)

Do you suffer from constipation or stool incontinence?
(RATIONALE: A decrease in intestinal motility characteristically accompanies aging; constipation also may be related to poor dietary intake, physical inactivity, or emotional stress, or may occur as an adverse reaction to drugs. Elderly clients often consume nutritionally inadequate diets of soft, refined foods that are low in residue and dietary fiber. Laxative abuse, another common problem in elderly clients, moves foods rapidly through the GI tract and subsequently decreases periods of digestion and absorption.)

Has your diet changed as you have grown older? If so, how?
(RATIONALE: Individual protein, vitamin, and mineral requirements usually remain the same during aging, while caloric needs decrease. Decreased activity may lower energy requirements about 200 calories/day for men and women age 51 to 75, 400 calories/day for women over age 75, and 500 calories/day for men over age 75. Other physiologic changes can affect nutrition in an elderly client. For example, decreased renal function can cause greater susceptibility to dehydration and formation of renal calculi. A decreased salivary flow and diminished sense of taste may reduce the client's appetite and increase consumption of sweet and spicy foods. Other physiologic changes that can affect nutrition include loss of calcium and nitrogen [in nonambulatory clients], decreased enzyme activity and gastric secretions, and decreased intestinal motility.)

Health promotion and protection patterns

Which particular foods do you believe you should eat at this time? Which particular foods do you believe you should not eat at this time? How would these foods affect your body?

(RATIONALE: Different cultural health beliefs exist concerning food intake and its relationship to health.)

How would you describe your usual activity patterns? Do you exercise? If so, what specific type of exercise do you do? How often do you exercise and for how many minutes? What time of day do you usually exercise?
(RATIONALE: The response will reveal if the client is active or sedentary and will help you determine the client's caloric requirements.)

Do you use food or drink to help you get through stressful times?
(RATIONALE: Answers to this question will help identify whether the client uses food or drink as a coping mechanism. Individuals respond to stressful situations in different ways; they may increase or decrease food intake, or change the type of food they eat. The client may not be fully aware of an increase in stress, or may be reluctant to identify or discuss the situation because of its stressful nature.)

Where and how is your food prepared? Do you have access to adequate storage and refrigeration?
(RATIONALE: A client who must rely on others for food preparation may be at risk for nutritional deficiency if the food preparer is unavailable. Inadequate food storage and refrigeration can lead to nutritional problems.)

Do you receive food stamps, Social Security payments, supplemental Social Security payments, or assistance from welfare or the WIC (Women, Infant, Child) program? Do you participate in a community meal program for your main meals, or a "Meals On Wheels" program?
(RATIONALE: A change in economic status or the loss of a food program can alter meal planning and eliminate certain foods, thus placing the client at risk for a nutritional disorder.)

Role and relationship patterns

Are you content with your present weight?
(RATIONALE: The client's answer may reveal beliefs about weight that can lead to serious

Dietary recall methods

The nurse can use one of several diet recall methods to assess a client's dietary patterns, as described below.

For the *24-hour dietary recall,* ask the client to recall everything taken as food or drink within the past 24 hours (or yesterday), the time it was taken, the amount, and how it was prepared. If the client is an infant or small child, determine the feeding schedule and the types and amounts of food and drink taken. (Determine if intake is adequate.) If the client is hospitalized, the 24-hour recall will not provide information regarding the usual dietary pattern; ask this client to write down 24-hour food intake on a "typical day."

When completing the *3-day* or *7- to 14-day dietary inventory* or *diary,* have the client record everything taken as food or fluid; the time it was taken; the amount; and if cooked, how prepared—that is, broiled, fried (in what), baked, boiled, stir-fried, microwaved. Also have the client record the place in which it was consumed, whether it was taken when alone or with others, and whether it was taken in response to a felt personal need, such as hunger or thirst, or for some other reason. This type of inventory is considered very reliable; however, a client may consciously or unconsciously modify the dietary intake during the recorded time.

The *food frequency form* provides an overview of the quality and variety of the foods eaten. Using the list of foods, the client indicates how often a particular food is eaten.

Agency *dietary history questionnaires* usually combine dietary intake inventory with questions about factors that affect food intake.

When completing any of the diet recall intake forms, be sure to ask the client to indicate the addition of any seasoning to the food.

eating disorders, such as anorexia nervosa or bulimia.)

Do you eat alone or with others?
(RATIONALE: Single adults and elderly clients who are isolated from support systems may neglect nutrition. A person grieving over the recent loss of a spouse, a family member, a close friend, or a pet may lose interest in preparing food or eating.)

On a scale of 1 to 10, with 10 being most important to you, how would you rate mealtimes?
(RATIONALE: Use of the scale helps determine if meals are enjoyed or endured. If they are endured, the client could develop an eating disorder, such as bulimia.)

PHYSICAL ASSESSMENT

The nurse uses the following equipment and techniques when assessing nutritional status.

Equipment
• standing platform scale with height attachment
• infant scale and recumbent measuring board, when appropriate
• stature measuring device, when appropriate
• skinfold calipers
• measuring tape

Techniques
• inspection
• palpation

Inspection

Begin by inspecting the client's overall appearance, particularly the skin, hair, mouth (lips, teeth, gingivae, tongue, and mucous membranes), eyes, nails, posture, muscles, extremities, and thyroid gland. Generally, the skin should appear smooth, free of lesions, and appropriate for the client's age. The hair should be shiny. The mouth, mucous membranes, lips, tongue, and gingivae should be pink and free of lesions. The teeth should be intact, firmly attached to the gingivae, and contain few cavities. The eyes should be clear with pink conjunctiva. The nails should be smooth without cracks or fissures. The client's posture should be appropriate for age, and the movement of extremities and muscles should be symmetrical. The thyroid should not appear enlarged.

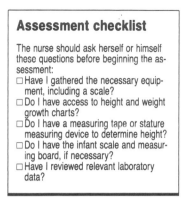

Assessment checklist

The nurse should ask herself or himself these questions before beginning the assessment:

☐ Have I gathered the necessary equipment, including a scale?

☐ Do I have access to height and weight growth charts?

☐ Do I have a measuring tape or stature measuring device to determine height?

☐ Do I have the infant scale and measuring board, if necessary?

☐ Have I reviewed relevant laboratory data?

Considering the client's height in relation to weight may provide clues to undernutrition or overnutrition. Comparison with standard measurements shows whether the client's weight, height, and body frame are above or below that standard, indicating whether the client is undernourished or overnourished.

Although an adult's self-report of height is usually correct, take a baseline measurement. Weigh the client yourself, if possible, to obtain an accurate baseline for comparison with ideal body weight, usual weight, and future weight.

To determine ideal body weight for an adult client (ages 18 and over), first determine body frame size. Then, based on body frame size, compare the client's height and weight with the values on a standard height-weight chart.

Palpation

Although less important than inspection for detecting nutritional deficiencies, palpation helps detect enlarged glands, including the thyroid, parotid, liver, spleen, and others that may indicate a nutrition-compromising disorder. Palpation may also reveal signs of deficiency when performed on the teeth and tongue.

Developmental considerations

Children require special techniques for physical assessment of nutritional status. In a child under age 2, measure length with the child supine. Weigh an infant nude, be-

cause diapers vary greatly in weight. Use growth charts to compare the height and weight measurements; these charts reflect measurements of the population of American children taken as a whole.

A healthy, growing child usually maintains the same relative position on the growth chart. Measure head and chest circumference in infants and children; as with height and weight, compare these measurements to standard growth charts.

Head circumference

To measure an infant's head circumference, wrap a nonstretching measuring tape around the head just above the supraorbital ridges and over the most prominent part of the occiput.

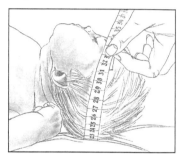

Chest circumference

To measure an infant's chest circumference, wrap the tape around the chest at the nipples. Take the measurement between inspiration and expiration.

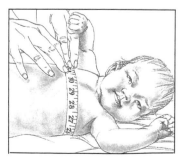

Common laboratory studies

For a client with signs and symptoms of a nutritional disorder, various laboratory studies can provide the nurse with valuable clues to the possible cause. This chart lists common laboratory studies along with normal values or findings. Remember that values differ among laboratories; check the normal value range for the specific laboratory.

BLOOD TESTS	NORMAL VALUES OR FINDINGS
Hemoglobin	*Males:* 14 to 18 g/dl *Females:* 12 to 16 g/dl *Children:* 11 to 13 g/dl
Hematocrit	Concentration varies with the client's age and sex *Males:* 42% to 54% *Females:* 38% to 46% *Children:* 36% to 40%
Red blood cell indices	*Mean corpuscular volume (MCV):* *84 to 99/mu³ /red cell*
	Mean corpuscular hemoglobin (MCH): 26 to 32 pg/red cell
	Mean corpuscular hemoglobin concentration (MCHC): 30% to 36%
Serum iron	*Males:* 70 to 150 mcg/dl *Females:* 80 to 150 mcg/dl
Serum albumin	3.3 to 4.5 g/dl
Serum transferrin (siderophilin)	250 to 390 mcg/dl (65 to 170 mcg usually bound to iron)
Total iron-binding capacity (TIBC)	*Males:* 300 to 400 mcg/dl *Females:* 300 to 450 mcg/dl
Total lymphocyte count (TLC)	1,500 to 3,000 mm³ (TLC value stems from differential white blood cell [WBC] count)
Total protein	6 to 8 g/dl

Advanced assessment skills: Anthropometric arm measurements

• Midarm circumference, triceps skinfold thickness, and midarm muscle circumference provide a way to determine the amount of skeletal muscle and adipose tissue—which indicate protein and fat reserves.

• Serial measurements reflect changes in nutritional status. Documenting the measurements on a graphic flow chart provides an excellent visual means of following a trend.

Selected nursing diagnosis categories

The nurse can use these diagnosis categories to formulate nursing diagnoses for a client with nutritional disorders.
- Altered growth and development
- Altered nutrition: Less than body requirements
- Altered nutrition: More than body requirements
- Body image disturbance
- Bowel incontinence
- Constipation
- Diarrhea
- Feeding self-care deficit
- Fluid volume deficit
- Fluid volume excess
- Impaired swallowing
- Impaired tissue integrity

DOCUMENTATION

The SOAPIE method of documentation includes the following components: subjective (history) data, objective (physical) data, assessment, planning, implementation, and evaluation. The following example shows how to document nursing care for a client with unexplained weakness and weight loss.

Case history

Mrs. Elsa Braun, age 72, was admitted to the hospital with a medical diagnosis of "unexplained weakness and weight loss."

S O A P I E

Client states, "I feel so tired and weak lately. I've had a poor appetite since my husband's death 3 months ago. I've been sleeping poorly since then, too."

S **O** A P I E

Client appears tired and close to tears.
Vital signs: BP 120/82; pulse 76, regular; respirations irregular. Weight: 122 lb. Height: 5'7". Body frame: medium. Triceps skinfold: 16 mm; midarm circumference, 25 cm; midarm muscle circumference, 20 cm. Dry, pale skin. Teeth in good repair.

S O **A** P I E

Altered nutrition: less than body requirements, related to decreased appetite after death of spouse. Client's measurements are at the 15th percentile, indicating mild depletion.

S O A **P** I E

Broaden dietary intake to include foods from the five basic food groups. Add bran to prevent constipation. Increase fluid intake. Increase body weight by 1 lb every 2 weeks for 5 weeks.

S O A P **I** E

Taught client about five food groups. Taught client to keep a food diary. Weighed client every 3 days.

S O A P I **E**

Client wants to eat properly and take care of herself. She understands the importance of writing down what she eats every day.

SUGGESTED READINGS

Cerrato, P. (1991). Assessing your patient's diet. *RN*, 54(1), 60-63.

Cerrato, P. (1992). Goodbye four food groups...Food guide pyramid. *RN*, 55(12), 61-62.

Cerrato, P. (1993). What diet can do to combat HIV infection. *RN*, 56(6), 71-72.

Charalambous, L. (1993). A healthy approach. *Nursing Times*, 89(20), 58-60.

Chernoff, R., and Ropka, M. (1993). The unique nutritional needs of the elderly patient with cancer. *Caring*, 12(2), 64-71.

Dean, D. (1993). Nutritional assessment of disadvantaged children. In R. Karp, *Malnourished children in the United States: Caught in the cycle of poverty* (pp. 59-67). New York: Springer Publishing.

Gerber, J. (1993). *Handbook of preventive and therapeutic nutrition.* Gaithersburg, MD: Aspen Publishers.

Gianino, S., and St. John, R. (1993). Nutritional assessment of the patient in the intensive care unit. *Critical Care Nursing Clinics of North America*, 5(1), 1-16.

Giotta, M. (1993). Nutrition during pregnancy: Reducing obstetric risk. *Journal of Perinatal and Neonatal Nursing,* 6(4), 1-12.

Gizis, F. (1992). Nutrition in women across the life span. *Nursing Clinics of North America,* 27(4), 971-982.

Houda, B. (1993). Evaluation of nutritional status in persons with spinal cord injury: A prerequisite for successful rehabilitation. *SCI Nursing,* 10(1), 4-7.

Huddleston, K. (1993). Nutritional support of the critically ill child. *Critical Care Nursing Clinics of North America,* 5(1), 65-78.

Kelly, K. (1993). Advances in perioperative nutritional support. *Medical Clinics of North America,* 77(2), 465-475.

Krause, M., and Mahan, L. (1992). *Food, nutrition, and diet therapy* (8th ed.). Philadelphia: W.B. Saunders Co.

Lee, M., Freeman, R., Cialone, J., and Lichtenwalter, L. (1993). Nutrition care for children with special health needs: A chart review. *Public Health Nursing,* 10(3), 177-182.

Lehmann, S. (1993). Nutritional support in the hypermetabolic patient. *Critical Care Nursing Clinics of North America,* 5(1), 97-103.

Loogman, E. (1992). Nutritional assessment in nursing. *Gastroenterology Nursing,* 14(4), 189-194.

Mairis, E. (1992). An appetite for life: Assessing and meeting nutritional needs. *Professional Nurse,* 7(11), 732-737.

Mancusi-Ungaro, H., et al. (1992). Caloric and nitrogen balances as predictors of nutritional outcome in patients with burns. *Journal of Burn Care Rehabilitation,* 13(6), 695-702.

Poole, S. (1993). A requirement not to be overlooked: Nutritional aspects of respiratory disease. *Professional Nurse,* 8(4), 252-256.

Schultz, T. (1993). Nutrition: Its role in wound healing. *Journal of Home Health Care Practice,* 5(3), 56-63.

Sidenvall, B., and Ek, A. (1993). Long-term care patients and their dietary intake related to eating ability and nutritional needs: Nursing staff interventions. *Journal of Advanced Nursing,* 18(4), 565-573.

Udine, L., and Capozza, C. (1993). Nutritional care of the HIV client. *Caring,* 12(5), 36-40.

Williams, S. (1993). *Nutrition and diet therapy* (7th ed.). St. Louis: Mosby, Inc.

UNIT THREE

Assessing Body Structures and Systems

5

Skin, Hair, and Nails

The largest body system, the skin and its appendages (the hair, nails, and certain glands) protect underlying structures, help regulate body temperature, and serve as a sensory organ. Because changes in the skin can indicate health changes, assessment of this system is an essential part of the total physical assessment.

HEALTH HISTORY

Skin assessment begins with a complete health history, which includes information that can tell the nurse a considerable amount about the client's skin, hair, and nails.

Three groups of sample questions follow. Those on *health and illness patterns* help the nurse identify actual or potential health problems; those on *health promotion and protection patterns* help the nurse determine how environment and life-style relate to the client's skin, hair, and nails; and those on *role and relationship patterns* help the nurse determine the client's social practices that relate to skin, hair, and nails.

Health and illness patterns

What aspect of your skin problem bothers you the most?
(RATIONALE: This question allows the client to identify the most important personal aspect of the problem, even though other concerns are apparent. For example, the client

may be more concerned with itching than with change in appearance.)

Where on your body did the skin problem begin?
(RATIONALE: Explain the importance of identifying the original site of the problem. Otherwise, a client who is too embarrassed to indicate an area considered private, such as the genitalia, may name another area as the origin of the problem instead.)

When did you first notice these changes?
(RATIONALE: Knowing the progression of the skin changes can provide important information.)

Please describe the initial problem in as much detail as possible, even if that problem has already disappeared. Can you also describe how the problem spread and in what order other areas were affected?
(RATIONALE: The shape, size, color, location, and distribution of the problem give clues to the cause of the disorder. So do the sensations associated with it and any pattern of migration. For example, chicken pox [varicella] spreads from the trunk to the limbs; shingles [herpes zoster] spreads in a distinct pattern along cutaneous nerve endings.)

Do you have other symptoms?
(RATIONALE: Symptoms in other body systems may be associated with certain skin

Anatomy review

The illustrations below show the anatomic structures of the skin, hair, and nails.

Skin

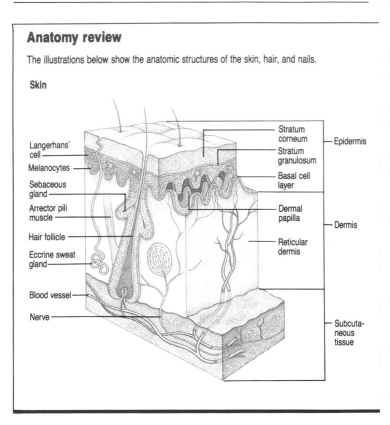

disorders. For example, systemic prodromal symptoms such as malaise and anorexia are associated with chicken pox.)

How does your skin feel?
(RATIONALE: Try to obtain the client's description before asking about specific sensations, such as itching, burning, stinging, tingling, numbness, pain, tenderness, malaise, or achiness.)

Does anything make the problem worse?
(RATIONALE: Aggravating factors are part of the diagnostic pattern for many skin disorders. Ask specifically about changes related to food, heat, cold, exercise, sunlight, stress, pregnancy, and menstruation. Shingles, for example, are frequently aggravated by sunlight, menstruation, or stress.)

Does anything make the problem better?
(RATIONALE: A positive answer, with specific drug or treatment description, helps the physician plan treatment and the nurse plan appropriate nursing interventions.)

Does the problem seem to be resolving or improving?
(RATIONALE: If the problem is resolving without treatment, the physician may want to watch and wait rather than treat it.)

Have you used any home remedies to try to resolve your problem, such as medications, compresses, lotions, creams, or ointments? Have you used any prescription or over-the-counter drugs?

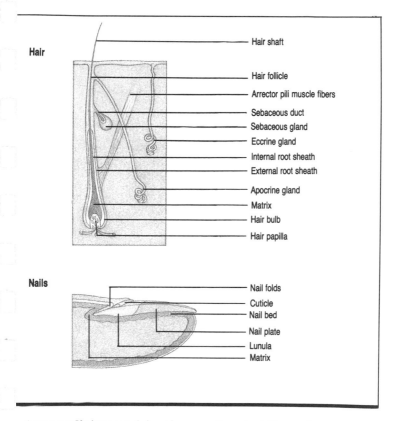

Hair

- Hair shaft
- Hair follicle
- Arrector pili muscle fibers
- Sebaceous duct
- Sebaceous gland
- Eccrine gland
- Internal root sheath
- External root sheath
- Apocrine gland
- Matrix
- Hair bulb
- Hair papilla

Nails

- Nail folds
- Cuticle
- Nail bed
- Nail plate
- Lunula
- Matrix

(RATIONALE: If a home remedy is not harmful and the client believes it helps, try to incorporate it into the care plan. Especially note the client's use of antibiotics or other drugs that may exacerbate the disorder.)

Have you noticed any unusual, overall, or patchy hair loss?
(RATIONALE: Overall hair loss may result from systemic illness or any treatment that affects the hair growth cycle, such as chemotherapy for cancer. Patchy hair loss may stem from hair care products, hairstyles, or infestations, such as lice [pediculosis].)

Have you noticed any changes in your nails?
(RATIONALE: Nail changes from aging are exacerbated by peripheral vascular disease;

other systemic illnesses also may cause negative changes.)

Have you recently experienced any fever, malaise, upper respiratory, or gastrointestinal problems?
(RATIONALE: Many common skin eruptions are related to viral infections. Recent infections and illnesses as well as treatment regimens may contribute to skin disorders.)

Have you had any allergic reactions to medications, foods, or other substances, such as cosmetics?
(RATIONALE: Past and present allergies, including those caused by cutaneous, ingested, or inhaled allergens, may predispose the client to other skin disorders.)

Has anyone in your family had a skin problem? If so, what was it and when did it occur?
(RATIONALE: Some skin disorders, such as allergic dermatitis, acne, or psoriasis, have familial tendencies; contagious skin problems, such as chicken pox and scabies, may be transmitted to the client from a family member.)

Has anyone in your family had an allergy? If so, what was it and how was it treated?
(RATIONALE: The client's problem may stem from an allergy that may be identified through knowledge of allergies in other family members.)

Pediatric client
Ask the parents of an infant or young child these types of questions:
Is the infant breast-fed or formula-fed?
(RATIONALE: Breast-fed infants have fewer allergies because they are not exposed to foreign proteins as early as formula-fed infants.)

Has the child had any skin problems related to a particular formula or food added to the diet?
(RATIONALE: Food allergies often manifest as skin problems in infants and young children.)

Has your infant had any diaper rashes that did not clear up readily with over-the-counter skin preparations?
(RATIONALE: Severe, unremitting diaper rashes may be caused by infection.)

What kind of diapers do you use? If cloth diapers, how do you wash them?
(RATIONALE: Severe, unremitting diaper rash may result from diapers that are not changed often enough or not washed properly.)

How often do you bathe your infant?
(RATIONALE: Too-frequent bathing can lead to skin problems, including dry skin with excessive desquamation. Conversely, infrequent bathing can lead to intertrigo [a superficial dermatitis in the skin folds] or cradle cap [a sebaceous hair and skin cell collection on the scalp].)

What products do you use on the infant's skin?
(RATIONALE: The infant may be allergic to soaps or other skin preparations, especially if they contain perfumes.)

Is your child attending nursery school? Do you have an older child in kindergarten or elementary school?
(RATIONALE: Contact with other children increases early exposure to communicable diseases with exanthems [skin eruptions accompanied by inflammation], such as measles or scarlet fever.)

Do you have pets in your home? Does the child sleep with stuffed animals?
(RATIONALE: Contact with pets and stuffed animals exposes the child to animal dander and collected dust, which may cause an allergic reaction.)

Has the child been scratching the scalp? Does the skin or scalp scale in circular patterns? Has the child lost an unusual amount of hair? Has the child been pulling his or her own hair?
(RATIONALE: The child may have pediculosis or ringworm [tinea capitis]. Both conditions injure the hair roots, weaken hair follicles, and may damage hair. A hair-pulling habit (trichotillomania) may cause patchy hair loss.

Has the child ever had warts? If so, on which body surfaces? How were they treated?
(RATIONALE: Warts are a viral condition. Warts on the soles of the feet may be painful. Warts on the genitalia may be a sign of sexual abuse by a person with venereal warts.)

Ask a school-age child or an adolescent these questions:
Do you play where you might come in contact with bugs, weeds, or bushes?
(RATIONALE: A child may develop transient or permanent hypersensitivity to insect bites or contact dermatitis from plant oils. The resulting itching can lead to scratching, excoriation, and possibly infection.)

Do you bite your nails? Do you twirl or otherwise play with your hair?

(RATIONALE: The client may develop nail infections from nail-biting and pattern baldness [alopecia] from playing with the hair.)

Does your face, upper back, or chest ever break out? If so, how do you feel about your skin appearance?
(RATIONALE: The adolescent may be self-conscious about acne and reluctant to talk about it until you establish a rapport. Knowing what exacerbates the problem, how the client feels about it, and what skin preparations are used can help establish an effective therapeutic regimen.)

Pregnant client
Have you noticed any changes in your skin during your pregnancy?
(RATIONALE: The answer provides an opportunity to discuss normal changes with the client and to explore abnormal changes more fully.)

Elderly client
How has your skin changed as you have aged?
(RATIONALE: The answer allows you to assess the client's perception of changes and provides an opportunity to discuss and clarify normal changes and explore abnormal ones.)

How do you feel about the skin changes you have noticed?
(RATIONALE: The changing body image may lower the client's self-image and self-esteem.)

Do external temperature changes, touch, pressure, or pain affect your skin?
(RATIONALE: With normal aging, these sensations decrease as the number of skin receptors transmitting sensations to the central nervous system decreases.)

Have you developed more moles recently? If so, where? Have any of your moles changed in appearance, become painful, developed a discharge, or bled?
(RATIONALE: The number of moles normally increases with age. Warts that rub against clothing may become painful. However,

changes in their appearance—including changes in color—drainage, or bleeding may indicate cancer.)

Health promotion and protection patterns
What do you do to try to keep your skin healthy? What things would you like to do for your skin but feel unable to do?
(RATIONALE: The answer helps reveal the client's skin care routine and beliefs).

What type of soap and skin creams or lotions do you use? Do you use ointment, oil, or styling spray on your hair? How often do you shampoo and what product do you use? Do you use makeup or scents? If so, what type? Do you shave with a blade or an electric razor? Do you use a depilatory? Do you color your hair?
(RATIONALE: Skin changes, contact dermatitis, or allergy may result from cosmetics and grooming practices. Information on personal habits such as grooming are pertinent for some skin disturbances, particularly those localized to a body area. For example, dying the hair may have preceded scalp or hair changes.)

How would you describe your usual skin exposure to the sun? Do you wear a sun block or cover your skin with clothing before going out in the sun?
(RATIONALE: This question investigates the client's sun protection practices and the potential for exacerbating age-related changes and skin cancers.)

How do you cut your nails?
(RATIONALE: Improper nail cutting can cause infections or ingrown nails. This question provides an opportunity to teach correct nail-cutting technique.)

What are your recreational activities? Do these activities expose you to sun or other light, chemicals or other toxins, animals, the outdoors, or foreign travel?
(RATIONALE: Recreational activities, such as craft work, gardening, camping, outdoor sports, and tanning, may expose the client

to sources of skin problems. Foreign travel may expose the client to skin diseases that are uncommon in North America.)

What concerns do you have about your skin problem and its treatment?
(RATIONALE: Many treatments for skin disorders are expensive and time consuming, limiting the client's ability to carry out the regimen. The client may express concern about the cost of medications.)

Role and relationship patterns

How has your skin problem affected your daily activities?
(RATIONALE: This line of questioning may provide information on limitations related to physical or emotional discomfort or distress. For example, gloves may be required because pain occurs when water contacts the affected area.)

How does the affected area look to you?
(RATIONALE: Skin appearance is important to the client because it provides an initial impression to others. The client's perception of this appearance can affect self-image, self-esteem, and participation in activities.)

How does this rash or skin lesion make you feel? How have these skin changes affected your relationships with others? How do you feel about going out socially?
(RATIONALE: A client with noticeable skin lesions may report that others make unkind remarks or move away, making the person feel unclean, embarrassed, and isolated. Such a client may choose to limit social contact to avoid emotional discomfort.)

PHYSICAL ASSESSMENT

The nurse uses the following equipment and techniques when assessing the skin, hair, and nails.
Equipment
• bright, even light source
• penlight
• tongue depressor
• centimeter rule

• magnifying glass
• flashlight with a transilluminator
• Wood's lamp
• gloves
Techniques
• inspection
• palpation

Assessing related body structures

To assess the client's skin, hair, and nails thoroughly, the nurse must evaluate features that reflect skin composition and function, such as body weight, fluid balance, general appearance, and related body systems.
• Weight—recent weight changes (over the previous 48 hours) reflect changes in fluid status rather than body mass and may affect skin turgor (resiliency).
• General appearance—long-term, excessive sun exposure, acute or chronic illness, and long-term smoking can cause a client to look older than his or her actual age.
• Mucous membranes—pale mucous membranes may indicate anemia; a blue tinge may indicate excess carbon dioxide in the blood. Dry mucous membranes suggest dehydration. Other mucous membrane conditions and lesions may be caused by pressure; burns; actinic (sun) damage; contact with tobacco, chemicals, and allergens; drug reactions; infections with viruses, bacteria, spirochetes, fungi, or animal parasites; or systemic causes, including leukemia, thrombocytopenia, pernicious anemia, metabolic disorders, collagen vascular disease, autoimmune disease, and underlying cancers.

Inspecting the skin, hair, and nails

The nurse continues physical assessment by inspecting the client's skin, hair, and nails.

Skin inspection
• Observe the client's overall appearance from a distance of 3' to 6', noting complexion, general color, color variations, and general appearance.
• Note any body odor, especially unusual odors, such as mustiness or sourness. Keep in mind that a client's cultural background may influence standards of hygiene and grooming.

• Note disturbances in pigmentation, freckles, moles, and tanning. Remember that skin color varies from person to person, depending on race and ethnic origin. Skin color also varies normally in different parts of the body, although overall coloring should remain fairly even—especially within a body region.

• Observe and document any lesion according to the following considerations:

Morphology (clinical description) of the lesion—Note size (measure and record its dimensions), shape or configuration, color, elevation or depression, pedunculation (connection to the skin by a stem or stalk), and texture. Note odor, color, consistency, or amount of exudate. Use a flashlight to assess the color of the lesion and elevation of its borders. Use a transilluminator to assess fluid in a lesion by darkening the room and placing the tip of the illuminator against the side of the lesion; a fluid-filled lesion glows red, whereas a solid lesion does not. Use a Wood's lamp to assess fungal lesions and a magnifying glass to inspect tiny lesions.

Distribution—Lesion distribution may vary with the disease progression or external factors. Note the pattern on first inspection; many skin disorders involve specific skin areas. Assessment of distribution includes the extent of involvement; the pattern of involvement (such as photodistribution or symmetry); and characteristic locations, such as dermatomes (along cutaneous nerve endings), flexor or extensor surfaces, intertriginous areas, or palms or soles.

Location (related to total skin area)—Note whether the pattern of lesions is local (in one small area), regional (in one large area), or general (over the entire body). Also note which areas they affect, such as flexor or extensor surfaces, along cutaneous nerve endings, along clothing or jewelry lines, or if they appear randomly.

Configuration or pattern (arrangement of lesions in relation to each other)—Configuration may help determine the cause. Note whether lesions are discrete (separate and distinct), coalesced or confluent (fused or blended), grouped (positioned close to-

---

Assessment checklist

The nurse should ask herself or himself these questions before beginning the assessment:

☐ Is the examination room warm and adequately lit?

☐ Have I gathered all necessary equipment, including culture materials?

☐ Have I washed my hands? Do I have gloves?

☐ Have I reviewed relevant laboratory data?

---

gether), diffuse (scattered), linear (arranged in a line), annular (distributed in a ring), or arciform (arranged in a curve or arc). Also note gyrate or polycyclic (concentric), herpetiform (along the course of cutaneous nerves), and iris configurations. (For more information, see *Assessing lesion distribution and configuration,* page 60.)

When inspecting a client's skin, keep in mind the following normal cultural and developmental variations, as appropriate:

A dark-skinned client may have *Futcher's lines* (pigmented lines running diagonally from the shoulders to the elbows) and deep pigmentation lines on the palms and soles.

An *infant* with less subcutaneous fat may appear redder than an infant with more subcutaneous fat. A dark-skinned infant may appear lighter at birth than at age 2 or 3 months. A normal physiologic jaundice may occur 2 to 3 days after birth; this should resolve in about 1 week. Normal skin lesions in infants include port-wine stain, hemangiomas, and Mongolian spots.

An *adolescent client* often has acne lesions and increased body odor.

A *pregnant client* may display chloasma, linea nigra, spider angiomas, varicose veins, and striae.

Hair and scalp inspection

• When assessing the hair, note its quantity, texture, color, and distribution. Keep in mind that these factors vary greatly among individuals and are affected by race and ethnic origin. Variations in hair growth and distribution, including hereditary baldness

Assessing lesion distribution and configuration

When a client has skin lesions, the nurse must assess their distribution and configuration. This information may help pinpoint the cause of the lesion. This chart shows possible distribution patterns and configurations.

Distribution patterns

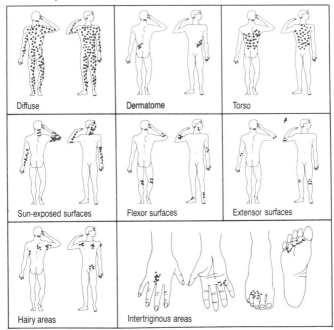

Diffuse

Dermatome

Torso

Sun-exposed surfaces

Flexor surfaces

Extensor surfaces

Hairy areas

Intertriginous areas

Configurations

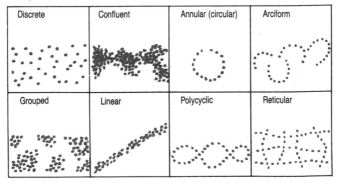

Discrete	Confluent	Annular (circular)	Arciform

Grouped	Linear	Polycyclic	Reticular

and excessive facial hair, occur naturally and are not preventable.
• Assessment of the scalp should reveal a clean surface, free of debris, with equal distribution of hair follicles.
• Keep in mind these normal developmental variations:

An *infant* normally sheds his birth hair within 3 months.

In an *adolescent,* axillary and pubic hair develops. A male adolescent develops facial hair and often profusion, darkening, and thickening of body hair.

In an *elderly client,* hair grays and thins.

Nail inspection

• Inspect the nails for color, consistency, smoothness, symmetry, and freedom from ridges and cracks as well as for length, jagged or bitten edges, and cleanliness. An *elderly client's* toenails may appear yellowed, thickened, and fragile.
• Assess the angle between the fingernail and the nail base (usually about 160 degrees) by placing the lucite ruler across the dorsal surface of the finger and the nail, and observing the angle formed where the proximal nail fold meets the nail plate.

Palpating the skin, hair, and nails

Palpation allows assessment of skin texture, consistency, temperature, moisture, and turgor and permits evaluation of changes or tenderness of particular lesions. Skin texture refers to smoothness or coarseness; consistency refers to changes in skin thickness or firmness and relates more to changes associated with lesions. (*Note:* Remember to wear gloves when palpating moist skin lesions.)

Skin palpation

• Note the general texture of the skin and the location of any changes, such as roughness.
• Assess temperature by using the dorsal surfaces of your fingers or hands, which are most sensitive to temperature perception. The skin should feel warm to cool, and areas should feel the same bilaterally.
• Assess for moisture with the relatively dry dorsal surface of your hands and fingers to

prevent confusing the client's moisture with yours. Moisture normally varies in different parts of the body. The greatest amounts are found on the palms, soles, and skin folds (intertriginous areas). A *pregnant client* commonly has increased skin moisture. In an *elderly client,* decreased numbers of functioning sebaceous and sweat glands cause skin dryness.
• Assess skin turgor by gently grasping and pulling up a fold of skin, releasing it, and observing how quickly it returns to normal shape. Normal skin usually resumes its flat shape immediately. This technique also assesses skin mobility, which may be diminished in connective tissue disorders. Keep in mind that an *elderly client* normally has decreased skin turgor and mobility.

Hair and nail palpation

• To palpate the client's hair, rub a few strands between the index finger and thumb. Feel for dryness, brittleness, oiliness, and thickness.
• When palpating the nails assess the nail base for firmness and the nail for firm adherence to the nail bed; sponginess and swelling accompany clubbing. Remember that a *pregnant client* commonly has brittle nails.

DOCUMENTATION

The SOAPIE method of documentation includes the following components: subjective (history) data, objective (physical) data, assessment, planning, implementation, and evaluation. The following example shows how to document nursing care for a client with skin changes.

Case history

Ms. Julie Roman, age 21, is a single Caucasian female law student. She has noted changes in her skin over the last 4 months.

S   O   A   P   I   E

Client states, "The doctor told me I have psoriasis and I'll have it forever! It started with redness, and now I have these ugly silver patches on my elbows, knees, and buttocks." Client reports severe itchiness (8 on

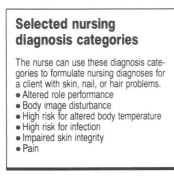

Selected nursing diagnosis categories

The nurse can use these diagnosis categories to formulate nursing diagnoses for a client with skin, nail, or hair problems.
- Altered role performance
- Body image disturbance
- High risk for altered body temperature
- High risk for infection
- Impaired skin integrity
- Pain

a severity scale of 1 to 10). Says she started law school 6 months ago and finds it harder than she expected. She feels depressed about her appearance.

S **O** A P I E

Skin: Large (12 x 5 cm) erythematous plaques with silver scales over knees and elbows, with multiple plaques (4 x 5 cm) over buttocks and on right thigh. Multiple scratch marks around lesions. Nails pitted, onycholysis in four nails (right index and middle, left index and ring fingers). Tearful at present. Earlier in visit, mentioned interest in learning relaxation response.

S O **A** P I E

Ineffective individual coping related to change in body image. Client is depressed about changes in appearance and stressed about school.

S O A **P** I E

Allow time for client to discuss feelings about skin appearance. Provide emotional support. Assist client with stress-reduction measures. Reinforce that psoriasis is a disease characterized by remissions and exacerbations. Make referral to psoriasis support group.

S O A P **I** E

Gave client information about relaxation-response class and psoriasis support group being held at the hospital. Explained signs and symptoms, causes, and treatment of psoriasis.

S O A P I **E**

Client enjoyed relaxation response, reported having used a variation of it in past. Will encourage continued use.

SUGGESTED READINGS

Agency for Health Care Policy and Research. (1992). How to predict and prevent pressure ulcers...clinical practice guidelines (standards). *American Journal of Nursing, 92*(7), 52-60.

Campbell, L. (1993). Assessing pediatric rashes. *RN, 56*(4), 58-65.

Coulter, J. (1991). ABCD's of assessing skin lesions. *Advancing Clinical Care, 6*(6), 18-19.

Flory, C. (1992). Perfecting the art: Skin assessment. *RN, 55*(6), 22-27.

Irwin, M. (1991). Assessing color changes for dark skinned patients. *Advancing Clinical Care, 6*(6), 8-11.

McConnell, E. (1992). Clinical do's and dont's: Assessing the skin. *Nursing92, 22*(4), 86.

McGovern, M., and Kuhn, J. (1992). Skin assessment of the elderly client. *Journal of Gerontological Nursing, 18*(4), 39-43.

6

Head and Neck

The head and neck support and protect the brain, sensory organs, and other structures. Because of these functions, they are among the first structures to evaluate in the assessment process.

The health history has particular importance in a head and neck assessment because of the wide range of disorders that can affect these structures. Normal head and face appearance varies greatly between individuals and between age-groups. Differences require careful evaluation to distinguish between actual abnormalities and normal variations.

HEALTH HISTORY

Because of the many structures involved in the head and neck, the nurse should construct health history questions that elicit information on topics as diverse as headaches and oral hygiene.

When assessing a client with recent head or neck trauma, the nurse should gather information about the chief complaint and current status but postpone taking the complete health history until X-rays have been taken, to prevent further injury from head or neck movement.

Three groups of sample questions follow. Those on *health and illness patterns* help the nurse identify actual or potential health problems; those on *health promotion and protection patterns* help the nurse assess any behaviors that may affect the client's health; and those on *role and relationship patterns*

help the nurse determine if the client has a head or neck problem that relates to roles and relationships with others.

Health and illness patterns

Have you ever had head trauma, skull surgery, or jaw or facial fractures? If so, when? What events came before and what happened afterward?
(RATIONALE: Head trauma, skull surgery, or jaw or facial fractures can change the configuration of the skull or face, producing abnormalities that should be fully evaluated during physical assessment. Events before and after the trauma or surgery—for instance, common sequelae such as frequent headaches or blurred vision—provide clues for further questioning.)

Do you have frequent headaches? If so, how often do they occur? What precedes them and what relieves them? Do they occur at a particular time of day? What part of your head do they affect? How would you describe the pain?
(RATIONALE: Answers to these questions can help differentiate one type of headache from another. For example, muscle contraction headaches usually produce a tight sensation in the occipital or temporal areas and are relieved by mild analgesics. Vascular headaches produce a throbbing, typically unilateral pain that is not relieved by analgesics. Headaches from brain tumors are typically

Anatomy review

The illustrations below show the anatomic structures of the head and neck.

Head and neck

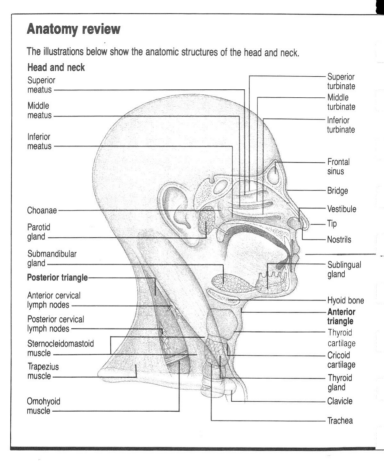

intermittent, deep-seated, and dull at the tumor site. They may be especially intense in the morning.)

Have you ever had any swelling over your face, jaws, or mastoid process? (Point out the mastoid area, located just behind the client's ear.) *If so, when did it occur?*
(RATIONALE: Jaw swelling suggests an abscessed tooth or other dental problem. Facial swelling may be caused by a local problem, such as an abscessed tooth, sinusitis, or salivary gland cancer; or by a systemic problem,

such as an allergic reaction or nephrotic syndrome. Mastoid swelling may arise from lymph node infection.)

Do you have a history of sinus infections or tenderness?
(RATIONALE: Sinus infections tend to recur in those persons susceptible to such infections. Tenderness usually accompanies sinus infections.)

Do you have any nasal discharge or postnasal drip? If so, describe it. When does it occur?

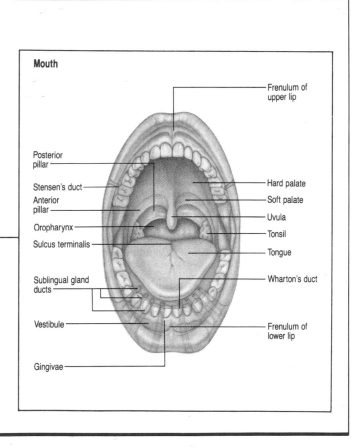

Mouth

- Frenulum of upper lip
- Posterior pillar
- Stensen's duct
- Anterior pillar
- Oropharynx
- Sulcus terminalis
- Sublingual gland ducts
- Vestibule
- Gingivae
- Hard palate
- Soft palate
- Uvula
- Tonsil
- Tongue
- Wharton's duct
- Frenulum of lower lip

(RATIONALE: Nasal discharge and postnasal drip typically result from infections, allergies, or environmental irritants. Thick, tenacious, purulent discharge suggests infection; a watery discharge suggests an allergy or irritant. Certain types of allergies, such as hay fever, occur only at specific times of the year.)

Do you have frequent or prolonged nosebleeds?
(RATIONALE: Epistaxis [nosebleed] can occur with overuse of nasal sprays, from elevated blood pressure, and from other

problems such as hematopoietic disorders, including leukemia and thrombocytopenia. Analyzing the symptoms can help identify the probable cause.)

Have you had any mouth lesions, ulcers, or cold sores? If so, how would you describe them? How long have you had them? Do they recur?
(RATIONALE: Among the various disorders causing mouth lesions are: the fungal infection candidiasis, which produces soft, white, elevated plaques; herpes simplex, which produces vesicles [cold sores] that

rupture and leave a painful, crusting ulcer that often recurs; and gonorrhea, which causes painful lip ulcerations and rough, red, bleeding gingivae.)

Do you have any difficulty swallowing or chewing? If so, how would you describe this difficulty? Does it occur all the time, or only when you eat or drink?
(RATIONALE: Calculi in the parotid gland interfere with normal salivation and cause difficult swallowing [dysphagia]. Painful swallowing accompanied by hoarseness may indicate cancer of the larynx or esophagus. Difficult chewing and swallowing may result from dental problems, such as malocclusion, or from neuromuscular disorders, such as myasthenia gravis.)

Have you experienced any hoarseness or noticed any changes in the sound of your voice?
(RATIONALE: A positive response warrants further investigation; these signs can occur with numerous disorders, ranging from a sinus or tonsil infection to a tumor.)

Do you have any allergies that cause breathing difficulty and a sensation that your throat is closing? If so, when do these symptoms typically occur and how do you deal with them?
(RATIONALE: Documenting any known allergies and effective treatment measures will be valuable if the client is subsequently exposed to the offending allergen.)

Have you ever had a neck injury or experienced difficulty moving your neck in any direction? If so, how would you describe the problem? When did it occur and what, if anything, helped relieve it?
(RATIONALE: Disorders as diverse as neck sprain and cervical lymphadenitis [inflamed lymph nodes in the neck] can cause pain and tenderness and restrict the range of motion in the neck.)

Have you ever had neck surgery? If so, when and why?
(RATIONALE: In a client who has had unilateral carotid endarterectomy, expect to

hear bruits [low-pitched sounds caused by turbulent blood flow] when auscultating the opposite side.)

Pediatric client
Ask a child's parent or guardian these types of questions.
Is your drinking water treated with fluoride?
(RATIONALE: Fluoride helps prevent dental caries, especially in children. If the water is unfluoridated, ask what other measures the family takes to prevent caries.)

Does the child use a pacifier or suck his thumb?
(RATIONALE: These habits misalign the upper teeth as they erupt.)

When did the child begin teething?
(RATIONALE: If the child's dentition is progressing slowly, check for other developmental lags.)

Does the child have tonsils? If not, when were they removed?
(RATIONALE: A child with intact tonsils is at greater risk for frequent streptococcal throat infections, which could lead to chronic tonsillitis.)

Elderly client
Do you wear dentures? If so, how well do they fit?
(RATIONALE: Ill-fitting dentures can cause reluctance to speak, difficulty with eating, or gingival lesions in an elderly client.)

Health promotion and protection patterns
Do you smoke a pipe?
(RATIONALE: Pipe smoking increases the risk of lip and mouth cancer.)

Do you chew tobacco or use snuff?
(RATIONALE: These practices greatly increase the risk of mouth cancer.)

If you suffer from headaches or tightness in the neck or jaw, what do you do for relief? Does relaxation, exercise, or massage help you? Does headache or neck or jaw tightness correlate with lack of sleep, missed meals, or stress?

(RATIONALE: Inadequate sleep, nutrition, or relaxation can produce stress, which can cause headaches or tightness in the neck or jaw.)

Does your job require long hours of sitting, such as at a computer terminal?
(RATIONALE: Sitting in a particular position for long hours can cause headaches and tightness in the neck or jaw.)

Do you grind your teeth?
(RATIONALE: Bruxism [grinding of teeth, especially while asleep] can be a sign of stress. The client may benefit from learning stress-reduction techniques, which may eliminate bruxism.)

Does your job put you at risk for head injury? If so, do you wear a hard hat? Do you participate in any sports that require a helmet? Do you wear a seat belt when you are in an automobile?
(RATIONALE: The answers to these questions will show how highly the client regards personal safety.)

What are your mouth-care habits? How often do you brush and floss your teeth? When was your last dental examination?
(RATIONALE: These questions elicit information about the client's dental health habits.)

Role and relationship patterns
Does your head or neck problem affect the way you feel about yourself or the way you relate to your family?
(RATIONALE: Chronic headaches or neck or jaw tightness may result from family stress. The chronic discomfort can then trigger further stress by lowering the client's self-esteem and interfering with family and social activities. More symptoms then follow. Stress-reduction techniques may help relieve the problem, breaking the cycle of stress-symptoms-stress.)

Has your head or neck problem interfered with your activities of daily living or normal sexual activity?

(RATIONALE: If activities of daily living or sexual activity are affected, exercises that strengthen the head and neck may help the client.)

PHYSICAL ASSESSMENT
The nurse uses the following equipment and techniques when assessing the head and neck.
Equipment
● stethoscope
● tape measure
● glass of water
● tongue depressor
● gloves
● 4″ × 4″ gauze pad
● flashlight
● nasal speculum or ophthalmoscope handle with nasal attachment
Techniques
● inspection
● palpation
● percussion
● auscultation

Inspecting the head and face
● Note the client's spontaneous facial expression. Inspect the head and face for any abnormalities in size, shape, contour, or symmetry.
● Observe the client's head; it should be erect and midline, and the client should be able to hold it still.
● Inspect the face for symmetry, paying particular attention to the palpebral fissures and nasolabial folds.
● Check that the eyes are equidistant both midline and laterally and that they align horizontally with the helix, the prominent outer rim of the ear.
● Look for facial lesions, rash, swelling, or redness. Note any tics, twitching, or other abnormal movements.
● Note facial color.

Palpating the head and face
● Use your fingertips to discriminate skin surface textures and the pads of your fingers to determine the configuration and consistency of bony structures or skin lesions.

Assessment checklist

The nurse should ask herself or himself these questions before beginning the assessment:
☐ Have I gathered the necessary equipment?
☐ Have I tested the bulb and batteries in the flashlight?
☐ Do I have gloves?
☐ Do I have water for the client's swallowing test?
☐ Have I reviewed relevant laboratory data?

• Palpate the head for symmetry and contour; then palpate the scalp, using a gentle rotary movement of the fingertips.
• Gently palpate the face to assess skin tone and facial contours. Palpate bilaterally, using both hands simultaneously.
• Evaluate facial muscle tone by palpating the skin of the cheeks for recoil.
• Palpate the muscles on both sides of the face while the client smiles, frowns, grits the teeth, and puffs out the cheeks.
• Check the temporal artery pulses; they should be of equal strength and rhythm.

Temporomandibular joint palpation
To palpate this area, place the middle three fingers of each hand bilaterally over each joint, then gently press on the joints as the client opens and closes the mouth. Evaluate the joints for movability, approximation (drawing of bones together), and discomfort. Normally, this process should be smooth and painless for the client.

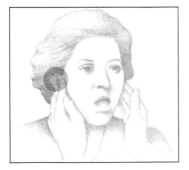

Developmental considerations
To assess the head and neck of a neonate or child, the nurse will need to modify some assessment techniques.
• Inspect the neonate's head; asymmetry may result from molding during vaginal delivery.
• Inspect and gently palpate the fontanels, which should feel soft, yet firm and be flush with the scalp.
• To assess a child under age 2, measure the head circumference.

Auscultating the head
Auscultate over the major vessels of the head—the periorbital, temporal, and occipital arteries—using the bell of the stethoscope.

Inspecting and palpating the nose
• Inspect the nose for symmetry and contour, noting any areas of deformity, swelling, or discoloration.
• The septum should be aligned with the bridge of the nose. With the head in the same position, evaluate flaring of the nostrils. Some flaring during quiet breathing is normal, but marked flaring may indicate respiratory distress.
• Note the character and amount of any drainage from the nostrils.
• Next, palpate the nose, checking for patency, any painful or tender areas, swelling, or deformities.

Palpating and percussing the sinuses
Although the head contains four paranasal sinuses, only two—the frontal and maxillary sinuses—can be assessed.

Sinus palpation
To palpate the frontal sinuses, place the thumbs above the eye just under the bony ridge of the upper orbit. Place the fingertips on the forehead and apply gentle pressure as shown. Then palpate the maxillary sinuses by applying gentle pressure with the index and middle fingers (or thumbs) on each side of the nose in the area immediately below the zygomatic bone (cheekbone).

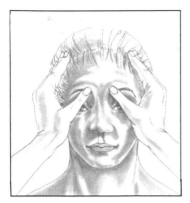

Sinus percussion

Percuss the frontal sinuses by gently tapping the index or middle finger just above the eyebrows. Then percuss the maxillary sinuses by tapping the index or middle finger on both sides of the nose beneath the eye in line with the pupils as shown below.

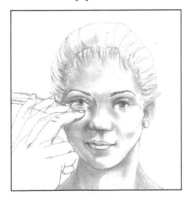

Advanced assessment skills: Direct inspection

Perform direct inspection with a nasal speculum and a small flashlight, or an ophthalmoscope handle with a nasal tip. A nasal speculum is not used to assess infants or toddlers, because their nostrils are too small for the sharp speculum blades. A flashlight will do.

• Facing the seated client, insert the tip of the closed speculum into the nostril up to the point at which the blade widens.

• Then slowly open the speculum as wide as possible (without causing the client discomfort) to allow visibility.

• To improve visibility, ask the client to tilt the head back. Move your head as necessary to examine the structures. Shine a small flashlight into the nostril to illuminate the area.

• Examine one nostril at a time. The mucosa should be moist, pink to red, and free of lesions and polyps. You will also see the choana (posterior air passage), variable amounts of cilia, the middle and inferior turbinates, and a groovelike meatus below each turbinate. The nasolacrimal duct drains into the inferior meatus; most paranasal sinuses drain into the middle meatus. Direct inspection should disclose no excessive drainage, edema, or inflammation of the nasal mucosa — although some tissue enlargement is normal in a pregnant client.

• Note the color, patency, and presence of any exudate in each nostril. When direct inspection is completed, close the speculum before removing it.

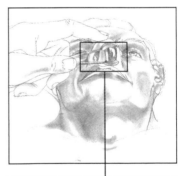

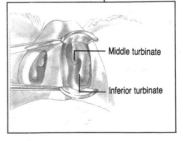

Middle turbinate

Inferior turbinate

Advanced assessment skills: Sinus transillumination

If sinus palpation and percussion cause tenderness, transillumination of the frontal and maxillary sinuses will help the nurse fully evaluate these structures. This technique, which may be performed on clients over age 8, requires a small flashlight or an ophthalmoscope handle with a transilluminator head.

• Darken the room and place the flashlight against the orbital bone immediately below the eyebrow.

• Hold one hand over the end of the transilluminator and the skin surface being assessed. Usually, a reddish glow (illumination) will be visible above the sinus area. Lack of illumination may indicate frontal sinus congestion. Extreme illumination may occur in an elderly client because of reduced subcutaneous facial fat.

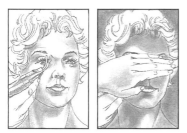

• Repeat this procedure to assess the other frontal sinus.

• To transilluminate the maxillary sinuses, place the transilluminator beneath the center of the eye, lateral to the nose.

• Ask the client to open the mouth. A soft glow should illuminate the hard palate and allow you to see the sinuses above.

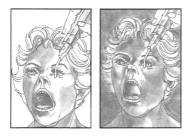

Inspecting and palpating the mouth and oropharynx

• Inspect the oral mucosa by inserting a tongue depressor between the teeth and the cheek to examine the membranous tissue. Note the color of the mucosa; it is usually pink, although some dark-skinned clients may have bluish-tinted or patchily pigmented mucosa.

• Observe the gingivae and teeth. Gingival surfaces should appear pink, moist, and slightly irregular, with no spongy or edematous areas. The edges of the teeth should be clearly defined, with a shallow crevice visible between the gingivae and teeth.

• Check tooth color, which normally varies from bright white to ivory.

• Assess for occlusion of the upper and lower jaw, by asking the client to close the mouth gently. The upper teeth should extend slightly beyond and over the lower teeth.

• Inspect the tongue, which should appear pink and slightly rough with a midline depression and a V-shaped division.

• Ask the client to stick out the tongue, and observe for midline positioning, voluntary movement, and tremors.

• Next, ask the client to touch the tip of the tongue to the roof of the mouth, and observe the underside for any lesions or other abnormalities. Also, inspect the lingual frenulum and the Wharton's ducts.

• Inspect the hard and soft palates. They should appear pink to light red, with symmetrical lines.

• Observe the tonsils for unilateral or bilateral enlargement. Grade tonsil size on a scale of 0 to +4. A grade of 0 (normal) indicates that both tonsils are behind the pillars (the supporting structures of the soft palate); +1, that the tonsils are peaking from the pillars; +2, that the tonsils are between the pillars and the uvula; +3, that the tonsils are touching the uvula; and +4, that one or both tonsils are extending to the midline of the oropharynx.

• Palpate the upper and lower lips and the tongue.

• Examine the oropharynx, using a tongue depressor and a flashlight, if necessary. Observe the position, size, and overall appearance of the uvula and the tonsils. Then, place the tongue depressor firmly on the midpoint of the tongue, almost far enough back to elicit the gag reflex, and ask the client to say "ah." The soft palate and uvula should rise symmetrically.

● The last step of the basic mouth and oropharynx assessment involves evaluating the gag reflex. With the tongue depressor, gently touch the posterior aspect of the tongue. Gagging during this maneuver indicates that cranial nerves IX and X (the glossopharyngeal and vagus nerves) are intact.

Inspecting and palpating the neck

● Inspect the skin of the neck for lesions.
● Palpate along the chains of lymph nodes for masses.
● Have the client slowly and carefully rotate the neck through the entire range of motion, then shrug the shoulders and lift the arms. The neck should be supple, moving easily and without discomfort. Many elderly clients experience decreased range of motion in the neck and pain on neck movement.
● Inspect the midline of the neck for thyroid gland swelling. Then, carefully palpate the trachea.
● Determine the position of the trachea by placing your index finger or thumb along each side of the trachea and assess the space between the trachea and the sternocleidomastoid muscle. The space should be equal on each side; narrowing on either side indicates tracheal deviation to that side. A client with a short, thick, muscular neck is more difficult to examine; apply slightly more pressure during palpation.
● Assess the ability to swallow by having the client sip from a glass of water with the head tipped back slightly. Normally, the larynx, trachea, and thyroid will rise with swallowing.
● Palpate down the posterior neck over the bony prominences of the cervical vertebrae, checking for any tenderness. Then, palpate on either side of the bony prominences to assess alignment.

Auscultating the neck

Using the bell of the stethoscope, auscultate over the major vessels in the neck, particularly the carotid arteries. Pay particular attention to any arteries that feel hard, rope-like, or tender on palpation. Normally, auscultation of these vessels detects no sounds.

Selected nursing diagnosis categories

The nurse can use these diagnosis categories to formulate nursing diagnoses for a client with head or neck disorders.
● Altered oral mucous membrane
● Altered parenting
● Anxiety
● Impaired physical mobility
● Impaired swallowing
● Ineffective airway clearance
● Ineffective breathing pattern
● Pain
● Sexual dysfunction

DOCUMENTATION

The SOAPIE method of documentation includes the following components: subjective (history) data, objective (physical) data, assessment, planning, implementation, and evaluation. The following example shows how to document nursing care for a client with neck pain.

Case history

Janet Wilson, age 26, has come to the outpatient clinic complaining of neck pain with any movement. Ms. Wilson grimaces in pain and holds her neck.

S O   A   P   I   E

Client came to walk-in nursing clinic complaining of neck pain of 36-hour duration. Has not had fever or noticed "lumps" in neck. Was passenger in stopped car that was rear-ended by another car going 10 miles an hour. Client denies hitting dashboard or windshield.

S   **O**   A   P   I   E

Range of motion severely limited because of pain. Unable to flex and rotate neck. Palpation reveals tenderness and muscle spasm with passive range of motion. Cervical vertebrae nonmovable with palpation. Temperature 98.6° F.

S   O   **A**   P   I   E

Knowledge deficit related to cause and self-care of neck symptoms.

S   O   A   **P**   I   E

Teach client about physiologic causes and proper self-care of neck symptoms.

S   O   A   P   **I**   E

Instructed client to apply warm compresses t.i.d. and to take 600 mg of aspirin every 4 hours. Recommended cervical collar. Will call in 48 hours for follow-up.

S   O   A   P   I   **E**

Client repeated aspirin dosage instructions and potential adverse reactions without difficulty. Understands need for physician evaluation if symptoms not reduced in 48 hours.

SUGGESTED READINGS

Barnett, J. (1991). A reassessment of oral healthcare. *Professional Nurse*, 6(12), 703-708.

Boyle, S. (1992). Assessing mouth care. *Nursing Times*, 88(15), 44-46.

Henry, R. (1991). Pediatric dental emergencies. *Pediatric Nursing*, 17(2), 162-167.

Muhrer, J. (1991). Diagnostic considerations in the evaluation and treatment of sore throat. *Nurse Practitioner*, 16(9), 33-41.

Sherman, J., and Fields, S. (1991). Patient evaluation: What's causing Jean's "sore throat"? *Nursing91*, 21(2), 32.

7

Eyes and Ears

Although the eyes and ears differ in structure and function, they share several important features. For example, they are two of the main sources of perception, responsible for the senses of sight and hearing. They usually are assessed sequentially. Clients with an inflamed or injured eye, a foreign body in the eye, or an earache can be any age and usually are not acutely ill. However, eye and ear disorders can signal a serious neurologic problem, such as a brain tumor or an acoustic nerve (cranial nerve VIII) damaged by an adverse drug reaction. Regardless of the cause, the nurse should keep in mind that, because vision and hearing are vital, a client may be especially anxious about an eye or ear disorder.

HEALTH HISTORY: THE EYE

To obtain an accurate and complete health history, adjust questions to the client's specific complaint and compare the answers with the results of the physical assessment. In the case of a well client, ask more general history questions about the eye.

Three groups of sample questions follow. Those on *health and illness patterns* help the nurse identify actual or potential eye or vision problems; those on *health promotion and protection patterns* help the nurse assess any behaviors that may affect the client's eyes or vision; and those on *role and relationship patterns* help the nurse determine the extent to which vision disturbances influence the client's roles and relationships with others.

Health and illness patterns

Do you have any problems with your eyes?
(RATIONALE: Besides indicating visual disturbances, problems with the eyes can indicate other conditions, such as diabetes, hypertension, or neurologic disorders.)

Do you wear or have you ever worn corrective lenses? If so, when and for how long?
(RATIONALE: This establishes how long the client has had a vision disorder and informs the nurse of the client's need to wear corrective lenses during the visual acuity check.)

If you wear corrective lenses, are they glasses or hard or soft contact lenses?
(RATIONALE: Improperly fitted contact lenses or prolonged wearing of contact lenses can cause eye inflammation and corneal abrasions. Wearers of soft lenses are especially vulnerable to conjunctival inflammation and infection because the lenses, worn for long periods of time, can irritate the eye.)

If you once wore corrective lenses and have stopped wearing them, why and when did you stop?
(RATIONALE: Eyestrain or excessive tearing may occur if the client is not wearing necessary lenses.)

Anatomy review

The illustrations below show the anatomic structures of the eye.

Central retinal artery and vein
Retina
Choroid layer
Sclera
Conjunctiva (bulbar)
Iris
Pupil
Cornea
Lens
Canal of Schlemm
Ciliary body
Posterior chamber (filled with aqueous humor)
Anterior chamber (filled with aqueous humor)
Vitreous humor
Optic nerve

Retina (left eye)

Superonasal arteriole and vein
Vein
Optic disk
Arteriole
Inferonasal arteriole and vein
Superotemporal arteriole and vein
Macular area
Fovea centralis
Physiologic cup
Inferotemporal arteriole and vein

When did you last have your lenses changed?
(RATIONALE: A recent lens change with continued visual disturbances could indicate an underlying health problem, such as a brain tumor.)

Have you ever had blurred vision?
(RATIONALE: Blurred vision can indicate a need for corrective lenses or suggest a neurologic disorder, such as a brain tumor, or an endocrine disorder, such as diabetic retinopathy.)

Have you ever seen spots, floaters, or halos around lights? If yes, is this a sudden change or has it occurred for a while?
(RATIONALE: The sudden appearance of spots, floaters, or halos may indicate a retinal detachment or glaucoma. Chronic appearance of spots or floaters is a common normal occurrence in elderly and myopic clients.)

Do you suffer from frequent eye infections or inflammation?
(RATIONALE: Frequent infections or inflammation can indicate low resistance to infection, eyestrain, allergies, or occupational or environmental exposure to an irritant.)

Have you ever had eye surgery or injury?
(RATIONALE: A history of eye surgery may indicate glaucoma, cataracts, or injuries—such as detached retina—that may appear as abnormalities on ophthalmoscopic examination.)

Do you often have styes?
(RATIONALE: Styes [hordeolums], infected meibomian or zeisian glands, tend to recur.)

Do you have a history of high blood pressure or diabetes?
(RATIONALE: High blood pressure can cause arteriosclerosis of the retinal blood vessels and visual disturbances. Diabetes can cause retinopathy.)

Are you currently taking any prescription medications for your eyes? If so, which medications and how often?
(RATIONALE: Prescription eye medications should alert the nurse to an eye disorder.

For example, a client who is taking pilocarpine probably has glaucoma.)

Has anyone in your family ever been treated for cataracts, glaucoma, or blindness?
(RATIONALE: These conditions have a familial tendency.)

Pediatric client

Ask a child's parent or guardian these types of questions.
Does your infant gaze at you or other objects and blink at bright lights or quick, nearby movements?
(RATIONALE: Failure to gaze and blink appropriately could indicate impaired vision.)

Are the child's eyes ever crossed or do both eyes ever move in different directions?
(RATIONALE: These abnormal movements suggest impaired eye muscle coordination.)

Does the child often squint or rub his eyes?
(RATIONALE: Frequent squinting or rubbing could indicate visual disturbances, eye inflammation, or light sensitivity.)

Does the child often bump into, or have difficulty picking up, objects?
(RATIONALE: A positive response indicates astigmatism. Astigmatism distorts or blurs vision because of an irregularly shaped lens.)

If school-age, does the child have to sit at the front of the room to see the chalkboard? Does the child sit close to the television at home?
(RATIONALE: If so, the child could be nearsighted.)

If school-age, how is the child's progress in school?
(RATIONALE: Poor progress in school could indicate a visual disturbance.)

Elderly client

Do your eyes feel dry?
(RATIONALE: Dry eyes or a feeling of sand or grittiness is common in elderly clients because of decreased lacrimal gland secretion.)

Do you have difficulty seeing in front of you but not to the sides?
(RATIONALE: In macular degeneration, which is common in elderly clients, central vision deteriorates, but peripheral vision remains intact.)

Do you have problems with glare?
(RATIONALE: As the lens thickens and yellows with age, excessive light becomes an irritant.)

Do you have any problems discerning colors?
(RATIONALE: The thickening and yellowing of the lens also makes blues and purples look green.)

Do you have difficulty seeing at night?
(RATIONALE: Lens opacity that occurs with cataracts causes night blindness.)

Health promotion and protection patterns

When was your last eye examination? What were the results?
(RATIONALE: Besides suggesting the importance of eye examinations to the client, the question may reveal changes that caused the client to have an examination. If that examination was more than 2 years ago, suggest another one.)

Does your health insurance cover eye examinations and lenses?
(RATIONALE: If not, the client may forgo eye examinations or buying lenses for economic reasons.)

Does your occupation require close use of your eyes, such as long-term reading or prolonged use of a video display terminal?)
(RATIONALE: These activities can cause severe eyestrain and dryness. Instruct the client to take periodic breaks to rest the eyes.)

Does the air where you work or live contain anything that causes you eye problems?
(RATIONALE: Cigarette smoke, formaldehyde insulation, or occupational materials such as glues or chemicals can cause eye irritation.)

Do you wear goggles when working with power tools, chain saws, or table saws, or when engaging in sports that might irritate or endanger the eye, such as swimming, fencing, or playing racquetball?
(RATIONALE: Serious eye irritation or injury can occur with these activities. If the client does not wear goggles, provide instruction about eye safety.)

Role and relationship patterns

If you wear glasses, are they a problem for you?
(RATIONALE: Some clients, especially children and adolescents, may feel less attractive with glasses and may not wear them as prescribed. If this is so, provide instruction about eye health.)

If you are visually impaired, do you have difficulty fulfilling home or work obligations?
(RATIONALE: Visual impairment can seriously affect the client's ability to carry out a role. For example, a homemaker may have to depend on another person to help with housework. If this is the case, refer the client to an occupational health therapist, who can help the client make necessary adjustments in the environment.)

PHYSICAL ASSESSMENT: THE EYE

The nurse uses the following equipment and techniques when assessing the eye.
Equipment
- Snellen eye chart
- a piece of newsprint
- eye occluder or 3 × 5 card
- penlight
- wisp of cotton
- pencil or other narrow cylindrical object
- ophthalmoscope

Techniques
- inspection
- palpation

Testing vision

Prepare for the assessment by washing your hands. Then test visual functions, including near and distance visual acuity, color perception, and peripheral vision. Perform the vision tests in a room that is well-lit, but where you can control the amount of light.

Distance vision test

To test the distance vision of a client who can read English, use the Snellen alphabet chart containing various-sized letters. For clients who are illiterate or who cannot speak English, use the Snellen E chart, which displays the letter in varying sizes and positions. The client indicates the position of the E by duplicating the position with his or her fingers.

• Test each eye separately by covering first one eye and then the other with an opaque 3 x 5 card or an eye occluder. Afterward, test the client's binocular vision by having the client read the chart with both eyes uncovered. The client who normally wears corrective lenses for distance vision should wear them for the test.

• Start with the line marked 20/20. If the client reads more than two letters incorrectly, go up to the next line (20/25). Continue until the client can read a line correctly with no more than two errors. That line indicates the client's distance visual acuity.

Near vision test

Test the client's near vision by holding either a Snellen chart or a card with newsprint 12″ to 14″ (30.5 to 35.5 cm) in front of the client's eyes. The client who normally wears reading glasses should wear them for the test. As with distance vision, test each eye separately and then together.

Color perception test

Ask the client to identify patterns of colored dots on colored plates. The client who cannot discern colors will miss the patterns.

Testing extraocular muscle function

To assess a client's extraocular muscle function, the nurse should perform three tests: the six cardinal positions of gaze test, the cover-uncover test, and the corneal light reflex test.

Six cardinal positions of gaze test

• Sit directly in front of the client, and hold

a cylindrical object, such as a pencil, directly in front of, and about 18″ (46 cm) away from, the client's nose.

• Ask the client to watch the object as you move it clockwise through each of the six cardinal positions—superior medial, superior lateral, lateral, inferior lateral, inferior medial, and medial—returning the object to midpoint after each movement.

• Throughout the test, the client's eyes should remain parallel as they move. Note any abnormal findings, such as nystagmus or the deviation of one eye away from the object.

Cover-uncover test

• Have the client stare at an object on a distant wall directly opposite. Cover the client's left eye with an opaque card and observe the uncovered right eye for movement or wandering.

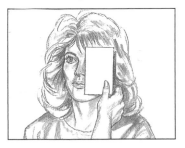

• Next, remove the card from the left eye. That eye should remain steady and fixed on the object, without moving or wandering. Repeat the process on the right eye.

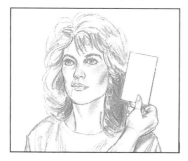

Corneal light reflex test

• Ask the client to stare straight ahead while you shine a penlight on the bridge of the client's nose from a distance of 12″ to 15″ (30.5 to 38 cm). Check to make sure that the cornea relects the light in exactly the same place in both eyes. An asymmetrical reflex indicates a muscle imbalance causing the eye to deviate from the fixed point.

Testing peripheral vision

• Sit facing the client, about 2′ (60 cm) away, with your eyes at the same level as the client's. Have the client stare straight ahead.

• Cover one of your eyes with an opaque cover or your hand and ask the client to cover the eye directly opposite your covered eye.

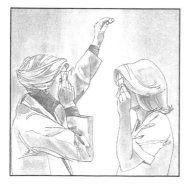

• Next, bring an object, such as a pencil, from the periphery of the superior field toward the center of the field of vision, as shown in the illustration. The object should be equidistant between you and the client.

• Ask the client to tell you the moment the object appears. If your peripheral vision is intact, you and the client should see the object at the same time.

• Repeat the procedure clockwise at 45-degree angles, checking the superior, inferior, temporal, and nasal visual fields, as shown in the diagram. When testing the temporal field, you will have difficulty moving the pencil far enough out so that neither person can see it. So test the temporal field by placing the pencil somewhat behind the client and out of the client's visual field. Slowly bring the pencil around until the client can see it.

Inspecting the eye

After performing vision testing, perform the following assessment techniques. Inspect the eyelids, eyelashes, eyeball, and lacrimal apparatus. Also inspect the conjunctiva, sclera, cornea, anterior chamber, iris, and pupil. Use an ophthalmoscope to assess the vitreous humor and retina.

Eyelid, eyelashes, eyeball, and lacrimal apparatus inspection

• Eyelids should be consistent with client's complexion, with no edema or lesions. The palpebral folds should be symmetrical with no lid lag.

• Eyelashes should be equally distributed along the lids.

• Eyeballs should be bright and clear.

• Lacrimal apparatus should not have any inflammation, swelling, or excessive tearing.

• An *elderly client* may experience decreased tear production.

Conjunctivae inspection

• Check the palpebral conjunctiva only if you suspect a foreign body or if the client complains of eyelid pain. To examine this part of the conjunctiva, have the client look down while you gently pull the medial eyelashes forward and upward with your thumb and index finger.

- While holding the eyelashes, press on the tarsal border with a cotton-tipped applicator to evert the eyelid. This technique requires skill to avoid client discomfort. Hold the lashes to the brow and examine the conjunctiva, which should be pink and free from swelling.
- To return the eyelid to its normal position, release the eyelashes and ask the client to look upward. If this does not invert the eyelid, grasp the eyelashes and gently pull them forward.
- To inspect the bulbar conjunctiva, gently separate the eyelids with your thumb or index finger. Ask the client to look up, down, left, and right as you examine the entire lower eyelid.

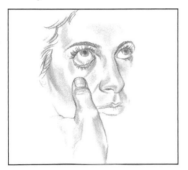

Cornea, anterior chamber, and iris inspection

- To inspect the cornea and anterior chamber, shine a penlight into the client's eye from several side angles (tangentially). Normally, the cornea and anterior chamber are clear and transparent. Calculate the depth of the anterior chamber from the side by figuring the distance between the cornea and the iris. The iris should illuminate with the side lighting. The surface of the cornea normally appears shiny and bright without any scars or irregularities. In an *elderly client*, arcus senilis (a gray-white ring around the edge of the cornea) is normal.
- Test for corneal sensitivity, which indicates intact functioning of cranial nerve V

(trigeminal nerve) by lightly stroking a wisp of cotton across the corneal surface. The lids of both eyes should close when you touch either cornea. Use a separate piece of cotton for each eye to avoid cross-contamination.
- Inspect the iris for shape, which should appear flat when viewed from the side, and color.

Pupil inspection

- Examine the pupil of each eye for equality of size, shape, reaction to light, and accommodation. To test pupillary reaction to light, darken the room, and, with the client staring straight ahead at a fixed point, sweep a beam from a penlight from the side of the left eye to the center of its pupil. Both pupils should respond; the pupil receiving the direct light constricts directly, while the other pupil constricts simultaneously and consensually.
- Now test the pupil of the right eye. The pupils should react immediately, equally, and briskly (within 1 to 2 seconds). If the results are inconclusive, wait 15 to 30 seconds and try again. The pupils should be round and equal before and after the light flash.
- To test for accommodation, ask the client to stare at an object across the room. Normally, the pupils should dilate. Then ask the client to stare at your index finger or at a pencil held about 2′ (60 cm) away. The pupils should constrict and converge equally on the object. To document a normal pupil assessment, use the abbreviation *PERRLA* (which stands for: pupils equal, round, reactive to light, and accommodation) and the terms *direct* and *consensual*. Keep in mind that in an *elderly client*, accommodation may be decreased.

Palpating the eye

- Gently palpate the eyelids for swelling and tenderness. Next, palpate the eyeball by placing the tips of both index fingers on the eyelids over the sclera while the client looks down. The eyeballs should feel equally firm.
- Next, palpate the lacrimal sac by pressing the index finger against the client's lower

orbital rim on the side closest to the client's nose. While pressing, observe the punctum for any abnormal regurgitation of purulent material or excessive tears, which could indicate blockage of the nasolacrimal duct.

Advanced assessment skills: Ophthalmoscopic examination

● To perform an ophthalmoscopic examination, place the client in a darkened or semidarkened room, with neither you nor the client wearing glasses unless you are very myopic or astigmatic. Contact lenses may be worn by you or the client.

● Sit or stand in front of the client with your head about 18″ (45 cm) in front of and about 15 degrees to the right of the client's line of vision in the right eye. Hold the ophthalmoscope in your right hand with the viewing aperture as close to your right eye as possible. Place your left thumb on the client's right eyebrow to prevent hitting the client with the ophthalmoscope as you move in close. Keep your right index finger on the lens selector to adjust the lens as necessary, as shown here.

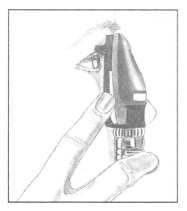

● Instruct the client to look straight ahead at a fixed point on the wall at eye level. Also instruct the client that, although blinking during the examination is acceptable, the eyes must remain still. Next, approaching from an oblique angle about 15″ (38 cm) out and with

the diopter at 0, focus a small circle of light on the pupil, as shown here. Look for the orange-red glow of the red reflex, which should be sharp and distinct through the pupil. The red reflex indicates that the lens is free from opacity and clouding.

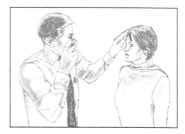

● Move closer to the client, changing the lens with your forefinger to keep the retinal structures in focus, as shown here.

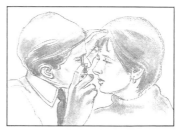

● Change to a positive diopter to view the vitreous humor, observing for any opacity.

● Next, view the retina, using a strong negative lens. Look for a retinal blood vessel, and follow that vessel toward the client's nose, rotating the lens selector to keep the vessel in focus. Because focusing depends on both your and the client's refractive status, the lens diopters may differ for almost every client. Carefully examine all the retinal structures, including the retinal vessels, the optic disk, the retinal background, the macula, and the fovea.

● Examine the vessels and retinal structures for their color, the size ratio of arterioles to veins, the arteriole light reflex, and the arteriovenous crossing. The physiologic cup is normally yellow-white and readily visible.

• Examine the macula last because it is very light-sensitive.

HEALTH HISTORY: THE EAR

Before beginning the interview, ascertain if the client hears well. If a hearing problem exists, look directly at the client and speak clearly when interviewing. Keep in mind that hearing problems can seriously affect the client's ability to carry out activities of daily living and can adversely affect every aspect of the client's life.

Three groups of sample questions follow. Those on *health and illness patterns* help the nurse identify actual or potential ear or hearing problems; those on *health promotion and protection patterns* help the nurse assess any behaviors that may affect the client's ears and hearing; and those on *role and relationship patterns* help the nurse determine the extent to which ear disorders affect the client's roles and relationships with others.

Health and illness patterns

Have you recently noticed any difference in your hearing in one or both ears?
(RATIONALE: The pattern of hearing loss gives clues about its cause. For example, unilateral hearing loss could be caused by a polyp on the affected side. Sudden hearing loss may be caused by a rupture of the tympanic membrane. Unilateral, intermittent hearing loss could be caused by Ménière's disease.)

Do you have ear pain?
(RATIONALE: Ear pain can indicate a middle or inner ear infection, an ear canal obstruction by earwax [cerumen] or a foreign body, or temporomandibular joint infection.)

Do you ever have trouble with earwax? If so, what do you do for it?
(RATIONALE: Using cotton-tipped swabs to clear the ear canal can cause injury. Also, the overuse of home remedies or over-the-counter products can cause skin abrasion in the external ear canal and lead to infection.)

Have you had an ear injury? If so, describe the injury and treatment.
(RATIONALE: Some injuries can cause permanent hearing impairment.)

Have you ever experienced ringing or crackling in your ears?
(RATIONALE: Tinnitus can result from hypertension, ossicle dislocation, or a blockage by cerumen, whereas crackling occurs because of fluid in the middle ear.)

Have you recently had a foreign body in your ear?
(RATIONALE: A recent history of a foreign body in the ear may explain an infection. Also, if the foreign body caused trauma to the external canal, an otoscopic assessment can be very painful, so proceed carefully.)

Do you suffer from frequent ear infections?
(RATIONALE: Chronic otitis media can cause a gradual hearing loss.)

Have you had drainage from your ears? If so, when and how was it treated?
(RATIONALE: Cloudy otorrhea [drainage from the ear] could be caused by serous fluid pressure buildup from an allergy, which ruptures the tympanic membrane. Clear, watery otorrhea could be cerebrospinal fluid from a basilar skull fracture. Bloody, purulent otorrhea could be caused by otitis media.)

Have you had problems with balance, dizziness, or vertigo?
(RATIONALE: Vertigo can indicate a neurologic or otologic disorder. Dizziness may not be caused by an ear disorder but may be caused by inadequate blood flow and blood supply to the brain.)

Have you been taking any prescription or over-the-counter medications or home remedies for your ears or for any other conditions? If so, which medications and how often?
(RATIONALE: Certain medications, such as aspirin, taken for other conditions can affect hearing.)

Anatomy review

The illustrations below show the anatomic structures of the ear.

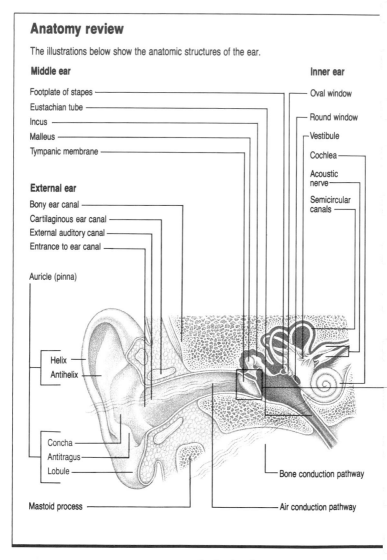

Middle ear

Footplate of stapes

Eustachian tube

Incus

Malleus

Tympanic membrane

Inner ear

Oval window

Round window

Vestibule

Cochlea

Acoustic nerve

Semicircular canals

External ear

Bony ear canal

Cartilaginous ear canal

External auditory canal

Entrance to ear canal

Auricle (pinna)

Helix

Antihelix

Concha

Antitragus

Lobule

Mastoid process

Bone conduction pathway

Air conduction pathway

Has anyone in your family had hearing problems?
(RATIONALE: Otosclerosis is a hereditary disorder that begins between ages 20 and 30 as unilateral conductive hearing loss and progresses to bilateral mixed hearing loss.)

Pediatric client
Ask a child's parent or guardian these types of questions.
Does the infant respond to loud or unusual noises?

The tympanic membrane separates the middle ear from the external ear at the proximal portion of the auditory canal. Composed of layers of skin, fibrous tissue, and mucous membrane, the tympanic membrane appears pearly gray, shiny, and translucent. The auditory canal stretches most of the membrane, called the pars tensa, tightly inward; however, a superior portion of the membrane, called the pars flaccida, hangs loosely and covers the short process of the malleus. The center of the membrane (the umbo) covers the long process of the malleus. Around the outer border of the membrane is a pale, white, fibrous ring called the annulus.

Otoscopic view of the tympanic membrane (right ear)

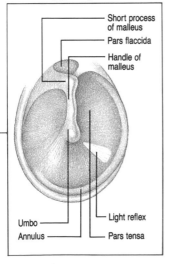

- Short process of malleus
- Pars flaccida
- Handle of malleus
- Light reflex
- Umbo
- Annulus
- Pars tensa

(RATIONALE: A negative response could indicate a hearing loss. In this case, refer the infant to a specialist for further evaluation.)

If over age 6 months, does the infant babble?
(RATIONALE: Failure to babble after 6 months could indicate a hearing impairment. Refer the infant to a specialist for further evaluation.)

If over age 15 months, does the toddler rely on gestures and make no attempt at sound?
(RATIONALE: Making no attempt to speak beyond the appropriate developmental age could indicate a hearing loss. Refer such a toddler to a specialist for further evaluation.)

Is the toddler speaking appropriately for his or her age?
(RATIONALE: Problems with speech development can indicate a hearing impairment.)

Have you noticed the child tugging at either ear?
(RATIONALE: This is often a sign of an ear infection.)

Have you noticed any coordination problems?
(RATIONALE: Inner ear infections can affect equilibrium.)

Has the child had meningitis, recurrent otitis media, mumps, or encephalitis?
(RATIONALE: Any of these conditions can cause hearing loss.)

Elderly client
Have you noticed any change in your hearing recently?
(RATIONALE: Elderly clients commonly develop presbycusis—a physiologic hearing loss that usually affects those over age 50.)

Do you wear a hearing aid? If so, for how long? How do you care for it?
(RATIONALE: If the client wears a hearing aid, be especially careful to speak clearly and directly. Also, some clients who hear poorly refuse to wear a hearing aid because they do not want to accept that they have a hearing problem.)

Health promotion and protection patterns
When was your last ear examination or hearing test? What were the results?
(RATIONALE: The answer to this question could suggest the importance of preventive health care to the client. The last exami-

Ototoxic drugs

When assessing a client's ears, the nurse should ask the client about current drug use. Many drugs can cause adverse reactions that can mimic signs or symptoms of various diseases or damage the cochlea or vestibule of the ear, resulting in tinnitus, vertigo, or hearing loss.

DRUG CLASS	DRUG	POSSIBLE ADVERSE REACTION
Aminglycosides	All aminoglycosides	Tinnitus, vertigo, hearing loss
Anti-inflammatory agents	All nonsteroidal anti-inflammatory agents (such as diflunisal, ibuprofen, and indomethacin)	Tinnitus, vertigo, hearing loss
Antimalarials	Quinine	Tinnitus, vertigo, hearing loss
Diuretics	Furosemide and bumetanide	Tinnitus, vertigo, hearing loss (with too-rapid I.V. administration)
Nonnarcotic analgesics and antipyretics	All salicylates and all combination products containing salicylates	Tinnitus, dizziness, hearing loss (with high dose of long-term therapy)
Miscellaneous agents	Capreomycin, cisplatin, ethacrynic acid, quinidine sulfate, and vancomycin	Tinnitus, vertigo, hearing loss

nation date also can serve for assessing recent changes.)

Do you take any prescription or over-the-counter medications or home remedies for your ears or for any other conditions? If so, which medications and how often?
(RATIONALE: Certain medications, such as aspirin, taken for other conditions can affect hearing. For more information, see *Ototoxic drugs.)*

Do you have any other concerns about your ears or other symptoms that I haven't asked you about?
(RATIONALE: The client may have a different perception of the ear problem. This open-ended question gives the client the opportunity to discuss it with the nurse.)

Do you work around loud equipment, such as heavy machinery, airguns, or airplanes? If so, do you wear ear protectors?
(RATIONALE: Working around loud machinery for long periods of time can cause hearing loss. However, the client can prevent this type of loss by using ear protectors. Teach the client the importance of wearing them.)

Role and relationship patterns
Does your hearing difficulty interfere with your activities of daily living?
(RATIONALE: A client who has a hearing problem may not want to work or perform regular chores, such as shopping. If so, refer the client to an occupational therapist.)

Does your hearing difficulty affect your relationships with other people? If so, how?
(RATIONALE: The spouse or friends of a client

with a hearing loss may become impatient with the hearing-impaired person. Many times, the client will feel left out of conversations, especially if background noise makes hearing even more difficult. The client may withdraw rather than try to understand the conversation.)

PHYSICAL ASSESSMENT: THE EAR

The nurse uses the following equipment and techniques when assessing the ear.
Equipment
● watch
● tuning fork
● otoscope
Techniques
● inspection
● palpation

Assessing auditory function

The most common causes of hearing loss result from conduction problems, neural problems, or problems with the auditory center from injury or damage.

Gross hearing screening

● For the voice test, have the client occlude one ear with a finger. Test the other ear by standing behind the client at a distance of 1' to 2' (30 to 60 cm) and whispering a word or phrase. A client with normal acuity should be able to repeat what was whispered.
● The watch tick test evaluates the client's ability to hear high-frequency sounds. Gradually move a watch until the client can no longer hear the ticking, which should occur when the watch is about 5" (13 cm) away. These are crude methods, so use these tests with other forms of auditory screening.

Weber's test

● This test evaluates bone conduction. Perform the test by placing a vibrating tuning fork on the top of the client's head at midline or in the middle of the client's forehead. The client should perceive the sound equally in both ears.
● If the client has a conductive hearing loss, the sound will be heard in (will lateralize to) the ear that has the conductive loss be-

cause the sound is being conducted directly through the bone to the ear. If the client has a sensorineural hearing loss in one ear, the sound will lateralize to the unimpaired ear because nerve damage in the impaired ear prevents hearing.

Rinne test

● This test compares bone conduction to air conduction in both ears. Assess bone conduction by placing the base of a vibrating tuning fork on the mastoid process, noting how many seconds pass before the client can no longer hear it. Then, quickly place the still-vibrating tuning fork with the tines parallel to the client's auricle near the ear canal (to test air conduction). Hold the tuning fork in this position until the client no longer hears the tone. Note how many seconds the client can hear the tone. Repeat the test on the other ear. Normally, sound traveling through air remains audible twice as long (a 2:1 ratio) as sound traveling through bone.
● If the client reports hearing the sound longer through bone conduction, the client has a conductive loss. In a sensorineural loss, the client will report hearing the sound longer through air conduction, but the ratio will not be a normal 2:1.

Inspecting the ear

● Seat the adult client and begin inspecting the external ear structures. The auricle should cross a line approximated from the outer canthus of the eye to the protuberance of the occiput. The ear position should be almost vertical, with no more than a 10-degree lateral-posterior slant.
● Next, inspect the ear for color and size. The ears should be similarly shaped, colored the same as the face, and sized in proportion to the head. However, ear shape and size vary greatly within the population, so obtain information about what other family members' ears look like before concluding that an abnormality exists.
● Inspect the ear for drainage, nodules, or lesions. Some ears normally drain large amounts of cerumen. Also check behind the ear for inflammation, masses, or lesions.

Palpating the ear

• Palpate the external ear and the mastoid process to discover any areas of tenderness, swelling, nodules, or lesions, and then gently pull the helix of the ear backward to determine the presence of pain or tenderness.

Advanced assessment skills: Otoscopic examination

• Before inserting the speculum into the ear, inspect the canal opening for a foreign body or discharge. Palpate the tragus and pull up the auricle to assess for tenderness. If tenderness is present, the client may have external otitis media; therefore, do not insert the speculum because pain is likely to result. Also inspect the external auditory canal before proceeding.

• After determining that inserting the otoscope is safe, tip the adult client's head to the side opposite from the ear being assessed. Straighten the canal by grasping the superior posterior auricle between your thumb and index finger and pulling it up and back as shown here.

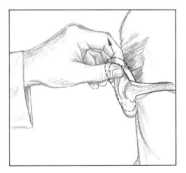

• Then grasp the otoscope in your dominant hand with the handle parallel to the client's head and the speculum at the client's ear. Hold the otoscope firmly against the client's head, as shown here, to prevent jerking the speculum against the external canal. Examination of the external canal normally reveals varying amounts of hair and cerumen because the distal third of the canal contains hair follicles and sebaceous and ceruminous glands. Note the color of the cerumen — old cerumen is usually dry and grayish brown in color. Excessive cerumen

can conceal the tympanic membrane and can also be a factor in reduced hearing ability or in a conductive hearing loss. Occasionally, hard, black cerumen plugs may require removal to allow you to see the tympanic membrane. The external canal should be free from inflammation and scaling.

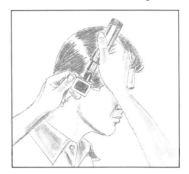

• The inner two-thirds of the canal is sensitive to pressure, so insert the speculum gently to avoid causing the client pain. Gently rotate the angle of the speculum as needed to gain a complete view of the tympanic membrane.

• Inspect the tympanic membrane at the end of the canal; it should be pearly gray in color and glisten, with the annulus appearing white and denser than the rest of the membrane. The inferior edge of the tympanic membrane is posterior to the outside, and the superior edge is anterior. Look for bulging, retraction, or perforations at the periphery of the tympanic membrane.

• Next, check the light reflex, which is in the anterior inferior quadrant in the 5 o'clock position in the right tympanic membrane and in the 7 o'clock position in the left. The light reflex usually appears as a bright cone of light with its point directed at the umbo and its base at the periphery of the tympanic membrane.

• Also examine the malleus. The handle of the malleus originates in the superior hemisphere of the tympanic membrane and, when viewed through the membrane, looks like a dense whitish streak. The malleus attaches to the center of the tympanic membrane at the umbo. At the top portion of the handle are the malleolar folds, where you can normally see the small white projection of the short process of the malleus.

• Prepare a toddler or preschooler for an otoscopic examination by allowing the child to hold the equipment and "blow out" the light. Stroking the child's arm with the speculum can also reduce the fear of pain and facilitate the otoscopy. However, for some children, the examination will be difficult despite the preparation and distraction. In these instances, perform the examination as quickly as you can while the parent restrains the child.

• To perform an otoscopic examination on an infant or toddler, pull the auricle down and back to straighten the canal, as shown here.

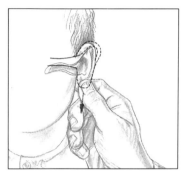

• Brace your hand against the child's head, as shown here, to avoid traumatizing the canal with the speculum in case the child moves. The tympanic membrane and its landmarks will have the same norms as in an adult, except for the light reflex, which is diffuse in an infant. If an infant is crying, the increased intracranial pressure will cause the membrane to turn pink or even red. Only

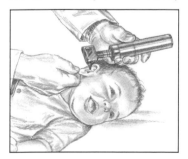

Selected nursing diagnosis categories

The nurse can use these diagnosis categories to formulate nursing diagnoses for a client with eye or ear disorders.
• Altered parenting
• Altered role performance
• Anticipatory grieving
• Anxiety
• Bathing or hygiene self-care deficit
• Dressing or grooming self-care deficit
• Fear
• High risk for injury
• Impaired physical mobility
• Impaired verbal communication
• Pain
• Powerlessness
• Sensory or perceptual alterations (visual or auditory)

experienced examiners can rule out tympanic membrane disease under those conditions. Talking softly and distracting the infant may reduce the likelihood of crying.

DOCUMENTATION

The SOAPIE method of documentation includes the following components: subjective (history) data, objective (physical) data, assessment, planning, implementation, and evaluation. The following example shows how to document nursing care for a client with visual changes.

Case history

James Curran, age 52, is a married Caucasian male who works as a middle manager for a computer manufacturing firm. A known diabetic, Mr. Curran has come to the clinic complaining of difficulty seeing objects to the side.

S   O   A   P   I   E

Client states, "I can't see things from the side as well as I used to." Client states he has had diabetes for 22 years and that, "I only take insulin when I've eaten too much sugar." Family history of diabetes and glaucoma. Last eye examination 12 years ago. No complaints of eye pain, discharge, infection, or injury. Wears glasses to read.

S **O** A P I E

Temperature 99° F.; pulse 92 and regular; respirations 24 and regular; blood pressure 170/100. PERRLA direct and consensual. Cover-uncover test, six cardinal positions of gaze, corneal light reflex revealed no abnormalities. Peripheral vision revealed visual field deficits laterally in each eye. Visual acuity 20/30 O.D., O.S., and together. Ophthalmoscopic examination demonstrated 2:4 AV ratio with nicking. Exudates of 3 DD from disk at 1 and 4 o'clock bilaterally. Maculas have several white exudates bilaterally.

S O **A** P I E

Knowledge deficit related to relationship between vision changes and diabetes.

S O A **P** I E

Teach client about the need to see a physician and about the eye complications that can result from diabetes. Instruct the client in the use of a glucometer. Instruct client that nurse will follow up with a phone call and a visit.

S O A P **I** E

Called client's physician and scheduled appointments. Taught client how to use glucometer to test blood glucose levels. Instructed client on the potential complications of noncompliance. Will follow up with phone call in 1 week.

S O A P I **E**

Client verbalized fear, anger, and frustration with health care system and at having a chronic illness. Able to relate the effects of diabetes on vision.

SUGGESTED READINGS

Abrahamson, I., and Abrahamson, R. (1993). Eye signs of systemic diseases. *Emergency Medicine,* 25(2), 94-108.

Cochrane, D., et al. (1991). Ear emergencies. *Patient Care,* 25(13), 90-113.

Hunt, L. (1992). Ophthalmic nursing assessment. *Insight,* 17(3), 9-11.

Schremp, P. (1992). Ophthalmic nursing. *Nursing Clinics of North America,* 27(3), 703-816.

Vader, L. (1992). Vision and vision loss. *Nursing Clinics of North America,* 27(3), 705-714.

8

Respiratory System

Because the body depends on the respiratory system to survive, respiratory assessment constitutes a critical aspect of a client's health evaluation. The respiratory system functions primarily to maintain the exchange of oxygen and carbon dioxide in the lungs and tissues and to regulate the acid-base balance (stable concentration of hydrogen ions in body fluids). Any change in this system affects every other body system. In chronic respiratory disease, changes in pulmonary status occur slowly, allowing the client's body time to adapt to the gradual hypoxia. However, acute respiratory changes—such as a pneumothorax or aspiration pneumonia—create a sudden hypoxia. Because this does not allow the body time to adapt, death may result.

Environmental factors, such as air pollution and cigarette smoke, may also cause or exacerbate respiratory changes. Even second-hand cigarette smoke can cause respiratory problems, especially in very young and very old clients.

HEALTH HISTORY

Before beginning, quickly assess the client for signs of acute respiratory distress, such as restlessness, anxiety, inability to follow conversation, or noisy or labored respirations. If the client displays these signs, obtain help and, if possible, question the client's family about the current problem. Then, when the client is breathing comfortably, proceed with the full health history.

Three groups of sample questions follow. Those on *health and illness patterns* help the nurse identify actual or potential respiratory-related health problems; those on *health promotion and protection patterns* help the nurse determine how the client's life-style and behavior affect respiratory function; and those on *role and relationship patterns* help the nurse evaluate how the client's respiratory problem affects his life-style and relationships with others.

Health and illness patterns

Do you have shortness of breath? If so, is it constant or intermittent? Does position, medication, or relaxation relieve it? Do your lips or nail beds ever turn blue? Does body position, time of day, or a particular activity affect your breathing? How many stairs can you climb, or blocks can you walk, before you feel short of breath?

(RATIONALE: A distressing symptom, dyspnea can result from various respiratory disorders. Although dyspnea may begin suddenly in relation to a specific activity, it usually develops gradually and insidiously. The client may have unconsciously made life-style changes to compensate for dyspnea, making the exact time of onset difficult to determine.)

Anatomy review

The illustration below shows the anatomic structures of the respiratory system.

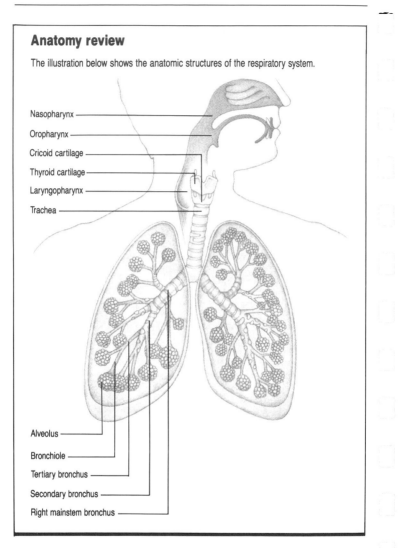

Nasopharynx

Oropharynx

Cricoid cartilage

Thyroid cartilage

Laryngopharynx

Trachea

Alveolus

Bronchiole

Tertiary bronchus

Secondary bronchus

Right mainstem bronchus

Do you have a cough? If so, does it sound dry, hacking, barking, or congested? Does it usually occur at a certain time of day? (RATIONALE: Cough, whether productive or nonproductive, usually indicates a respiratory disorder. Severe cough may disrupt activities of daily living, cause chest pain, or result in acute respiratory distress. Early-morning cough may result from a chronic airway inflammation caused by smoking; late-afternoon cough may indicate exposure to irritants at work; evening cough may suggest chronic postnasal drip, sinusitis, or gastric reflux with nocturnal aspiration. Dry cough may signal a cardiac condition; barking cough, croup or influenza; hacking cough, pneumonia; and congested cough, a cold, pneumonia, or bronchitis.)

Do you cough up sputum? If so, how much do you cough up each day? What color is it? How does it smell? Is it thick or thin? What time of day do you cough up the most sputum?

(RATIONALE: Sputum production accompanies a cough when the hairlike processes of the mucous membranes [cilia] attempt to clear debris from the airway by a wavelike, upward motion. In small amounts and with sufficient fluidity, sputum production serves to maintain airway hygiene and patency. Normal mucus is thin, clear to white, tasteless, odorless, and scant. Mucoid sputum may suggest tracheobronchitis or asthma; yellow or green sputum, bacterial infection; rust-colored sputum, pneumonia, pulmonary infarction, or tuberculosis [TB] ; pink and frothy sputum, pulmonary edema.)

Do you have chest pain? If so, is it constant or intermittent? Is it localized? Does any activity produce pain? Does pain occur when you breathe normally or when you breathe deeply?

(RATIONALE: Chest pain may have a cardiac, pulmonary, or musculoskeletal origin. The characteristics of the pain help determine the probable origin. For example, pain that increases with deep breathing may be pulmonary [pleuritic] in origin. Musculoskeletal chest pain may mimic lung dysfunction. The lungs themselves have no pain-sensitive nerve endings, but the thoracic muscles, parietal pleura, and tracheobronchial tree do. Therefore, pulmonary chest pain may be a late sign of lung disease.)

Have you had any lung problems, such as asthma or tuberculosis? If so, what type? How long did they last and what treatment did you receive?

(RATIONALE: Frequent upper respiratory infections may indicate an underlying respiratory problem.)

Have you had chest surgery or any diagnostic study of the pulmonary system? If so, what type, and why did you have it?

(RATIONALE: Previous diagnostic studies—such as bronchoscopy, arterial blood gas analysis, and sputum cultures—or a thoracotomy or other chest surgery can reveal a history of, or predisposition to, respiratory disorders.)

How many pillows do you sleep on? Does this number represent a change in your previous number?

(RATIONALE: The need for more than one pillow could indicate nocturnal dyspnea that has developed over time. The client may not realize that using more than one pillow relates to a breathing problem.)

Do you have allergies that flare up in different seasons? If so, what causes them? Do they cause runny nose, itching eyes, congestion, or other symptoms? What do you do to relieve these symptoms?

(RATIONALE: A client with allergies may use over-the-counter [OTC] drugs and inhalers, which could interact with medications ordered by the physician. Answers to these questions also reveal the use of common household remedies, and whether they are successful.)

Do you smoke tobacco? If so, for how long have you been smoking, and how much do you smoke?

(RATIONALE: Cigarette, cigar, or pipe smoking can predispose a smoker to various respiratory disorders. Information about pack years [the number of packs smoked per day multiplied by the number of years of smoking] can indicate the severity of the problem.)

Do you ever use over-the-counter nasal sprays or inhalers? If so, how frequently?

(RATIONALE: A client who uses OTC nasal sprays and inhalers too frequently may develop a tolerance and may have to use the spray more often for relief. Overuse of nasal inhalers may also cause rebound nasal congestion, characterized by red, swollen nasal mucosa.)

Do you use a nebulizer or other breathing treatment? If so, what is it used to treat, what dose of medication do you use, and how often do you take a treatment? Do you ever have any side effects from the treat-

(Text continues on page 95.)

The mechanics of respiration

The muscles of respiration help the chest cavity expand and contract. The air pressure differences between the outside air and the lungs help produce air movement. Together, these actions allow inspiration and expiration.

Anterior view

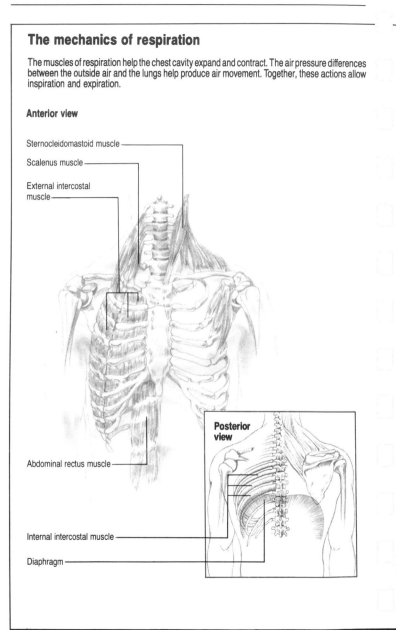

Sternocleidomastoid muscle

Scalenus muscle

External intercostal muscle

Abdominal rectus muscle

Internal intercostal muscle

Diaphragm

Posterior view

Air pressure differences

During inspiration and expiration, pressure differences allow the bellows-like movement of air in and out of the lungs. All gases move from an area of greater pressure to one of lesser pressure.

Resting phase

During the resting phase (occurring at the end of inspiration and expiration), no pressure difference exists between the atmosphere and the alveoli, and, thus, no airflow occurs. The negative intrapleural pressure prevents the lungs from collapsing.

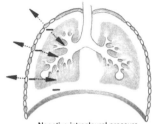

Negative intrapleural pressure

Inspiration

On inspiration, as the diaphragm descends and the chest cavity expands, intrapulmonary negative pressure builds. Then, as the lungs expand, the negative pressure transfers to the alveolar spaces, creating a pressure difference between the atmosphere and the alveoli. Because gas moves from an area of greater to lesser concentration, this pressure difference—called the transairway pressure gradient—moves gas through the upper airways and into the top of the lower airways, creating the first step in ventilation.

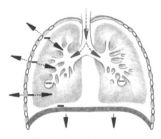

Negative intrapulmonary pressure

Expiration

On expiration, the diaphragm rises and the chest cavity contracts. Intrapleural pressure rises, but remains negative. As the chest cavity further compresses the lungs, lung pressure rises above atmospheric pressure. This creates a positive intrapulmonary pressure, forcing air out of the lungs, into the trachea, and into the atmosphere.

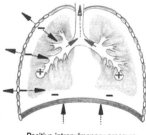

Positive intrapulmonary pressure

Chest contours of different age-groups

The following illustrations compare the chest contours of an infant, toddler, adult, and elderly adult. An infant has a rounded thorax, with an anteroposterior diameter equal to or slightly greater than the lateral diameter. By the time the infant has grown into a toddler, the lateral diameter of the chest has grown broader than the anteroposterior diameter. By adulthood, the lateral diameter of the chest is broader by up to twice the anteroposterior diameter. Then, in the elderly adult, the chest again exhibits an increased anteroposterior diameter as the result of changes in the spine from aging.

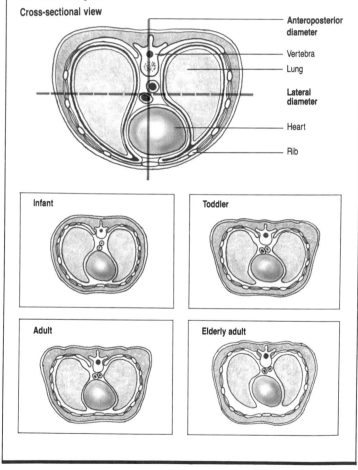

Cross-sectional view

Anteroposterior diameter

Vertebra

Lung

Lateral diameter

Heart

Rib

Infant

Toddler

Adult

Elderly adult

ment? Do you follow special instructions for using therapy? When did you last have a treatment?
(RATIONALE: Use of a nebulizer or other breathing treatment at home may indicate a chronic respiratory disorder. If hospitalized, the client would probably require continuation of the same home breathing treatments.)

Do you use oxygen at home? If so, do you use a cannula or mask? Do you use it continuously or intermittently? What is the liter flow rate at rest and with activity? Must you follow any special instructions for use?
(RATIONALE: Use of oxygen therapy at home may indicate a chronic respiratory disorder. Learn the client's maintenance amount as a baseline for future adjustments, and determine the client's awareness of necessary precautions.)

How long have you been on home oxygen? Who is your supplier? Does your insurance cover the cost of oxygen therapy?
(RATIONALE: Sometimes economics prevents clients from complying with ordered treatments. If financial considerations prevent proper oxygen supply, refer the client to a social worker.)

Have you ever been vaccinated against flu or pneumonia?
(RATIONALE: Expect the very young, very old, and those with chronic respiratory disease to have been vaccinated. If such a client has not been vaccinated, plan to educate the client about the protection that vaccinations provide.)

Has any member of your family had emphysema, asthma, respiratory allergies, or tuberculosis?
(RATIONALE: A family predisposition to emphysema and allergies may exist. If a family member has had TB, find out when the client may have been exposed to determine the need for a tuberculin skin test.)

In the last 1 to 2 months, have you had fever, chills, fatigue, or night sweats?
(RATIONALE: These signs and symptoms are associated with TB.)

Have you ever had a blood test that showed you had anemia? If so, when?
(RATIONALE: Anemia decreases the ability of the blood to carry oxygen because of reduced red blood cells and hemoglobin. This, in turn, leads to fatigue, dyspnea, and orthopnea.)

Do you periodically suffer from sinus pain, nasal discharge, or postnasal drip?
(RATIONALE: These signs and symptoms may suggest allergies or sinus infection.)

Do you suffer from a bad taste in your mouth or bad breath?
(RATIONALE: These signs and symptoms could indicate a sinus or pulmonary infection, such as an abscess or bronchiectasis.)

Pediatric client
Ask the parent or guardian the following questions:
Did the infant have respiratory problems at birth? If so, how were they treated?
(RATIONALE: The nurse should know if problems were temporary, which the parent may forget about unless asked, or if residual respiratory difficulty continues and how it is treated.)

Does the infant suffer from frequent congestion, runny nose, or colds?
(RATIONALE: If yes, ask about the parents' smoking habits. Second-hand smoke can cause frequent congestion and other respiratory problems in infants.)

Does shortness of breath interfere with the infant's ability to suck a bottle?
(RATIONALE: If yes, the infant will require referral to a physician.)

Does the child cough at night? If so, does the cough awaken the child?
(RATIONALE: A hacking cough could mean tracheobronchitis with epiglottitis, which could lead to airway obstruction.)

Does coughing or shortness of breath interfere with the child's play or school activities?
(RATIONALE: Asthma and dyspnea may interfere with the child's usual activities.)

Elderly client
Are you aware of any changes in your breathing patterns? Do you become easily fatigued when climbing stairs? Do you have trouble breathing when lying flat? Do you seem to have more colds that last longer?
(RATIONALE: Elderly clients are susceptible to breathing problems from limited chest wall and respiratory muscle strength. Their altered immune systems may increase their susceptibility to colds and respiratory infections.)

Health promotion and protection patterns
When was your last chest X-ray? Tuberculosis test?
(RATIONALE: Preventive and screening behaviors provide information about the client's self-care patterns and possible teaching opportunities.)

Which home remedies do you use for respiratory problems?
(RATIONALE: Using the client's belief system aids compliance and healing. For example, a client's care plan could include a simple, traditional home remedy, such as herbal tea with honey.)

Have your sleep patterns changed because of breathing problems?
(RATIONALE: Changes in sleep patterns could lead to fatigue. In a client with chronic obstructive pulmonary disease [COPD], such changes could make breathing even more tiring.)

Does your breathing problem affect your daily activities? Which activities can you manage without assistance? Which activities can you manage with assistance? Which activities are you unable to manage? What or who provides assistance when you need it? How do your current activities compare with those before your breathing problems?
(RATIONALE: These questions uncover the client's perceived need for help and also provide information that might suggest the need for follow-up care and services.)

Do you have any hobbies that expose you to respiratory irritants, such as glues, paints, and sprays?
(RATIONALE: The client who engages in such hobbies may need to increase the ventilation in the room when working with these agents. Also instruct the client to wear a protective mask.)

Do you have any breathing difficulty when eating? Do you eat three large meals or several small meals?
(RATIONALE: Clients with chronic respiratory disorders often eat small, frequent meals to reduce dyspnea and effortful breathing.)

Does stress at home or work affect your breathing?
(RATIONALE: Asthmatics and others may be able to identify an action-reaction cycle that includes stress and dyspnea.)

Can you afford the medication, equipment, and oxygen required for your health?
(RATIONALE: Often, noncompliance occurs because of economic reasons, not a lack of interest or understanding. If finances are a problem, refer the client to a social worker.)

How many people live with you? Do you have pets? Does the fur, or do the feathers, bother you? What type of home heating do you have? Is anything in your home a respiratory irritant, such as fresh paint, cleaning sprays, or heavy cigarette smoke?
(RATIONALE: The home environment is of special importance to a client with a respiratory problem. Data gathered from these questions can help the nurse and client plan for positive changes in the environment.)

What is your current occupation? What were your previous occupations? Are you exposed to any known respiratory irritants at work? Do you use safety measures during exposure?
(RATIONALE: Certain occupations, such as mining, chemical manufacturing, and working in a smoke-filled office, can expose a client to respiratory irritants. If the client

does not have adequate protection, plan to provide information about job safety and regulations.)

Role and relationship patterns

How have family members reacted to your respiratory illness? Whom among family and friends can you count on in time of need?
(RATIONALE: Many clients with chronic respiratory illness need a great deal of assistance. Learn whether the client will require outside help, and, if so, help the client make the necessary plans. Many clients with chronic breathing problems often feel depressed and isolated from their family. Explore these concerns with the client during the health history.)

How has your breathing problem affected your sexual activity? Have you found ways to decrease the effect of breathing problems on sexual activity? Would you care to discuss them?
(RATIONALE: A client with a breathing problem may be overwhelmed during sexual activity. To help the client overcome this problem, discuss alternate ways to obtain sexual satisfaction, such as using less tiring positions and touching.)

PHYSICAL ASSESSMENT

The nurse uses the following equipment and techniques when performing a respiratory system assessment.
Equipment
- stethoscope
- felt-tipped marking pen
- ruler
- tape measure

Techniques
- inspection
- palpation
- percussion
- auscultation

Assessing related body structures

To assess for central cyanosis (which results from prolonged hypoxia), inspect the following:
- buccal mucosa

Assessment checklist

The nurse should ask herself or himself these questions before beginning the assessment:
- ☐ Have I gathered all the necessary equipment, including a sputum specimen container?
- ☐ Have I washed my hands?
- ☐ Have I warmed the stethoscope's bell and diaphragm between my hands?
- ☐ Using a quick survey to evaluate the client's breathing difficulty, have I decided how extensive the examination should be?
- ☐ If examining a child, do I have a pediatric-size bell and diaphram for the stethoscope?
- ☐ Do I have sufficient drapes to cover the client?
- ☐ Have I reviewed relevant laboratory data?

- tongue
- lips
- nail beds.

To assess for peripheral cyanosis (which results from vasoconstriction, vascular occlusion, or reduced cardiac output), inspect these body structures:
- nail beds
- lips.

Inspecting the thorax

Basic assessment of respiratory function requires evaluation of the rate, rhythm, and quality of respirations, as well as inspection of chest configuration, chest symmetry, skin condition, and accessory muscle use. It also should include assessment for nasal flaring. Accomplish these steps by evaluating the client's breathing and inspecting the anterior and posterior thorax, and by noting any abnormal findings.

Anterior thorax inspection
- Inspect the thorax for structural deformities, such as a concave or convex curvature of the anterior chest wall over the sternum. In the normal adult thorax, the ratio of an-

Common chest deformities

Normally, the anteroposterior diameter is less than the lateral diameter. The illustrations below demonstrate three common deformities. For each deformity, a cross sectional view compares the anteroposterior and lateral diameters of the normal chest to that of the deformed chest (as indicated by the dotted line).

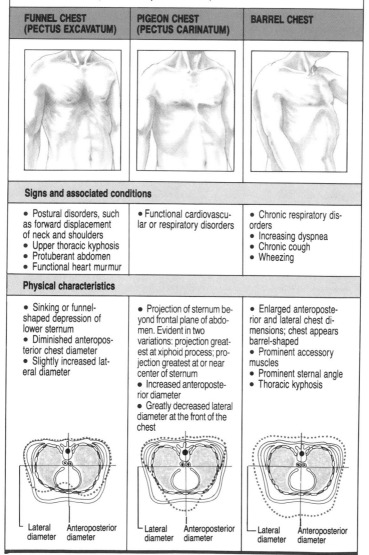

FUNNEL CHEST (PECTUS EXCAVATUM)	PIGEON CHEST (PECTUS CARINATUM)	BARREL CHEST
Signs and associated conditions		
• Postural disorders, such as forward displacement of neck and shoulders • Upper thoracic kyphosis • Protuberant abdomen • Functional heart murmur	• Functional cardiovascular or respiratory disorders	• Chronic respiratory disorders • Increasing dyspnea • Chronic cough • Wheezing
Physical characteristics		
• Sinking or funnel-shaped depression of lower sternum • Diminished anteroposterior chest diameter • Slightly increased lateral diameter	• Projection of sternum beyond frontal plane of abdomen. Evident in two variations: projection greatest at xiphoid process; projection greatest at or near center of sternum • Increased anteroposterior diameter • Greatly decreased lateral diameter at the front of the chest	• Enlarged anteroposterior and lateral chest dimensions; chest appears barrel-shaped • Prominent accessory muscles • Prominent sternal angle • Thoracic kyphosis

teroposterior to lateral diameter is about 1:2. For a *pediatric* or *elderly client,* this ratio is 1:1.
• Inspect between and around the ribs for visible sinking of soft tissues (retractions).
• Assess the client's respiratory pattern for symmetry, and look for any abnormalities in skin color or alterations in muscle tone.
• Note the angle between the ribs and the sternum at the point immediately above the xiphoid process. The normal costal angle is < 90 degrees. A *pregnant client* may exhibit an increased costal angle.
• To inspect the anterior chest for symmetry of movement, have the client lie in a supine position. Stand at the foot of the bed and carefully observe the client's quiet and deep breathing for equal expansion of the chest wall.
• Next, check for the use of the accessory muscles of respiration by observing the sternocleidomastoid, scalenus, and trapezius muscles in the shoulders and neck. Also observe the position the client assumes to breathe.
• Observe the client's skin on the anterior chest for any unusual color, lumps, or lesions, and note the location of any abnormality.
• Further inspect the chest for the location of the underlying ribs and other bones, cartilage, and lung lobes.
• Inspection may reveal structural deformities of the chest wall resulting from defects of the sternum, rib cage, or vertebral column. These deformities have many variations and may be congenital, acute or progressive. (See *Common Chest Deformities.*)

Posterior thorax inspection

• To inspect the posterior chest, observe the client's respiration and assess the posterior chest wall for the same characteristics as the anterior: chest structure, respiratory pattern, symmetry of expansion, skin color and muscle tone, and accessory muscle use.

Palpating the trachea and thorax

Palpation of the trachea and the anterior and posterior thorax can detect structural and skin abnormalities, areas of pain, and chest asymmetry.

Trachea palpation

• First, palpate the trachea for position. It should be midline.
• Next, palpate the suprasternal notch. In most clients, the arch of the aorta lies close to the surface just behind the suprasternal notch. Use your fingertips to gently evaluate the strength and regularity of the client's aortic pulsations there.

Anterior thorax palpation

• Palpate the thorax to assess the skin and underlying tissues for density. Check for masses, crepitus, or skin irregularities. Gentle palpation should not cause the client any pain; be sure to assess any complaints of pain for localization, radiation, and severity.
• Be especially careful to palpate any areas that appeared abnormal during inspection.
• If necessary, support the client during the procedure with one hand while using your other hand to palpate one side at a time, continuing to compare sides. Note any unusual findings, such as masses, crepitus, skin irregularities, or painful areas.
• To palpate the anterior thorax, begin in the supraclavicular area ¾" to 1½" (2 to 4 cm) above the inner aspect of the clavicle; then progress to the infraclavicular, sternal, xiphoid, rib, and axillary areas.
• Next, palpate the costal angle. The xiphoid process area contains many nerve endings, so be gentle to avoid causing pain. If a client frequently uses the internal intercostal muscles to breathe, these muscles will eventually pull the chest cavity upward and outward. If this has occurred, the costal angle will be greater than normal.

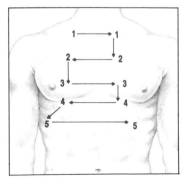

Anterior respiratory excursion

• Respiratory excursion assessment, performed anteriorly and posteriorly, provides information about chest wall expansion during inspiration and chest wall contraction during expiration.

• Assess respiratory excursion in three areas on the client's anterior thorax. For all three areas, stand in front of the client, who may either sit or stand.

• To assess the first area, place your hands on the anterior chest wall, thumbs equidistant from the sternum, with the rest of your fingers spread over the lateral thorax. To identify equal thumb placement, locate the second rib on either side of the client's sternum, and place your thumbs on the tissue directly below those ribs in the second intercostal space. Do not apply pressure, as this may alter the client's inspiration effort.

• Instruct the client to take a deep breath. During the inspiration, observe the separation of your thumbs; they should separate simultaneously and equally to a distance several centimeters from the sternum.

• To assess respiratory excursion in the second area, place your thumbs at the fifth intercostal space and repeat the procedure.

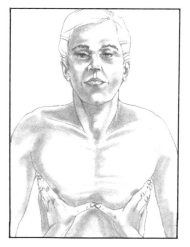

• To assess respiratory excursion in the third area, place your thumbs at the sixth intercostal space as shown and repeat the procedure. In a female client with pendulous

breasts, thumb placement may be difficult to evaluate; therefore, perform posterior respiratory excursion in this instance.

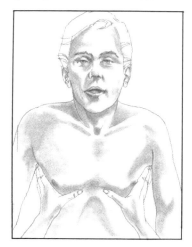

Posterior thorax palpation

• Palpate the posterior thorax similarly to the anterior thorax, using the palmar surface of the fingertips of one or both hands. Begin posterior palpation in the area above the scapulae (suprascapular), move to the area between the scapulae (interscapular), then below the scapulae (infrascapular), and down to the lateral walls of the thorax. During the process, identify bony structures, such as the vertebrae and the scapulae.

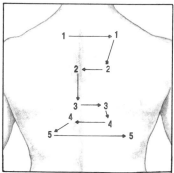

Posterior respiratory excursion

• Stand behind the client and place your thumbs in the infrascapular area on either side of the spine at the level of the tenth rib. Grasp the lateral rib cage and rest your palms gently over the lateroposterior surface. Avoid applying excessive pressure to prevent restricting the client's breathing.

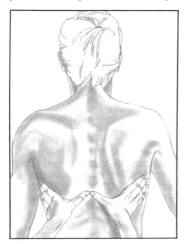

• As the client inhales, the posterior chest should move upward and outward and your thumbs should move apart. When the client exhales, your thumbs should return to midline and again touch.

• Repeat the procedure after placing your thumbs equally lateral to the vertebral column in the interscapular area, with your fingers extending into the axillary area. Instruct the client to take a deep breath while you watch for simultaneous, equal separation of your thumbs.

Percussing the thorax

Percussion helps determine the boundaries of the lungs and how much gas, liquid, or solid exists in the lungs. Percussion can effectively assess structures as deep as 1¾" to 3" (4.5 to 8 cm).

• To percuss the anterior chest, have the client sit facing forward, hands resting at the side of the body. Following the anterior percussion sequence, percuss and compare sound variations from one side to the other. Anterior chest percussion should produce resonance from above the clavicle to the fifth intercostal space on the right (where dullness occurs close to the liver) and to the third intercostal space on the left (where dullness occurs near the heart).

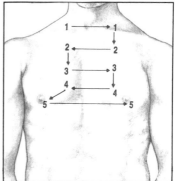

• Next, percuss the lateral chest to obtain information about the left upper and lower lobes, and about the right upper, middle, and lower lobes. The client's left arm should be positioned on the client's head. Repeat the same sequence on the right side. Lateral chest percussion should produce resonance to the sixth or eighth intercostal space.

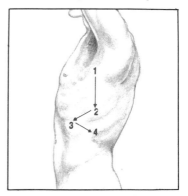

Abnormal breath sounds

Abnormal (adventitious) breath sounds occur when air passes through narrowed airways or moisture, or when the membranes lining the chest cavity and the lungs become inflamed.

TYPE	LOCATION
Abnormal breath sounds in adult and pediatric clients	
Crackles (rales)	Anywhere; in lung bases initially, usually heard during inspiration. Also in dependent lung portions of bedridden clients. If crackles clear with coughing, they are not pathologic.
Wheezes	Anywhere; heard during inspiration or expiration. If wheezes clear with coughing, they may be coming from the trachea or larger upper airways.
Rhonchi (gurgles)	Central airways; heard during inspiration and expiration; coughing may affect sound
Pleural friction rub	Lateral lung field; heard during inspiration and expiration (with client in upright position); coughing does not affect sound
Additional abnormal breath sounds in pediatric clients	
Grunting	Central airways; heard during expiration
Stridor	Trachea; heard during inspiration

• Finally, percuss the posterior thorax according to the percussion sequence. Posterior percussion should sound resonant to the level of T10.

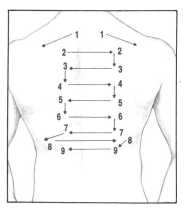

Auscultating the thorax

Auscultate the anterior, lateral, and posterior thorax to detect normal as well as abnormal breath sounds. Listen for tracheal sounds over the trachea; bronchial sounds over the manubrium; bronchovesicular sounds over the upper third of the sternum anteriorly and between the scapula posteriorly; and vesicular sounds in the lung periphery. To auscultate the thorax of an adult, first warm the stethoscope between your hands and then place the diaphragm of the stethoscope directly on the client's skin. Clothing or linen interferes with accurate auscultation.

Anterior thorax auscultation
• Begin at the upper lobes, and move from side to side and down. Auscultate a point first on one side of the chest and then auscultate the same point on the other side of

CAUSE	DESCRIPTION
Air passing through moisture, especially in the small airways and alveoli, with pulmonary edema	Light crackling, popping, nonmusical sound, like hairs being rubbed together. Further classified by pitch: high, medium, or low
Fluid or secretions in the large airways or airways narrowed by mucus or bronchospasm	Whistling sound; can be described as sonorous, bubbling, moaning, musical, sibilant and rumbling, crackling, groaning
Air passing through fluid-filled airways, as in upper respiratory tract infection	Bubbling sound
Inflamed parietal and visceral pleural linings rubbing together	Superficial squeaking or grating sound, like pieces of sandpaper being rubbed together
Physiologic retention of air in lungs to prevent alveolar collapse	Grunting noise
Forced movement of air through edematous upper airway	Crowing noise

the chest, comparing findings. Always assess one full breath (inspiration and expiration) at each point. Follow the same sequence as that used for percussion.

Lateral thorax auscultation
● To assess the right middle lung lobe, auscultate breath sounds laterally at the level of the fourth to the sixth intercostal spaces, following the lateral auscultation sequence, which is the same as the lateral percussion sequence.

Posterior thorax auscultation
● The auscultation sequence for the posterior thorax follows the same pattern as the percussion sequence. During auscultation, remain aware of the client's breathing pattern. Breathing too rapidly or deeply causes an excessive loss of carbon dioxide that may result in vertigo or syncope.

● In a normal adult, adolescent, or older child, bronchovesicular sounds should occur over the interscapular area; vesicular breath sounds should occur in the suprascapular and infrascapular areas.

Developmental considerations
When assessing a pediatric, pregnant, or elderly client, modify assessment techniques to accommodate developmental differences. Follow these guidelines.
● Before inspecting an infant's respiratory system, inspect the skin. Infants have a thin layer of subcutaneous tissue, making cyanosis a more reliable sign of respiratory distress in them than in adults.
● Inspect the chest wall to gain further information about respiratory status. More cartilage than bone composes a child's thoracic cage and, because less subcutaneous tissue is present to mask findings, chest wall

movement should be more visible during breathing.

• Infants and children often exhibit abdominal breathing or paradoxical breathing. Paradoxical breathing, which occurs when the chest and abdomen do not work together to expand and contract during inspiration and expiration, results because of the child's immature respiratory center and weak chest muscles.

• Next, observe for changes in thoracic structures, which are also easier to evaluate in an infant or child than in an adult. Assess an infant's chest circumference by snugly wrapping a tape measure around the chest at the nipple line. Rather than drawing a conclusion based on a single measurement, consider several measurements taken during the child's first 2 years to detect a trend.

• The mean chest circumference at birth is about 13″ (33 cm), usually ¾″ to 1⅛″ (2 to 3 cm) smaller than the head circumference; it is about 18½″ (47 cm) at 1 year.

• Normally, infants demonstrate a basically round thoracic structure; however, the ratio of chest width to chest depth varies with age from 1:2 to 5:7.

• Infants and children seldom exhibit hypertrophy of the accessory muscles of respiration. However, they may exhibit bulging or retractions during inspiration and expiration—a sign of breathing difficulty. The intercostals often bulge during infant respiratory distress, while the suprasternal, substernal, and abdominal muscles retract.

• Infants commonly use only the abdominal muscles to breathe until age 6 or 7, when the thoracic intercostal muscles take over.

• Infants and toddlers have small chest surfaces; therefore, limit palpation to an assessment of the suprasternal notch. Chest palpation becomes appropriate around age 4 or 5.

• Percussion is usually unreliable because of the disproportionate size between an infant's chest and an adult's fingers.

• Use a stethoscope with an appropriately sized diaphragm to auscultate a child. Because of a child's small chest size, fewer auscultation sites exist.

• To auscultate a child's anterior chest, begin just below the right clavicle, as shown.

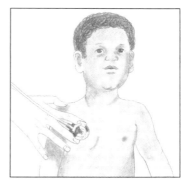

• Continue to auscultate the anterior chest, following the illustrated auscultation sequence.

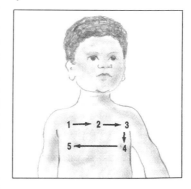

• Then auscultate the posterior chest, following the illustrated auscultation sequence.

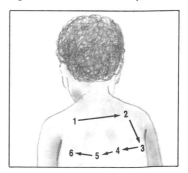

● Breath sounds travel easily throughout a child's chest, making differentiation difficult. For example, bronchovesicular sounds may appear throughout an infant's or child's chest. Also, an infant's chest is thinner and more resonant than an adult's, making breath sounds harsher or more bronchial. Otherwise, normal breath sounds for this age-group are identical to those for adults. Grunting (deep, low-pitched sounds at the end of each breath) and stridor (loud, harsh, musical sounds resulting from tracheal or laryngeal obstruction) also may be heard, sometimes even without equipment.

Pregnant client

● These clients normally exhibit an increased costal angle, up to 103 degrees by the third trimester. As a result, the lower rib cage appears to flare out. As the uterus enlarges, the woman's breathing becomes more thoracic than abdominal.

● The internal organs become crowded, which causes deeper respirations, increased sighing, and increased dyspnea.

● The respiratory rate and depth may increase during the second and third trimesters to meet the growing oxygenation and ventilation needs of the mother and fetus.

Elderly client

● These clients' thoracic structure typically becomes rounder, and the anteroposterior chest increases in relation to the lateral diameter. This is caused by changes in the thoracic and lumbar spine. Also, because of calcification of the rib articulations, elderly clients may use accessory muscles to breathe.

● Percussion may produce hyperresonant sounds because of the decreased distensibility of the lung tissue.

● Also, for clients with suspected atelectasis, begin auscultation at the base of the lungs rather than at the apices; atelectic crackles may disappear as the client repeatedly takes deep breaths.

● Keep in mind that a decreased cough reflex also increases the risk of aspiration for this age-group.

Advanced assessment skills: Palpation for tactile fremitus

Because sound travels more easily through solid structures than air, assessing tactile fremitus – which is the palpation of voice vibrations – provides valuable information about the contents of the lungs.

● Place your open palm flat against the client's chest without touching the chest with your fingers.

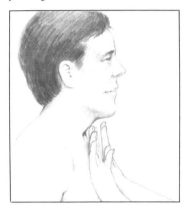

● Ask the client to repeat a resonant phrase like "ninety-nine" as you systematically move your hands over the client's chest from the central airways to the lung periphery and back.

● Repeat this procedure on the posterior thorax. You should feel vibrations of equal intensity on either side of the chest. The fremitus normally occurs in the upper chest, close to the bronchi, and feels strongest at the second intercostal space on either side of the sternum. Little or no fremitus should occur in the lower chest. The intensity of the vibrations varies according to the thickness and structure of the client's chest wall as well as the client's voice intensity and pitch.

Advanced assessment skills: Measurement of diaphragmatic excursion

● Instruct the client to take a deep breath and hold it while you percuss down the right side of the posterior thorax. Begin at the lower

Common laboratory studies

For a client with respiratory signs and symptoms, various laboratory studies can provide valuable clues to possible causes. This chart lists common studies along with normal values or findings. Remember that values differ among laboratories; check the normal value range for the specific laboratory.

TEST	NORMAL VALUES OR FINDINGS
Blood tests	
Arterial blood gas analysis	*Pao₂:* 75 to 100 mm Hg *Paco₂:* 35 to 45 mm Hg *pH:* 7.35 to 7.42 *HCO₃⁻:* 22 to 26 mEq/liter *O₂ saturation:* 94% to 100%
Red blood cell count	*Males:* 4.5 to 6.2 million/µl venous blood *Females:* 4.2 to 5.4 million/µl venous blood *Children:* 4.6 to 4.8 million/µl venous blood *Newborns:* 4.4 to 5.8 million/µl capillary blood
Total hemoglobin	*Males:* 14 to 18 g/dl *Females:* 12 to 16 g/dl *Children:* 11 to 13 g/dl *Newborns:* 17 to 22 g/dl
Sputum tests	
Sputum culture and sensitivity	Normal throat flora, such as alphahemolytic streptococci or diphtheroids

border of the scapula and continue until the percussion note changes from resonance to dullness, which identifies the location of the diaphragm. Using a washable, felt-tipped pen, mark this point with a small line.

• Instruct the client to take a few normal breaths. Then ask the client to exhale completely and hold it while you percuss again to locate the point where the resonant sounds become dull. Mark this point with a small line.

• Repeat this entire procedure on the left side of the posterior thorax. Keep in mind that the diaphragm usually sits slightly higher on the right side than on the left because of the position of the liver.

• Next, using a tape measure or ruler, measure the distance between the two marks on each side of the chest. The distance between these two marks reflects diaphragmatic excursion—the distance that the diaphragm travels between inhalation and exhalation.

Advanced assessment skills: Voice resonance

• To assess voice resonance, instruct the client to say "ninety-nine." As the client speaks, auscultate in the usual sequence. The voice normally sounds muffled and indistinct during auscultation. The sound appears loudest medially and softest in the lung periphery. However, conditions causing lung tissue consolidation cause bronchophony and the increased resonance that allows you to hear "ninety-nine" clearly during auscultation.

• To test any increased resonance further, ask the client to repeat the letter "e," which should sound muffled and indistinct on auscultation. If the letter sounds like "a" and the voice sounds nasal or bleating, you have heard egophony.

• To perform another test for increased resonance, ask the client to whisper the words "one-two-three." On auscultation, these words should be barely audible. If the words sound distinct and understandable, you have heard whispered pectoriloquy, which suggests lung tissue consolidation resulting from conditions such as a lung tumor, pneumonia, or pulmonary fibrosis. It occurs because sound vibrations travel with greater intensity through a solid structure than through a normal, air-filled lung.

Selected nursing diagnosis categories

The nurse may use these diagnosis categories to formulate nursing diagnoses for a client with a respiratory problem.
• Activity intolerance
• Altered peripheral tissue perfusion
• Altered role performance
• Anxiety
• Bathing or hygiene self-care deficit
• Decreased cardiac output
• Dressing or grooming self-care deficit
• High risk for infection
• Impaired gas exchange
• Ineffective airway clearance
• Ineffective breathing pattern
• Sleep pattern disturbance

DOCUMENTATION

The SOAPIE method of documentation includes the following components: subjective (history) data, objective (physical) data, assessment, planning, implementation, and evaluation. The following example shows how to document nursing care for a client complaining of chronic dyspnea.

Case history

Joseph Jones, age 66, a retired store manager, comes to the clinic with a major complaint of dyspnea (shortness of breath). Mr. Jones states that the dyspnea has become progressively worse over the past month.

S   O   A   P   I   E

Client states, "I get short of breath when I try to do anything. Why is this happening to me?"

S   **O**   A   P   I   E

Respiratory rate 26 per minute with prolonged expiratory phase. Facial grimacing, foot shuffling, chain smoking, and speaking in short sentences. Hypertrophy of accessory muscles of ventilation. Barrel chest. Assumes "tripod" position in chair. Decreased tactile fremitus and hyperresonance to percussion throughout both lungs. Decreased vesicular breath sounds and scattered wheezes bilaterally. Expiratory phase

prolonged with expiratory wheezes in both bases. Arterial blood gas analysis: PaO_2 60 mm Hg, $PaCO_2$ 55 mm Hg.

S   O   **A**   P   I   E

Ineffective breathing pattern related to decreased lung compliance and air trapping. Client compensating with position and pursed lip breathing.

S   O   A   **P**   I   E

Client showing interest in learning patterned breathing and understanding COPD. Initial history indicated that client can see well enough to read pamphlets and view audiovisuals. Client expresses the desire to have his family participate in learning about respiratory problems and therapy.

S   O   A   P   **I**   E

Began teaching about medications, activity, and breathing patterns. Reviewed physiology of respiratory system. Discussed causes and risk factors of respiratory disorders.

S   O   A   P   I   **E**

Reviewed current medications with client and family to maximize effectiveness. Suggested scheduling all daily activities to maximize oxygen conservation and allow for rest periods. Reviewed patterns of breathing and encouraged using the patterns, especially during activity, such as walking up stairs.

SUGGESTED READINGS

Brenner, M., and Welliver, J. (1990). Pulmonary and acid base assessment. *Nursing Clinics of North America*, 25(4), 761-770.

Finesilver, C. (1992). Respiratory assessment. *RN*, 55(2), 22-30.

Hagen-Moe, D. (1992). The ABCs of pediatric physical assessment. *Emergency*, 24(10), 32-35.

Kuhn, J., and McGovern, M. (1992). Respiratory assessment of the elderly. *Journal of Gerontological Nursing*, 18(5), 40-43.

West, A. (1992). The patient with bronchospasm: Assessment, triage, and teaching adjuncts. *Journal of Emergency Nursing*, 18(6), 511-518.

9

Cardiovascular System

Assessment of the cardiovascular system is important because cardiovascular disease is the most prevalent health care problem—and the most common cause of death—in the United States. Every year, more than 25,000 children are born with congenital heart disease, and more than 1.5 million adults experience myocardial infarctions (heart attacks). About 35 million Americans have hypertension (blood pressure measurements that consistently exceed 140/90 mm Hg).

HEALTH HISTORY

The cardiovascular health history that the nurse obtains should focus on client risk factors and any signs and symptoms of heart disease. The history should also assess client behaviors that promote cardiovascular health as well as those that jeopardize it. This part of the health history can uncover the need for teaching a client about behaviors that should be changed and can provide an opportunity to encourage the client to continue healthful behaviors.

Three groups of sample questions follow. Those on *health and illness patterns* help the nurse identify actual or potential cardiovascular-related health problems; those on *health promotion and protection patterns* help the nurse determine how the client's life-style and behavior affect cardiovascular

function; and those on *role and relationship patterns* help the nurse assess how the cardiovascular problem affects the client's self-image, life-style, and relationships with others. (See *Risk factors of cardiac disease* on pages 116 and 117.)

Health and illness patterns

Do you ever have chest pain or discomfort? If so, how would you characterize the pain? Where in your chest do you feel the pain? Does it radiate to any other area? How would you describe the pain? How long have you been having this chest pain? How long does an attack last?

(RATIONALE: Chest pain can result from many cardiac disorders, such as angina, myocardial infarction, and pericarditis [pericardial inflammation]. It can also result from pulmonary and gastroesophageal disorders. See *Evaluating chest pain* on pages 118 to 121 for more information.)

Do you ever experience shortness of breath? If so, is it accompanied by coughing?

(RATIONALE: Dyspnea commonly results from congestive heart failure. As the degree of heart failure increases, lung congestion occurs, leading to dyspnea and coughing. Dyspnea also may result from pulmonary disorders as well as other cardiovascular disorders, such as coronary artery disease, myocardial ischemia, and myocardial infarction. Dyspnea may occur with mild,

Anatomy review

The illustration below shows the anatomic structures of the heart.

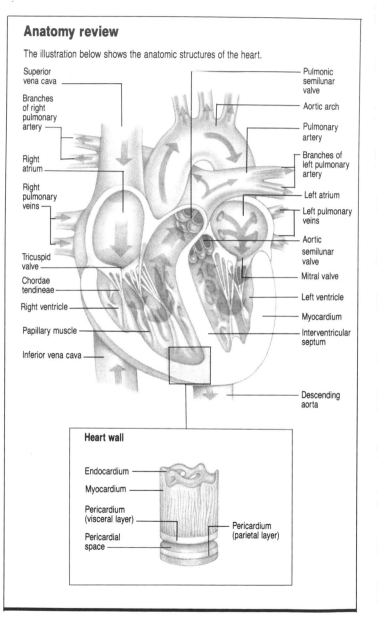

Superior vena cava

Branches of right pulmonary artery

Right atrium

Right pulmonary veins

Tricuspid valve

Chordae tendineae

Right ventricle

Papillary muscle

Inferior vena cava

Pulmonic semilunar valve

Aortic arch

Pulmonary artery

Branches of left pulmonary artery

Left atrium

Left pulmonary veins

Aortic semilunar valve

Mitral valve

Left ventricle

Myocardium

Interventricular septum

Descending aorta

Heart wall

Endocardium

Myocardium

Pericardium (visceral layer)

Pericardial space

Pericardium (parietal layer)

Events in the cardiac cycle

Basically, the cardiac cycle has two phases; systole, when the ventricles contract, ejecting blood into the aorta and the pulmonary artery; and diastole, when the ventricles relax and the atria contract.

At the beginning of systole, increasing ventricular pressure forces the mitral and tricuspid valves to shut. The closing of these atrioventricular (AV) valves produces the first heart sound, known as S_1 or the *lub of lub-dub*. The ventricular pressure builds until it exceeds that in the pulmonary artery and aorta. Then the aortic and pulmonic semilunar (SL) valves open and the ventricles eject blood into the arteries.

As the ventricles empty and relax, ventricular pressure falls below that in the

pulmonary artery and the aorta. The SL valves close, producing the second heart sound, S_2 or the *dub of lub-dub*, and marking the end of systole. As the ventricles relax during diastole, the pressure in the ventricles is less than that in the atria. The AV valves open and blood begins to flow into the ventricles from the atria. When the ventricles become full near the end of diastole, the atria contract to send the rest of the blood to the ventricles. Ventricular pressure is now greater than atrial pressure. The AV valves close, marking the beginning of systole and repetition of the cardiac cycle.

Events on the right side of the heart (lower pressure) occur a fraction of a second after events on the left side.

Systole

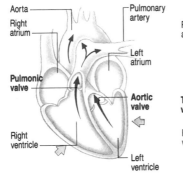

Diastole

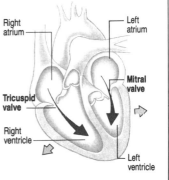

moderate, or extreme exertion; at rest; or even during sleep, when episodes of coughing and breathing difficulty may awaken the client [paroxysmal nocturnal dyspnea]).

Do you ever feel dizzy when you change positions?
(RATIONALE: Syncope develops when reduced cardiac output or vascular insufficiency deprives the brain of blood. It can accompany various cardiovascular problems, such as aortic stenosis [valve narrowing], mitral stenosis, certain dysrhythmias, and pacemaker failure.)

Do your shoes or rings feel tight? Do your ankles or feet feel swollen? If so, how long have you felt this way?
(RATIONALE: Swelling in the extremities signals edema. Edema indicates interstitial fluid collection and can occur when the heart fails to pump blood adequately, as in cardiac failure.)

Does your heart ever feel like it is pounding, racing, or skipping beats?
(RATIONALE: Palpitations may result from a dysrhythmia or from vigorous exercise.)

(Text continues on page 114.)

Circulatory system

The illustration below shows the anatomic placement of some vessels of the circulatory system.

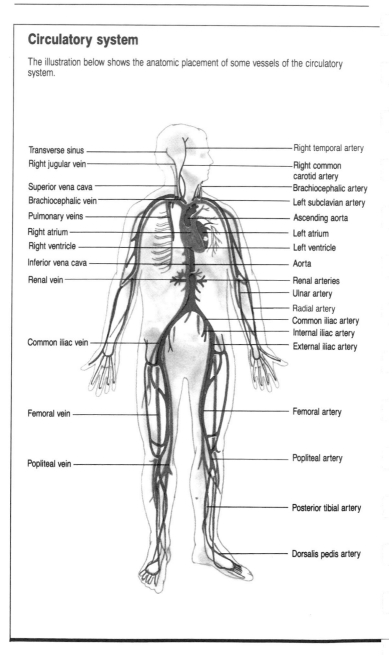

Transverse sinus

Right jugular vein

Superior vena cava

Brachiocephalic vein

Pulmonary veins

Right atrium

Right ventricle

Inferior vena cava

Renal vein

Common iliac vein

Femoral vein

Popliteal vein

Right temporal artery

Right common carotid artery

Brachiocephalic artery

Left subclavian artery

Ascending aorta

Left atrium

Left ventricle

Aorta

Renal arteries

Ulnar artery

Radial artery

Common iliac artery

Internal iliac artery

External iliac artery

Femoral artery

Popliteal artery

Posterior tibial artery

Dorsalis pedis artery

Schematic of blood circulation

The illustration below provides a schematic of the blood circulation, showing how the blood leaves the heart, reaches a body structure, exchanges nutrients and gases at the capillary level, and returns to the heart.

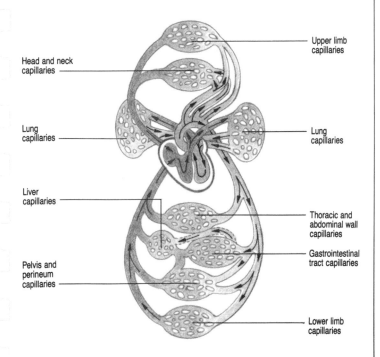

Head and neck capillaries

Lung capillaries

Liver capillaries

Pelvis and perineum capillaries

Upper limb capillaries

Lung capillaries

Thoracic and abdominal wall capillaries

Gastrointestinal tract capillaries

Lower limb capillaries

Do you tire more easily than you used to? What type of activity causes you to feel fatigued? How long can you perform this activity before you feel fatigued? Does rest relieve the fatigue?

(RATIONALE: Fatigue and weakness on mild exertion, especially if relieved by rest, may indicate early heart failure. In this disorder, the heart cannot provide enough blood to meet the slightly increased metabolic needs of the cells. However, few clients recognize fatigue as a cardiac symptom. When they feel fatigued during an activity, they stop and rest, preventing the occurrence of more obvious cardiac symptoms.)

Do you have any ulcers or sores on your legs? If so, are they healing? Do you notice any change in the feeling in your legs?

(RATIONALE: Decreased circulation to the lower extremities can cause ulcers that do not heal and can decrease sensation. Often, these changes occur so slowly that the client does not perceive them as a problem. In fact, the client may not offer information about these changes unless questioned.)

Were you born with a heart problem? If so, when and how was it treated?

(RATIONALE: Problems related to congenital heart disorders, such as tetralogy of Fallot and ventricular septal defect, may persist even after treatment or surgical correction.)

Have you had rheumatic fever? If so, when? Have any heart problems resulted from the rheumatic fever?

(RATIONALE: Rheumatic fever can lead to rheumatic heart disease, eventually causing valvular stenosis or insufficiency.)

Have you had a heart murmur? If so, who told you about it and when?

(RATIONALE: Many people have innocent, or functional, murmurs that are unrelated to structural heart disease. Other people have murmurs that are caused by permanent structural problems, such as septal defects or valvular stenosis or insufficiency caused by rheumatic fever.)

Do you have high blood pressure, high cholesterol, or diabetes mellitus? If so, when was the disorder first diagnosed? How do you manage it? Has it affected your lifestyle? If so, how?

(RATIONALE: Hypertension, hyperlipidemia, and diabetes mellitus are major risk factors of cardiac disease.)

Have you experienced chest pain, shortness of breath, fainting or dizziness, foot or ankle swelling, palpitations, or a bluish discoloration of your skin?

(RATIONALE: These are all major signs and symptoms of heart disease.)

Have you experienced confusion?

(RATIONALE: Confusion may be a sign of cardiac disease, especially in an elderly client. It typically results when a dysrhythmia decreases cardiac output. The decreased output, in turn, causes cerebrovascular insufficiency—and confusion.)

Have you felt fatigued in the past few months? What was the cause? How frequently has fatigue occurred?

(RATIONALE: Fatigue is a common symptom of heart disease. The frequency of fatigue and the circumstances surrounding it may provide clues to the severity of the heart disease. For example, fatigue at rest suggests a more severe disorder than fatigue after exertion.)

Have you had dental work done or undergone an invasive procedure, such as cystoscopy or endoscopy, within the last few weeks? If so, which procedure and when?

(RATIONALE: Invasive procedures can create an entry for organisms that can cause infective endocarditis, an endocardial infection from such bacteria as *Streptococcus, Pneumococcus,* or *Staphylococcus.*)

Has anyone in your family been treated for heart disease? If so, how was the person related to you? What was the disorder? At what age did it occur?

(RATIONALE: The incidence of cardiac disease in a blood relative increases the risk of cardiac disease in the client.)

Has anyone in your family died suddenly of an unknown cause?
(RATIONALE: The family member may have died from cardiac arrest. If so, this puts the client at a greater risk of cardiac disease.)

Does anyone in your family have high blood pressure, high cholesterol, or diabetes mellitus? If so, at what age did the disease develop? How is it treated?
(RATIONALE: The incidence of cardiac disease is higher in clients with a family history of hypertension, hyperlipidemia, or diabetes mellitus.)

Pediatric client

Try to involve the child in the interview along with the parent or guardian. The child's age will determine the degree of involvement and the terminology to use. For a thorough cardiovascular assessment of a child, ask the following questions.

Has the child experienced any growth delay?
(RATIONALE: Slow growth may result from impaired cardiac output.)

Does the child have any problems with coordination?
(RATIONALE: A poorly coordinated child who is unusually tall and thin may have Marfan's syndrome, a congenital disorder characterized by musculoskeletal disturbances, such as bone elongation and incoordination, and by cardiovascular abnormalities that may affect the aorta, aortic valve, and myocardium.)

Does the child turn blue when crying?
(RATIONALE: The bluish skin color signals cyanosis, which may indicate a congenital heart disease.)

Does the child stop frequently during play to sit or squat?
(RATIONALE: Frequent rest breaks during play suggest exercise intolerance, which frequently accompanies congenital cardiac disorders.)

Does the child have difficulty feeding?
(RATIONALE: Feeding difficulty may result from congestive heart failure or a congenital heart disease that causes dyspnea. In such

a child, the heart cannot increase its work load enough to provide the extra energy required during eating.)

Does the child tire easily or sleep excessively?
(RATIONALE: Poor exercise tolerance and fatigue may indicate congenital heart disease or congestive heart failure.)

Does the child frequently develop strep throat infections or a sore throat accompanied by fever?
(RATIONALE: Streptococcal infections may lead to rheumatic fever and rheumatic heart disease.)

Pregnant client

During this pregnancy, has any health care professional said that you have a heart murmur?
(RATIONALE: The increased blood volume associated with pregnancy can create an innocent, physiologic murmur. However, any murmur requires further study to exclude a pathologic cause.)

Do you ever feel dizzy when you change positions?
(RATIONALE: Early in pregnancy, vasodilation normally causes blood pressure to fall, which may result in syncope, especially with position changes.)

Have you noticed any swelling in your feet or ankles? Have you developed varicose veins in your legs or genitals? Have you developed hemorrhoids?
(RATIONALE: During pregnancy, increased venous pressure and venous pooling can result in edema and varicosities, including hemorrhoids. These effects usually subside after delivery.)

Elderly client

Does your heart pound after stress or exertion?
(RATIONALE: As the heart loses elasticity and muscle strength with age, it becomes less responsive to the body's increased oxygen demands caused by stress or exertion. Because of this, the heart seems to pound and takes longer to return to its normal rate.)

Risk factors of cardiac disease

Because a client can have coronary atherosclerosis for years without signs or symptoms, the nurse should carefully evaluate risk factors when obtaining a cardiovascular health history. Some risk factors can be altered to reduce the probability of a client's developing cardiac disease, but when two or more risk factors—whether unalterable or alterable—are present, the risk of disease is greater than the sum of the factors.

UNALTERABLE RISK FACTORS

Heredity
The occurrence of cardiac disease or hyperlipidemia in a blood relative before age 55 increases a client's risk of cardiac disease.

Sex
More men develop cardiac disease than women, and at a younger age. Before menopause, women have only one sixth the rate of cardiac disease as men in the same age-group. The difference narrows dramatically after a woman's menopause. By age 75, women become as likely as men to develop cardiac disease.

Race
Black women of all ages and Black men under age 45 have a higher incidence of hypertension than Causasian men and women of comparable ages, which increases the risk of cardiac disease in Blacks.

Age
The death rate from cardiac disease increases with age. Clients age 60 have three times the rate of disease found in clients age 45.

ALTERABLE RISK FACTORS

Hypertension
Hypertension (consistently high blood pressure exceeding 140/90 mm Hg) poses a major risk of cardiac disease. It is more prevalent in Black, elderly, and obese clients and in those who use oral contraceptives. It usually can be controlled with exercise, a low-sodium diet, stress reduction techniques, and antihypertensive agents.

Cigarette smoking
Men who smoke a pack of cigarettes daily run more than twice the risk of developing cardiac disease than nonsmoking men. Men who smoke two or more packs a day are four times as likely to get the disease. Women smokers also increase their risk of cardiac disease. Regardless of sex, the more a client smokes, the greater the risk. However, the effects of cigarette smoking seem reversible. Smokers who quit eventually return to the same risk level as people who have never smoked.

Hyperlipidemia
Hyperlipidemia refers to elevated lipid concentrations in plasma. Normally, total cholesterol (a component of lipoproteins) levels range from 160 to 180 mg/dl; a level above 180 mg/dl doubles the risk of cardiac disease. More men than women have abnormally high cholesterol levels. Serum cholesterol travels in lipoprotein fractions, including high-density lipoproteins (HDLs), which help remove cholesterol from the body, and low-density lipoproteins (LDLs), which promote cholesterol deposits in the body. Hyperlipidemia usually can be controlled with a low-fat diet, exercise, and antilipemic agents.

Diabetes mellitus
At age 45, diabetic men run twice the risk of cardiac disease as nondiabetic men; premenopausal diabetic women have six times the rate of cardiac disease as premenopausal nondiabetic women. Diabetes usually can be controlled with diet, insulin, and exercise.

Risk factors of cardiac disease continued

CONTRIBUTING FACTORS

Obesity
Obesity doubles the risk of congestive heart failure and cerebrovascular accident. It slightly increases the risk of coronary artery disease, probably because many obese individuals also have increased serum cholesterol and glucose levels as well as elevated blood pressure.

Inactivity
Lack of exercise seems to decrease HDL levels and promote atherosclerosis. Regular exercise increases HDL levels, lowers the resting heart rate, and may improve myocardial oxygenation.

Stress
Clients with type A personalities run twice the risk of cardiac disease as their more relaxed type B counterparts. Type A personalities typically exhibit chronic overreaction to stress; an exaggerated sense of urgency; excessive aggressiveness, competitiveness, and hostility; and compulsive striving for achievement. Stress contributes to cardiac disease by elevating catecholamine levels, which increase blood pressure and myocardial oxygen consumption. It can also lead to overeating and lack of exercise.

Diet
A diet high in cholesterol and saturated fats may promote hypertension and hyperlipidemia. High caffeine intake (more than the amount in six cups of coffee a day) may contribute to hypertension and dysrhythmias. Moderate alcohol consumption (one or two drinks a day) may reduce the risk of cardiac disease.

OTHER RISK FACTORS

Left ventricular hypertrophy (LVH)
A client with LVH greatly risks cardiac disease. Nearly half of all clients who die from cardiovascular disease first show signs of LVH.

Oral contraceptive use
In women who use oral contraceptives, the risk of hypertension is double or triple that of nonusers. Such women also have a higher risk of myocardial infarction, which increases with age, duration of oral contraceptive use, and smoking.

Gout
Twice as many men with gout develop cardiac disease as do men without gout. The higher risk may result from hyperlipidemia, hypertension, obesity, and glucose intolerance—common effects of gout.

Environmental factors
Cold, snowy regions have a higher mortality from cardiac disease. High-altitude regions and those with "hard" drinking water have a lower mortality.

Do you ever feel dizzy when changing position or exerting yourself?
(RATIONALE: Tortuous carotid arteries, a thickened endothelium, and a conduction system that has developed fibrosis can reduce an elderly client's blood supply to the brain, which can cause syncope.)

Do you suffer from shortness of breath? If so, is it ever accompanied by coughing or wheezing?
(RATIONALE: In an elderly client, a myocardial infarction or an ischemic episode may cause dyspnea, but no pain. A nonproductive cough, wheezing, or hemoptysis [coughing up of blood] may accompany the dyspnea.)

Health promotion and protection patterns

Do you smoke cigarettes, cigars, or a pipe or chew tobacco? If so, how long have you smoked? How many cigarettes, cigars, or pipes of tobacco do you smoke per day?
(RATIONALE: Smoking is a major risk factor for cardiac disease.)

(Text continues on page 122.)

Evaluating chest pain

If a client reports chest pain, the nurse should ask about its provocative (aggravating) factors and palliative (alleviating) actions, quality or quantity, region and radiation, sever-

PROVOCATIVE FACTORS AND PALLIATIVE ACTIONS	QUALITY OR QUANTITY
Cardiac cause: Angina	
Provocative factors: emotional stress, extreme weather, heavy meal, hot bath or shower, physical exertion, sexual intercourse, spontaneous (no apparent cause) *Palliative actions:* nitroglycerin, rest, high Fowler's position	Crushing or squeezing sensation; feeling of heaviness, pressure, or tightness; dull ache; or indigestion
Cardiac cause: Myocardial infarction	
Provocative factors: same as above *Palliative actions:* morphine, nitroglycerin	Crushing or squeezing sensation; feeling of heaviness, pressure, or tightness; dull ache; or indigestion
Cardiac cause: Postmyocardial syndrome	
Provocative factors: coughing, deep breathing, laughing, movement *Palliative actions:* aspirin, high Fowler's position, indomethacin (Indocin), nitroglycerin	Knifelike, sharp, or stabbing sensation
Cardiac cause: Pericarditis	
Provocative factors: coughing, deep breathing, laughing, lying down, movement *Palliative actions:* high Fowler's position, leaning forward	Knifelike, sharp, or stabbing sensation
Cardiac cause: Dissecting aortic aneurysm	
Provocative factors: lifting heavy weight, spontaneous *Palliative actions:* narcotic analgesic, surgery	Ripping or tearing sensation, throbbing of chest with heartbeat
Pulmonary cause: Pulmonary artery hypertension	
Provocative factors: anemia, carbon monoxide, chronic hypoxemia (acute flare-up), high altitude *Palliative action:* oxygen	Crushing or gripping sensation

ity, and timing. By using the PQRST method of symptom analysis, the nurse can determine if the pain is caused by cardiac, pulmonary, or gastroesophageal disorders.

REGION AND RADIATION	SEVERITY	TIMING
Substernal region: radiation to left shoulder, jaw, neck, arm, elbow, or wrist	Mild to severe	Gradual or sudden onset; 5 to 10 minutes duration
Substernal region: radiation to left shoulder, jaw, neck, arm, elbow, wrist, or fingers	Asymptomatic to severe	Gradual or sudden onset; constant duration during episode
Substernal region or at left sternal border; radiation to shoulders (but not down arms)	Severe	Sudden onset (typically occurs 1 week to 1 year after myocardial infarction; tends to recur); constant duration
Substernal region: radiation to back, neck, left shoulder, or arm	Mild to severe	Sudden onset; constant duration
Upper back (or upper anterior chest) region; radiation through back, abdomen, or thighs	Severe (especially at onset)	Sudden onset; few hours to days duration
Substernal region: does not radiate	Severe	Sudden onset; intermittent, nocturnal, or constant duration

continued

Evaluating chest pain continued

PROVOCATIVE FACTORS AND PALLIATIVE ACTIONS	QUALITY OR QUANTITY
Pulmonary cause: Pulmonary embolism	
Provocative factors: coughing, deep breathing, immobility *Palliative actions:* high Fowler's position, splinting of chest, position change	Gripping or stabbing sensation that worsens with deep breathing, or sensation of the inability to take a breath
Pulmonary cause: Pneumothorax	
Provocative factors: coughing, exertion, Valsalva maneuver, spontaneous (no apparent cause) *Palliative action:* chest tube insertion	Often described as sharp or tearing sensation
Pulmonary cause: Pneumonia	
Provocative factors: aspiration, hypoventilation (secondary to other disorders) *Palliative actions:* analgesic, rest	Burning, stabbing, or tearing sensation
Pulmonary cause: Rib fracture	
Provocative factors: chest compression during cardiopulmonary resuscitation, coughing, deep breathing, laughing, movement *Palliative actions:* analgesic, heat	Sore, stabbing, or sticking sensation
Gastroesophageal cause: Esophageal reflux	
Provocative factors: alcohol, aspirin, caffeine, constipation, spicy meal, lying down after meal, lifting heavy weight, obesity, smoking, straining, wearing clothing too tight at waist *Palliative actions:* antacid, food	Heartburn or dull, burning, or squeezing sensation
Gastroesophageal cause: Esophageal spasm	
Provocative factors: cold liquids, exercise, swallowing, spontaneous (no apparent cause) *Palliative action:* nitroglycerin	Dull, burning, crushing, gripping, or squeezing sensation or feeling of pressure

REGION AND RADIATION	SEVERITY	TIMING
Affected region; may radiate to neck or shoulder	Mild to severe	Sudden onset; few minutes to days duration
Lateral thorax; radiation to ipsilateral shoulder	Mild to severe	Sudden onset; few hours duration
Retrosternal region; usually does not radiate	Mild to severe	Gradual or sudden onset; days to weeks duration
Affected area (rib, sternum, or costochondral joint); does not radiate	Mild to severe	Onset during or after meal; intermittent duration (usually 10 minutes to 1 hour)
Epigastric and retrosternal region; mimics angina but rarely radiates to left shoulder, jaw, neck, arm, elbow, or wrist	Mild to severe	Onset during or after meal; intermittent duration (usually 10 minutes to 1 hour)
Retrosternal region and area across chest; radiation to left arm, neck, jaw, or back	Mild or severe	Sudden onset; seconds to minutes duration (with lingering ache); tends to recur

Do you drink alcoholic beverages? If so, what type? How often do you drink? How many drinks? Spread over how much time? (RATIONALE: In small amounts, alcohol may benefit some individuals because it is a vasodilator—it opens the vessels and increases the blood flow. However, alcohol can be habit-forming or addictive and can cause cardiomyopathy as well as problems in other body systems.)

Do you feel rested each morning? Do you feel tired later in the day? Do you take naps? (RATIONALE: Recently developed tiredness at any time of day and regular napping suggest fatigue, a common symptom of low cardiac output.)

Do you awaken during the night to urinate? (RATIONALE: Nocturia may occur in a client with low cardiac output.)

Do you experience episodes of shortness of breath or coughing during the night? If so, when and how frequently do they occur? (RATIONALE: Episodes of dyspnea and coughing at night are signs of paroxysmal nocturnal dyspnea, which results from congestive heart failure and interstitial pulmonary congestion.)

Do you become short of breath when you lie flat? How many pillows do you use at night? Has this number changed recently? (RATIONALE: Orthopnea, or shortness of breath that occurs in the supine position, may result from the pulmonary congestion that accompanies congestive heart failure.)

Do you exercise routinely? If so, what exercises do you perform? How would you describe the frequency, intensity, and length of time that you exercise? (RATIONALE: The degree of exercise tolerance reveals the client's cardiovascular response to increased metabolic demands.)

Has your exercise level changed from that of 6 months, 1 year, or 5 years ago? What caused this change? (RATIONALE: Exercise intolerance and a decreased activity level may be the first signs

that the cardiac output cannot meet the increased metabolic demands caused by exercise. These signs may indicate decreased cardiac output from a disorder such as coronary insufficiency or coronary artery disease.)

When you walk or exercise, do you experience leg pain? (RATIONALE: Leg pain may result from narrowed arteries that cannot provide the increased blood and oxygen needed.)

What have you eaten during the past 3 days? (RATIONALE: A 3-day diet recall may reveal patterns that contribute to the risk of cardiac disease, such as regular consumption of high-cholesterol foods or excessive caffeine.)

What causes you to feel stressed? How often does this occur? What physical feelings do you have when you are stressed? (RATIONALE: A risk factor of cardiac disease, stress increases the heart rate and blood pressure without providing an outlet for these responses.)

How is your house or apartment laid out physically? Must you climb steps to get inside? (RATIONALE: The physical layout of the client's house or apartment can provide an estimate of the energy needed to get around it.)

Do certain weather conditions affect your symptoms? If so, what conditions and how do they affect your symptoms? (RATIONALE: On extremely cold, windy, or hot days, a client may experience increased chest pain and dyspnea because the heart must work harder to regulate the body temperature.)

Role and relationship patterns

Do you think of yourself as a healthy or sick person? What makes you feel this way? Do you feel that your health problem has changed your life? (RATIONALE: Because many people think the heart is the seat of emotions, a cardiovascular dysfunction can negatively affect the client's sense of identity and self-esteem.)

Has your usual pattern of sexual activity changed in any way? If so, how would you describe this change? How do you feel about it?

(RATIONALE: Some clients with cardiac disease or their spouses may avoid sexual activity because they fear that it will cause further heart damage.)

PHYSICAL ASSESSMENT

The nurse uses the following equipment and techniques when performing a cardiovascular system assessment.

Equipment
- stethoscope
- sphygmomanometer
- scale
- ruler
- gown and drapes

Techniques
- inspection
- palpation
- percussion
- auscultation

Assessing related body structures

A client with a cardiovascular disorder may exhibit signs of illness in other parts of the body. The nurse should evaluate these areas in the physical inspection:

- skin color – for cyanosis, flushing, or pallor
- tongue, buccal mucosa, lips, and nail beds – for central cyanosis
- lips and nail beds – for peripheral cyanosis
- lower extremities – for arterial blood flow and perfusion
- skin – for temperature, moisture, turgor, and edema
- nails – for capillary refill, cyanosis, and clubbing
- eyelids – for xanthelasmas (small, slightly raised, yellowish plaques that usually appear around the inner canthus)
- retina – for nicking of vessels seen with hypertension.

Inspecting the cardiovascular system

After evaluating related body structures, assess the cardiovascular system. Expose the client's anterior chest and observe its general appearance. Normally, the lateral diameter is twice the anteroposterior diameter. Note any deviations from the typical chest shape.

Assessment checklist

The nurse should ask herself or himself these questions before beginning the assessment:

☐ Have I gathered all the necessary equipment?
☐ Have I washed my hands?
☐ Have I warmed the stethoscope's bell and diaphragm between my hands?.
☐ Has the client removed socks, stockings, or anti-embolism stockings so that I can check for edema and poor circulation in the legs?
☐ If examining a child, do I have a pediatric-size bell and diaphragm for the stethoscope?
☐ Do I have sufficient drapes to cover the client?
☐ Do I have adequate light to evaluate the neck veins?
☐ Have I reviewed normal pulse and blood pressure ranges for the client's age?
☐ Have I reviewed relevant laboratory data?

Jugular vein inspection

- To inspect the neck for jugular vein distention, place the client in semi-Fowler's position with the head turned slightly away from the side being examined. Use tangential lighting (lighting from the side) to cast small shadows along the neck, which allow you to see pulse wave movement better.
- If distention is present, characterize it as mild, moderate, or severe. Determine the level of distention in fingerbreadths above the clavicle or in relation to the jaw or clavicle.

Precordium inspection

- Before inspecting the precordium (the area over the heart), place the client supine with the head flat or elevated for respiratory comfort. Stand to the right of the client.

• Then identify the necessary anatomic landmarks.

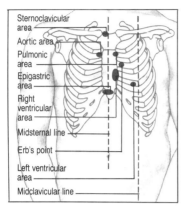

Sternoclavicular area
Aortic area
Pulmonic area
Epigastric area
Right ventricular area
Midsternal line
Erb's point
Left ventricular area
Midclavicular line

• Using tangential lighting to cast shadows across the chest, watch for chest wall movement, visible pulsations, and exaggerated lifts or heaves (strong outward thrusts palpated over the chest during systole) in all six areas of the precordium: sternoclavicular, aortic, pulmonic, right ventricular, left ventricular, and epigastric. Expect to detect the point of maximum impulse (PMI) in the left ventricular area.

• If pulsations are difficult to see in an obese client or a client with large breasts, perform inspection with the client sitting. This position brings the heart closer to the anterior chest wall and makes pulsations more noticeable.

Palpating the cardiovascular system

To continue the physical assessment, palpate the peripheral pulses and precordium according to the following guidelines. To aid palpation, ensure that the client is positioned comfortably, draped appropriately, and kept warm. Also, be sure to warm your hands and use gentle to moderate pressure for palpation.

Pulse palpation

• Palpate the carotid, brachial, radial, femoral, popliteal, dorsalis pedis, and posterior tibial pulses. These arteries are close to the body surface and lie over bones, making palpation easier. They should be equal (+ 2)

bilaterally. An elderly client may exhibit a weak pulse (+ 1); a pregnant client, a bounding pulse (+ 3). (See *Documenting pulse amplitude* and *Identifying normal and abnormal pulses,* pages 126 to 127.)

• *Caution:* Palpate only one carotid artery at a time; simultaneous palpation can slow the pulse or decrease the blood pressure, causing the client to faint.

Precordium palpation

• When palpating the precordium, use the pads of the fingers because they are especially sensitive to vibrations and can effectively assess large pulse sites.

• Be sure to follow a systematic palpation sequence that covers the sternoclavicular, aortic, pulmonic, right ventricular, left ventricular (apical), and epigastric areas.

• To locate the apical impulse, place your fingers over the apical area—a spot at the midclavicular line in the fifth intercostal space. For most clients, this is the PMI, the place where pulsations are felt best.

Percussing the cardiovascular system

The nurse may percuss the borders of the heart to estimate its size. However, most clients with cardiovascular signs and symptoms receive chest X-rays, which eliminate the need for percussion by providing more exact information about the heart. Also, many clients with cardiovascular disorders exhibit related lung problems, which reduce the accuracy of percussion.

• Beginning at the anterior left axillary line, percuss toward the sternum in the fifth intercostal space. The percussion note changes from resonance to dullness at the left border of the heart, usually near the PMI. On the right, the border of the heart lies under the sternum and cannot be percussed.

Auscultating the cardiovascular system

To complete the basic cardiovascular assessment, auscultate the precordium to detect heart sounds, and auscultate the central and peripheral arteries to detect vascular sounds.

Precordium auscultation

• Before auscultating a client's cardiovascular system, make sure that the room is as quiet as possible. If the client has special equipment, such as a suction device, try to schedule auscultation for a time when the equipment can be turned off temporarily.

• Use the diaphragm of the stethoscope to detect high-pitched heart sounds, such as the normal S_1 and S_2 sounds. Use the bell to identify low-pitched sounds, such as mitral stenosis murmurs, gallops, and S_3 and S_4 sounds.

• Help the client into a supine position, either flat or at a comfortable elevation. If you are right-handed, stand at the client's right side while performing auscultation. This position allows you to manipulate the stethoscope with your dominant hand and assist the client with your nondominant hand. Use alternative positions, such as the forward-leaning or left-lateral recumbent position, as needed.

• Now auscultate, listening for each cardiac cycle component. Move the stethoscope slowly and methodically over the four main auscultation sites. Follow the same sequence during every assessment.

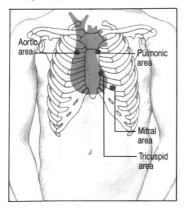

• Concentrate to hear the relatively quiet heart sounds; closing your eyes may help. Remember that stethoscope or client movement will interfere with your hearing cardiac sounds clearly.

Documenting pulse amplitude

To document pulse amplitude, the nurse may use a numerical scale or a descriptive term. Different health care facilities may use numerical scales that differ slightly. If you use a numerical scale, make sure it corresponds to the one used in your facility or by your colleagues. The scale shown here, along with the corresponding descriptions of pulse amplitude, is among the most commonly used. Remember, only +2 describes a normal pulse.

+3 = **bounding**—readily palpable, forceful, not easily obliterated by finger pressure

+2 = **normal**—easily palpable and obliterated only by strong finger pressure

+1 = **weak or thready**—hard to feel and easily obliterated by slight finger pressure

0 = **absent**—not discernible

• To assess heart sounds, begin by listening for a few cycles to become accustomed to the rate and rhythm of the sounds. Two sounds normally occur: the first heart sound (S_1) and the second heart sound (S_2), which are separated by a silent period.

• At each auscultatory site, use the diaphragm to listen closely to S_1 and S_2 and then compare them. Next, listen to the systolic period between S_1 and S_2 and the diastolic period between S_2 and the next S_1.

• Then, auscultate again, using the bell of the stethoscope. Both periods should be silent.

• At each site, note the rate, rhythm, intensity, pitch, timing, and duration of the heart sounds. Also note any extra sounds or splits.

• Normal auscultation findings include:
— Normal splits over site of second valve closure.

—In the aortic area: regular rate and rhythm; ⅔ intensity; high pitch; short duration; no radiation, splitting, or murmurs; S_2 greater than S_1.

Identifying normal and abnormal pulses

To identify various pulse abnormalities, the nurse should compare the client's peripheral pulse wave to the normal pulse wave shown here. Several common pulse abnormalities are associated with cardiovascular disorders, as described in the chart below.

NORMAL PULSE

As shown in this illustration, a normal pulse has two components: systole and diastole. Indicated by the initial upstroke, systole signifies the arterial pressure during ventricular contraction. Diastole, the downstroke, indicates the arterial pressure during ventricular relaxation when the heart fills.

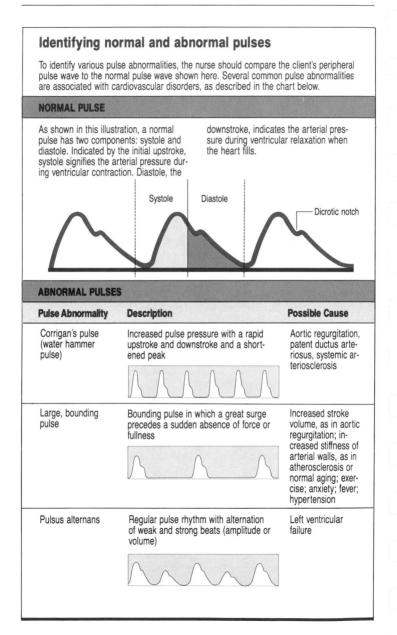

Systole | Diastole

Dicrotic notch

ABNORMAL PULSES

Pulse Abnormality	Description	Possible Cause
Corrigan's pulse (water hammer pulse)	Increased pulse pressure with a rapid upstroke and downstroke and a shortened peak	Aortic regurgitation, patent ductus arteriosus, systemic arteriosclerosis
Large, bounding pulse	Bounding pulse in which a great surge precedes a sudden absence of force or fullness	Increased stroke volume, as in aortic regurgitation; increased stiffness of arterial walls, as in atherosclerosis or normal aging; exercise; anxiety; fever; hypertension
Pulsus alternans	Regular pulse rhythm with alternation of weak and strong beats (amplitude or volume)	Left ventricular failure

Identifying normal and abnormal pulses continued

Pulse Abnormality	Description	Possible Cause
Pulsus bigeminus	Irregular pulse rhythm in which premature beats alternate with sinus beats	Premature ventricular beats caused by heart failure, hypoxia, or other condition
Pulsus bisferiens	A strong upstroke, downstroke, and second upstroke during systole	Aortic insufficiency, aortic regurgitation, aortic stenosis
Pulsus paradoxus	Pulse with a markedly decreased amplitude during inspiration Inspiration Expiration	Constrictive pericarditis, pericardial tamponade, advanced heart failure, severe lung disease
Small, weak pulse	Decreased pulse pressure with a slow upstroke and prolonged peak	Increased peripheral vascular resistance such as occurs in cold weather or severe congestive heart failure; decreased stroke volume such as occurs in hypovolemia or aortic stenosis

—In the pulmonic area: regular rate and rhythm; ⅜ intensity; high pitch; systolic short duration; no radiation or murmurs; split S_2 during inspiration; S_2 greater than S_1.

—In the tricuspid area: regular rate and rhythm; ⅜ intensity; high pitch; systolic short duration; no radiation; split S_1 possible; S_1 greater than S_2.

—In the apical area: regular rate and rhythm, ⅜ intensity; high pitch; systolic short duration; no radiation; S_1 greater than S_2.

Arterial auscultation

● Auscultate the carotid, femoral, and popliteal arteries and the abdominal aorta, using the stethoscope's bell to detect bruits.

● Over the carotid, femoral, and popliteal arteries, auscultation should reveal no sound.

● Over the abdominal aorta, auscultation may detect bowel sounds, but no vascular sounds.

Advanced assessment skills: Auscultation of extra heart sounds

Before performing advanced auscultation, prepare the environment, the equipment, and the client as for the basic assessment. During auscultation, follow the four-part auscultation sequence, moving the stetho-

Implications of abnormal heart sounds

The nurse must accurately identify abnormal heart sounds as well as their location and timing in the cardiac cycle. The location will provide baseline information; the other characteristics can help identify the possible causes, as shown below.

ABNORMAL HEART SOUND	TIMING	POSSIBLE CAUSES
Basic auscultation		
Accentuated S_1	Beginning of systole	Mitral stenosis; fever
Diminished S_1	Beginning of systole	Mitral regurgitation; severe mitral regurgitation with calcified immobile valve; heart block
Split S_1	Beginning of systole	Right bundle branch block
Accentuated S_2	End of systole	Pulmonary or systemic hypertension
Diminished or inaudible S_2	End of systole	Aortic or pulmonary stenosis
Persistent S_2 split	End of systole	Delayed closure of the pulmonic valve, usually from overfilling of the right ventricle, causing prolonged systolic ejection time
Reversed or paradoxical S_2 split that appears on expiration and disappears on inspiration	End of systole	Delayed ventricular stimulation; left bundle branch block or prolonged left ventricular ejection time
Advanced auscultation		
S_3 (ventricular gallop)	Early diastole	Normal in children and young adults; overdistention of ventricles in rapid-filling segment of diastole; mitral insufficiency or ventricular failure
S_4 (atrial gallop or presystolic extra sound)	Late diastole	Forceful atrial contraction from resistance to ventricular filling late in diastole; left ventricular hypertrophy, pulmonary stenosis, hypertension, coronary artery disease, and aortic stenosis
Pericardial friction rub (grating or leathery sound at left sternal border; usually muffled, high-pitched, and transient)	Throughout systole and diastole	Pericardial inflammation

Common laboratory studies

For a client with cardiovascular signs and symptoms, various laboratory studies can provide valuable clues to the possible cause. This chart lists common laboratory studies along with normal values or findings. Remember that values differ among laboratories; check the normal value range of the specific laboratory.

BLOOD TESTS	NORMAL VALUES OR FINDINGS
Creatinine phosphokinase (CPK)	Total CPK *Males:* 23 to 99 units/liter *Females:* 15 to 57 units/liter CPK-MB Less than 5% of total CPK
Lactic dehydrogenase (LDH)	Total LDH: 48 to 115 IU/liter LDH$_1$: 18% to 29% of total LDH LDH$_2$: 29.4% to 37.5% of total LDH
Serum glutamic-oxaloacetic transaminase (SGOT)	8 to 20 units/liter
Hydroxybutyric dehydrogenase (HBD)	114 to 290 units/liter
Triglycerides	Below 200 mg/dl
Total cholesterol	Below 200 mg/dl
Lipoprotein cholesterol fractionation	HDL: greater than 50 mg/100 ml LDL: less than 130 mg/100 ml

scope slowly between cardiac auscultation sites. Auscultation may reveal a third heart sound, a fourth heart sound, or both.

• Also known as S$_3$ or a ventricular gallop, the third heart sound is a low-pitched noise heard best with the bell of the stethoscope. Its rhythm resembles that of a horse galloping, and its cadence sounds like that of the word "Ken-tuc-ky" (lub-dub-by). Listen for S$_3$ with the client in the left lateral decubitus position or in the supine position.

• S$_3$ typically occurs during early to mid-diastole, at the end of the passive filling phase of either ventricle.

• Auscultation may reveal a fourth heart sound, or S$_4$, that occurs late in diastole, just before the pulse upstroke. This abnormal heart sound immediately precedes the S$_1$ of the next

cycle and is associated with acceleration and deceleration of blood entering a chamber that resists additional filling. S$_4$ is known as the atrial or presystolic gallop, because it occurs during atrial contraction.

• The fourth heart sound has the same cadence as the word "Ten-nes-see" (le-lub-dub). Heard best with the bell of the stethoscope and with the client supine, S$_4$ may occur in the tricuspid or mitral area, depending on which ventricle is dysfunctional.

Advanced assessment skills: Auscultation of murmurs

Advanced cardiac auscultation may reveal a murmur—a vibrating, blowing, or rumbling noise that is longer than a heart sound. Turbulent blood flow produces this abnor-

Grading murmur intensity

The intensity of murmurs varies greatly. To grade murmur intensity, use this standard scale, which ranks murmurs from I to VI.

Grade I
Very faint; barely audible even to the trained ear

Grade II
Soft and low; easily audible to the trained ear

Grade III
Moderately loud; about equal to the intensity of normal heart sounds

Grade IV
Loud with a palpable thrill at the murmur site

Grade V
Very loud with a palpable thrill; audible with the stethoscope in partial contact with the chest

Grade VI
Extremely loud with a palpable thrill; audible with the stethoscope over – but not in contact with – the chest

mal heart sound in the same way that turbulent water in a stream produces a rushing or babbling sound as it passes through a narrow point.

● If a murmur is present, identify the location where it is loudest, pinpoint the time when the murmur occurs during the cardiac cycle, and describe its pitch (frequency), pattern, quality, and intensity (loudness). (See *Grading murmur intensity.*) This information will help determine the cause of the murmur.

Advanced assessment skills: Auscultation of other abnormal heart sounds

During auscultation, three other abnormal sounds may occur: clicks, snaps, and rubs.
● Clicks (high-pitched abnormal heart sounds auscultated at the apex during midto late systole) result from tensing of the

chordae tendineae structures and mitral valve cusps.
● To detect the high-pitched click of mitral valve prolapse, place the stethoscope diaphragm at the apex and listen during midto late systole. To enhance the sound, change the client's position to sitting or standing, and listen along the lower left sternal border.
● Auscultation may detect an opening snap immediately after S_2.
● The snap resembles the normal S_1 and S_2 in quality and is heard medial to the apex along the lower left sternal border.
● To detect a pericardial friction rub, use the diaphragm of the stethoscope to auscultate at the third left intercostal space along the lower left sternal border.
● Listen for a harsh, scratchy, scraping, or squeaking sound that can occur throughout systole, diastole, or both. To enhance the sound, have the client sit upright and lean forward or exhale.

DOCUMENTATION

The SOAPIE method of documentation includes the following components: subjective (history) data, objective (physical) data, assessment, planning, implementation, and evaluation. The following example shows how to document nursing care for a client with chest pain.

Case history

Mrs. Sally Tate, age 52, was admitted to the coronary care unit (CCU) after experiencing the classic pain and dyspnea associated with a myocardial infarction. During her stay in the CCU, her pain was controlled with morphine and oxygen therapy. Mrs. Tate is now in the stepdown telemetry unit. If her progress continues, she will be discharged to home care after 72 hours.

S	O	A	P	I	E

Client states: "I get so weak and tired when I do anything. I even get short of breath." Client denies chest pain, dizziness, or palpitations with position change or activity. Client states: "I always thought men had heart attacks, not women. I don't understand this cholesterol stuff. I like to eat real food."

Selected nursing diagnosis categories

The nurse may use these diagnosis categories to formulate nursing diagnoses for a client with a cardiovascular problem.

- Activity intolerance
- Altered cardiopulmonary tissue perfusion
- Altered role performance
- Altered sexuality patterns
- Anxiety
- Bathing or hygiene self-care deficit
- Body image disturbance
- Decreased cardiac output
- Dressing or grooming self-care deficit
- Fear
- High risk for injury
- Ineffective breathing pattern
- Ineffective family coping: Compromised
- Ineffective individual coping
- Noncompliance
- Pain
- Powerlessness
- Spiritual distress

S **O** A P I E

Blood pressure 140/90 supine and sitting, 132/90 standing; temperature 97.8° F.; pulse 84 at rest, 96 after mild exertion, regular rhythm; respirations 18 at rest, 24 after mild exertion. Pulse and respirations return to normal within 5 minutes. Skin color and turgor normal. No pallor with standing or activity.

S O **A** P I E

Activity intolerance related to decreased cardiac output. Laboratory values show high cholesterol and LDL-cholesterol levels.

S O A **P** I E

Institute low-level (1 to 2 metabolic equivalent of a task [MET] level) activities and exercise plan for cardiac rehabilitation, progressing to 3 to 4 MET level by discharge, and evaluate response. Teach client about energy conservation and home rehabilitation program: activities, restrictions, reportable occurrences. Expect to arrange for low-level stress test before discharge and stress test 4 weeks after discharge.

S O A P **I** E

Taught client active range-of-motion exercises. Helped client walk to bathroom and sit at sink to wash. Returned client to bed to rest.

S O A P I **E**

Blood pressure, pulse, and respirations within normal limits 5 minutes after client returned to bed. Fatigue gone after short rest period. Client asked to learn what comes next.

SUGGESTED READINGS

Bright, L., and Georgi, S. (1992). Peripheral vascular disease: Is it arterial or venous? *American Journal of Nursing*, 92(9), 34-47.

Calloway, C. (1990). Zeroing in on chest pain. *Nursing90*, 20(4), 44-45.

Gawlinski, A., and Jensen, G. (1991). The complications of cardiovascular aging. *American Journal of Nursing*, 91(11), 26-32.

Gehring, P. (1992). Perfecting the art: Vascular assessment. *RN*, 55(1), 40-48.

McGovern, M., and Kuhn, J. (1992). Cardiac assessment of the elderly client. *Journal of Gerontological Nursing*, 18(8), 40-44.

Penckofer, S., and Holm, K. (1993). What you should know about women and heart disease. *Nursing93*, 23(6), 42-46.

Yacone-Morton, L. (1991). Perfecting the art: Cardiac assessment. *RN*, 54(12), 28-35.

10

Female and Male Breasts

The second leading cause of death in women, breast cancer currently affects one in ten women in the United States; only 1% of all breast cancers occur in men.

However, most breast tumors and related problems are not cancer, although they require careful assessment to rule out malignant conditions. The nurse can be a frontline promoter of breast care, teaching a client breast self-examination and encouraging routine breast assessment and mammography, when appropriate.

HEALTH HISTORY

Discussing the breast may be embarrassing and difficult for a female client, so ensure a comfortable interview environment that offers privacy and freedom from interruptions. Perform the interview before the physical assessment while the client is sitting up and dressed or covered with a gown.

Three groups of sample questions follow. Those on *health and illness patterns* help the nurse identify actual or potential breast-related health problems; those on *health promotion and protection patterns* help the nurse determine how the client's life-style and behavior affect breast health; and those on *role and relationship patterns* help the nurse determine how a breast problem may affect the client's self-image and sexual activity.

Health and illness patterns

What changes, if any, have you noticed in your breasts?
(RATIONALE: Breast changes may be menstrual-cycle related, or they may indicate cancer or benign breast disease, such as fibrocystic disease, which causes multiple, benign cysts of the breast. Approximately 80% of breast cancers occur in women over age 40.)

How would you describe the change?
(RATIONALE: A breast lump may indicate a benign cyst, a fibroadenoma, or a malignant tumor. Lumpy breasts may indicate fibrocystic disease, which occurs in about 58% of American women. The relationship between fibrocystic disease and breast cancer is uncertain. However, most researchers believe that fibrocystic disease is not a breast cancer precursor, unless the client shows evidence of epithelial hyperplasia [abnormal increase in epithelial cells], also called florid fibrocystic disease. An inverted nipple, skin swelling, skin dimpling, and superficial veins that are more prominent on one breast than the other may indicate cancer.)

Have you noticed any changes in your underarm (axillary) areas?
(RATIONALE: Any progressive swelling may indicate cancer. Dark pigmentation and a velvety-textured axilla also may indicate cancer.)

Anatomy review

The illustration below shows the anatomic structures of the female breast.

Lateral cross section of female breast

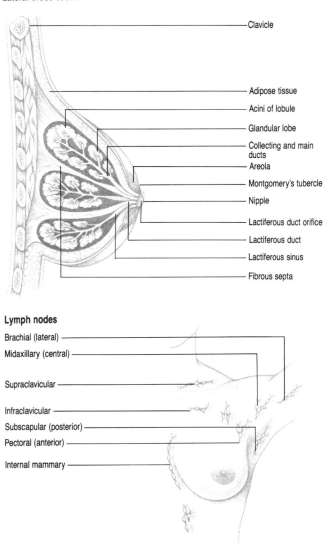

- Clavicle
- Adipose tissue
- Acini of lobule
- Glandular lobe
- Collecting and main ducts
- Areola
- Montgomery's tubercle
- Nipple
- Lactiferous duct orifice
- Lactiferous duct
- Lactiferous sinus
- Fibrous septa

Lymph nodes

- Brachial (lateral)
- Midaxillary (central)
- Supraclavicular
- Infraclavicular
- Subscapular (posterior)
- Pectoral (anterior)
- Internal mammary

If you have noticed a change, how long ago did you notice it?
(RATIONALE: Some changes relate to the menstrual cycle or to activities that involve strenuous chest movement.)

Do you have breast pain or tenderness?
(RATIONALE: Breast pain or tenderness is usually menstrual-cycle related.)

Have you noticed any nipple discharge?
(RATIONALE: Data about the discharge color and consistency, the number of ducts involved, and whether the discharge occurs spontaneously or manually or from one or both nipples can help diagnose the problem. Any discharge unrelated to childbirth or lactation needs evaluation.)

Do you have any rash or eczema on either nipple?
(RATIONALE: Paget's disease, a cancer of the nipple and areola that is usually associated with cancer in deeper breast structures, looks like eczema when it begins.)

Have you ever had breast surgery? If so, when and why?
(RATIONALE: Previous breast surgery could have been for cancer or benign fibroadenomas. If the client had breast cancer, breast changes could indicate another lesion.)

At what age did you begin to menstruate?
(RATIONALE: Onset of menses [menarche] before age 12 increases breast cancer risk because the breast is exposed to estrogen for a longer-than-normal time.)

If you have children, at what age did you bear them?
(RATIONALE: Having the first child before age 18 decreases a woman's risk of breast cancer; childlessness or bearing a first child after age 30 increases the risk.)

If you have children and did not breast-feed, did you take any medications to suppress lactation?
(RATIONALE: The use of estrogens or androgens to suppress lactation is no longer recommended. These drugs have been implicated in endometrial cancer.)

If you have gone through menopause, at what age did this occur?
(RATIONALE: Menopause [cessation of menses] after age 55 increases the risk of breast cancer because it exposes the breast to estrogen for a longer-than-normal time.)

Did you gain excess weight after menopause?
(RATIONALE: Postmenopausal weight gain increases estrogen levels, which increases breast cancer risk.)

Have you ever had a mammogram (breast X-ray)? If so, when?
(RATIONALE: Breast exposure to excessive ionizing radiation [such as that produced by early mammography machines] increases breast cancer risk.)

Have you had cancer, such as cancer of the uterine lining?
(RATIONALE: Previous or concurrent cancers, especially endometrial cancer, increase breast cancer risk.)

Have you had your uterus or ovaries removed, or have you had radiotherapy of your ovaries or uterus?
(RATIONALE: Breast cancer risk is decreased in women who have undergone any of these procedures.)

Did your mother or any siblings have breast cancer?
(RATIONALE: Breast cancer risk increases for a client who has a mother or sibling with a breast cancer history, especially if the cancer developed before menopause.)

If your mother or a sibling had breast cancer, was it in one breast or both breasts?
(RATIONALE: The risk of breast cancer increases further for a person whose mother or sibling had bilateral breast cancer.)

Pediatric client
If the child is over age 10, ask:
How do you think your breasts will change as you get older?
(RATIONALE: The premenarchal child needs to know what growth and development to

expect so that sexual maturity changes will not be frightening.)

Pregnant client
Do you wear a supportive brassiere?
(RATIONALE: Wearing a well-fitting, supportive brassiere can help prevent breast tone loss that may cause pendulous breasts later in life.)

Do you plan to breast-feed?
(RATIONALE: If the client plans to breast-feed, teach her how to roll the nipple gently between her thumb and index finger about 10 times twice a day to toughen it, and thereby decrease potential discomfort.)

Do you have any concerns about breast-feeding?
(RATIONALE: Many women are afraid that their breasts will be smaller when they stop breast-feeding.)

Elderly client
Do you wear a well-fitting, supportive brassiere?
(RATIONALE: Because breasts tend to sag with age, a good suppportive brassiere can prevent breast pain and discomfort.)

Health promotion and protection patterns
Do you perform breast self-examination? If so, how often? Please demonstrate how you do it.
(RATIONALE: The answer indicates the client's knowledge about breast care. If the client does not examine her breasts monthly, explain that breast self-examination is essential to early detection of cancer. A demonstration ensures that the client knows the correct technique, which is essential for maximum effectiveness.)

When was your last mammogram?
(RATIONALE: A client age 35 to 40 should have a baseline screening mammogram. A client age 40 to 49 should have one every 1 to 2 years; a client over age 50, once a year. A client with a family history of breast cancer may need mammography more frequently, as determined by the physician.)

If you have a breast change, can you relate it to a change in the type of brassiere you wear or a sudden blow to your breast?
(RATIONALE: Some breast changes are caused by constant irritation from a poorly fitting wire brassiere or other trauma, such as a blow to the breast.)

How much fat do you consume in your diet?
(RATIONALE: A high dietary intake of fat increases breast cancer risk.)

Have you experienced high stress levels for a long time?
(RATIONALE: Chronic psychological stress increases breast cancer risk.)

Role and relationship patterns
How important are your breasts to a positive view of yourself?
(RATIONALE: If a client has a breast lump that may need surgery, she may fear disfigurement, perhaps even more than the threat of cancer.)

If you have breast tenderness or pain related to lumpy breasts, how does it affect your sex life?
(RATIONALE: If breast pain or tenderness caused by fibrocystic disease affects a client's sexual relationships, suggest treatments to relieve the pain.)

PHYSICAL ASSESSMENT

The nurse uses the following equipment and techniques when performing a breast assessment.
Equipment
• flashlight
• small pillow
• folded sheet or towel
• ruler
• cytologic fixative
• slide for nipple discharge
Techniques
• inspection
• palpation

Assessment checklist

The nurse should ask herself or himself these questions before beginning the assessment:
□ Have I washed and warmed my hands?
□ Is the room warm?
□ Are drapes available?
□ Have I gathered culture materials?
□ Have I reviewed normal growth patterns for the client's age?
□ Do I have a breast model available to teach a female client breast self-examination?

Inspecting the breasts

Gentleness, privacy, warm hands, an objective approach, and explanations all contribute to client comfort during physical assessment.

The male client may question the need to assess his breasts and axillae. To help him understand the need for this assessment, explain that breast cancer occasionally occurs in men.

• Begin the assessment with the client seated, disrobed to the waist, and with the arms resting at each side.
• First, inspect the breasts for size, shape, and symmetry. In women, the breasts are normally symmetrical, convex, and similar in appearance. Usually, however, one breast is smaller than the other. The male breast usually is not convex unless the client is overweight.
• Look for obvious masses, flattening of the breast on one side, or retraction or dimpling. To inspect for hidden dimpling, ask the client to place her hands against her hips. Then, ask her to raise her arms slowly over her head. Inspect for equal and free breast movement without signs of dimpling.
• Ask the client with large or pendulous breasts to stand and lean forward with her hands or arms outstretched. Support the client's arms or use a chair or table. Both breasts should swing forward freely.
• Next, evaluate skin texture; it should look smooth and soft. The venous pattern on the skin should be similar bilaterally.
• Inspect the nipples and areolae for size, shape, and color.

• Montgomery's tubercles normally appear on male and female areolae. Inspect them for a discharge.
• Check the axillae for rashes, signs of infection such as boils, and unusual pigmentation.

Palpating the axillae and breasts

Palpate the male or female axillae with the client sitting or lying down. However, the sitting position provides easier access for palpation.

Axillae palpation

• Begin with the client's right axilla. Ask the client to relax the right arm while you use your left hand to support the client's elbow or wrist. With your right middle three fingers cupped, reach high into the central axilla. Sweep the fingers downward and against the ribs and serratus anterior to try to feel the central nodes. Palpating one or two small, nontender, freely movable nodes is normal.

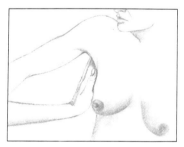

• Assess the anterior nodes by palpating along the anterior axillary fold.

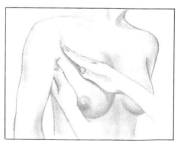

• Assess the posterior nodes by palpating along the posterior axillary fold.

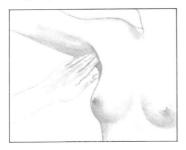

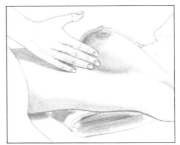

• Palpate the lateral nodes by pressing your fingers along the upper inner arm, trying to compress these nodes against the humerus. Repeat the assessment on the client's left side. Assess the infraclavicular and supraclavicular nodes if any axillary node findings appear abnormal.

• Palpate circularly from the center out or from the periphery in, making sure you palpate the tail of Spence.

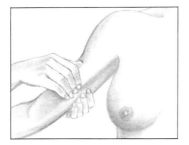

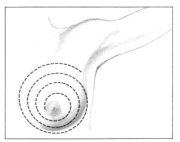

Breast palpation

• To palpate the breast, ask the client to lie supine with a small pad or pillow placed under the shoulder of the side being examined and with the arm on that same side placed above the client's head. This position allows the breast tissue to spread out evenly, facilitating the examination. Palpate a woman with large breasts in the supine and seated positions.

• Using the middle three finger pads, palpate the breast in a systematic pattern, rotating the fingers gently against the chest wall.

• Choosing to palpate across or down the breast is also satisfactory, especially on a client with pendulous breasts. This is best done with the client seated.

• As you palpate, feel for masses or areas of induration (hardness). If a mass is suspected, move or compress the breast gently to look for dimpling. Also palpate for consistency and elasticity. The youthful breast is firmly elastic, with the glandular tissue feeling like small lobules. The mature breast may feel more granular or stringy. More nodularity and fullness may occur premenstrually. The normal inframammary ridge at the lower edge of the breast is firm and may be mistaken for a tumor.

• Also assess for tenderness, which may be a normal finding because the breasts commonly are tender the week before the menstrual period. Note where the client is in the menstrual cycle when breast assessment data are recorded and interpreted.

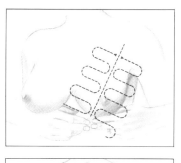

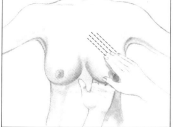

• Palpate the areola and nipple of male and female clients alike. Palpate the nipple by gently compressing it between your thumb and index finger. The nipple will become erect and the areola will pucker normally from the tactile stimulation.

• Gently milk the nipple for discharge by compressing it between the thumb and index finger. If discharge occurs, note the duct or ducts through which it appears. (*Note:* Some experts no longer check for discharge by squeezing the nipples because many women normally have a benign discharge on palpation. However, a spontaneous discharge is significant and needs physician referral.)

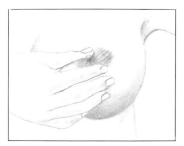

• Make a cytologic smear of any discharge not explained by pregnancy or lactation. Place a glass slide over the nipple, smear the discharge on it, and spray with fixative immediately.

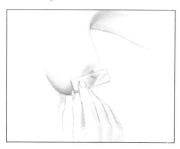

DOCUMENTATION

The SOAPIE method of documentation includes the following components: objective (history) data, objective (physical) data, assessment, planning, implementation, and evaluation. The following example shows how to document nursing care for a client with a lump in her breast.

Case history

Ms. Maria Moore, a 24-year-old copy editor, is a Native American whose clinic visit was prompted when her husband discovered a tender lump in her right breast last month.

S　O　　A　　P　　I　　E

Client states, "I cannot feel the lump my husband found last month, but I am afraid of cancer because my aunt had a mastectomy when she was 40." Client says she has taken oral contraceptives for 2 years; admits she knows little about breast anatomy and physiology or the menstrual cycle; recalls her last menstrual period was 3 weeks ago.

S　**O**　A　　P　　I　　E

Right breast slightly larger than left. Left nipple inverted but easily everted by gentle palpation. No masses or indurations felt. No breast dimpling or tissue retraction with arms lowered at side or raised overhead. No spontaneous discharge from nipple; no discharge on palpation.

Selected nursing diagnosis categories

The nurse may use these diagnosis categories to formulate nursing diagnoses for a client with a breast problem.
• Altered growth and development
• Anticipatory grieving
• Anxiety
• Body image disturbance
• Knowledge deficit
• Pain
• Sexual dysfunction

S   O   **A**   P   I   E

Knowledge deficit related to normal female physiology. Client shows an interest in learning by asking questions.

S   O   A   **P**   I   E

Review normal female anatomy and physiology and the influence of menstruation and oral contraceptives on breasts. Teach breast self-examination.

S   O   A   P   **I**   E

Reviewed normal breast anatomy and physiology and discussed menstruation as well as breast changes related to it. Taught client how to keep a menstrual-cycle calendar and to record breast changes associated with menstruation. Taught client breast self-examination.

S   O   A   P   I   **E**

Client explained how to keep menstrual-cycle calendar and discussed general breast changes related to the menstrual cycle.

SUGGESTED READINGS

Ali, N. (1991). Teaching early breast cancer detection strategies. *Advancing Clinical Care,* 6(4), 21-23.

Ellerhost-Ryan, J., et al. (1992). Women's health: Breast cancer. *Nursing Clinics of North America,* 27(4), 821-833.

Judkins, A., and Boutwell, W. (1991). A model program for teaching nurses breast assessment and cancer screening. *Journal of Continuing Education in Nursing,* 22(6), 233-236.

Knobf, T., and Gossage, J. (1990). Early-stage breast cancer. *American Journal of Nursing,* 90(11), 28-35.

Pinto, B., and Fugua, R. Training breast self-examination: A research review and critique. *Health Education Quarterly,* 18(4), 495-516.

11

Gastrointestinal System

Virtually everyone experiences some type of GI problem at one time or another. Besides being common, GI disorders have wide-ranging metabolic implications. For example, untreated vomiting and diarrhea can affect acid-base balance (the stable concentration of hydrogen ions in body fluids), and numerous disorders can interfere with nutritional status and normal body processes. For these reasons, the nurse should take a holistic approach to GI system assessment.

HEALTH HISTORY

A complete and accurate GI system assessment depends on the nurse asking the right health history questions, then relating the client's responses to physical assessment findings. Whether or not the client has an overt GI problem, questions should cover dietary intake, appetite, digestion, bowel elimination patterns, medication use, and history of past and present GI disorders.

Fully explore all GI complaints, even vague or seemingly mild ones, such as "heartburn," "upset stomach," and "too much gas." Although the client may dismiss them as unimportant, such complaints may signal a serious underlying problem.

Three groups of sample questions follow. Those on *health and illness patterns* help

the nurse identify actual or potential GI-related health problems; those on *health promotion and protection patterns* help the nurse determine how the client's life-style and behavior affect GI function; and those on *role and relationship patterns* help the nurse evaluate how the client's life-style or relationships with others may contribute to a GI problem.

Health and illness patterns

Do you have any pain in your mouth, throat, abdomen, or rectum? If yes, how would you describe it?
(RATIONALE: Pain is one of the most common GI symptoms; abdominal pain may signal a serious GI problem. GI pain is usually described as burning, squeezing, dull, or knotlike.)

Were you drinking alcohol before the stomach pain began?
(RATIONALE: Bouts of pancreatitis often occur or recur after weddings, holidays, and other celebrations where the client may have consumed a large amount of alcohol. Alcohol will also exacerbate an ulcer.)

What, if anything, reduces the pain?
(RATIONALE: Ulcer pain is often relieved by ingestion of food or antacids.)

Anatomy review

The illustration below shows the anatomic structures of the GI system.

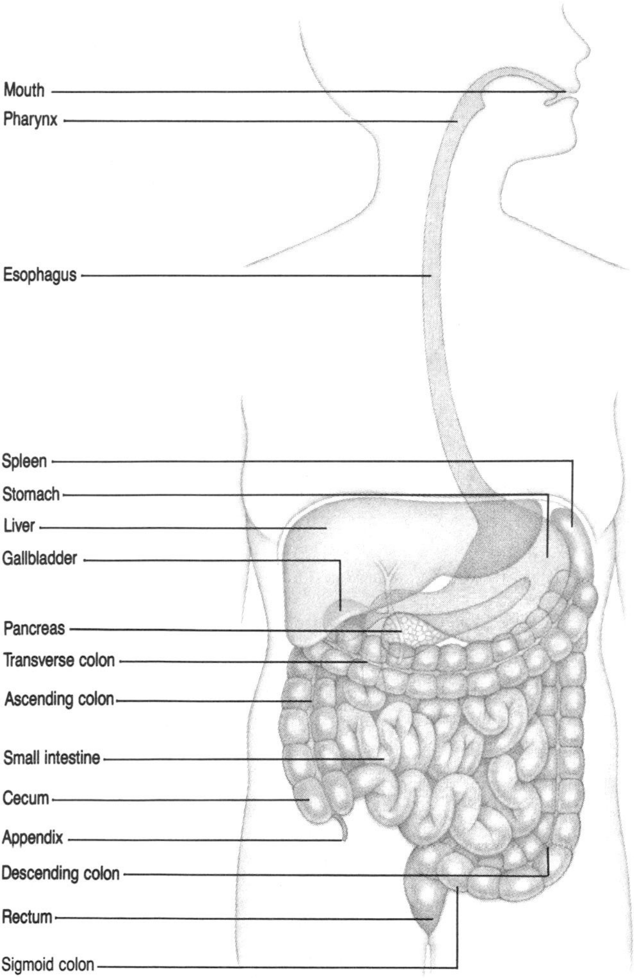

Mouth

Pharynx

Esophagus

Spleen

Stomach

Liver

Gallbladder

Pancreas

Transverse colon

Ascending colon

Small intestine

Cecum

Appendix

Descending colon

Rectum

Sigmoid colon

Is the pain confined to one specific area, or does it affect other parts of the abdomen?
(RATIONALE: Pain in an abdominal organ often radiates to other areas.

If you have abdominal pain, when does the pain occur in relation to eating?
(RATIONALE: Peptic ulcer pain usually occurs 2 hours after meals or when the stomach is empty. Insufficient blood flow to the bowel usually causes pain within 30 minutes after a meal.)

What other symptoms accompany this pain?
(RATIONALE: Fever, malaise, nausea, vomiting, redness, and swelling [such as in the mouth] may indicate a GI tract infection or inflammation.)

Do you have heartburn or indigestion?
(RATIONALE: These conditions usually are associated with ingestion of spicy foods. Dyspepsia also may occur in hiatal hernia, GI cancer, or as an adverse reaction to certain medications.)

Have you had nausea and vomiting along with the pain?
(RATIONALE: This may indicate appendicitis.)

If so, did you notice any blood in the vomit?
(RATIONALE: Hematemesis [vomiting of bright red blood] may indicate bleeding ulcer or esophageal bleeding.)

Did the vomited material have a fecal odor?
(RATIONALE: This may indicate a small-bowel obstruction.)

Is the pain related to constipation and swelling in the abdomen?
(RATIONALE: Such findings may indicate intestinal obstruction.)

Do any GI symptoms, such as cramping or pain, ever waken you during sleep?
(RATIONALE: Ulcer pain often occurs in the predawn hours when the stomach is empty, disrupting the client's normal sleep patterns.)

Do you have any difficulty swallowing?
(RATIONALE: Dysphagia [difficulty swallowing] may indicate a partial obstruction or

neurologic disease causing loss of motor coordination.)

When did you last have a bowel movement or pass flatus?
(RATIONALE: Inability to pass feces or gas [flatus] may indicate an obstruction. Diarrhea may indicate an infectious or inflammatory process.)

How often do you have bowel movements? Have you noticed any change in your normal pattern of bowel movements?
(RATIONALE: Normal bowel movement frequency ranges from three times a day to three times a week. A change in pattern must be explored; it could occur from bowel cancer, infection, or many other disorders.)

Do you have difficulty passing stools?
(RATIONALE: An affirmative answer may indicate constipation.)

What color are your stools?
(RATIONALE: Clay-colored or very lightly pigmented stools may indicate a liver or biliary tract problem. Black stools may indicate GI bleeding or may result from the use of iron supplements.)

Have you recently had an unintentional weight loss, appetite loss, unexplained fatigue, or recurrent fever?
(RATIONALE: These symptoms may indicate malabsorption, GI cancer, infection, or inflammation in the GI tract.)

Have you been depressed or felt anxious recently?
(RATIONALE: Emotional distress can cause symptoms of GI distress, such as diarrhea, nausea, and anorexia.)

Do you have any eye pain, tearing, redness, or a poor tolerance for light?
(RATIONALE: These symptoms suggest uveitis, which sometimes accompanies ulcerative colitis or Crohn's disease.)

Do you have any difficulty breathing? Have you noticed a change in the size of your abdomen?

(RATIONALE: Increased abdominal girth from ascites [collection of fluid in the abdominal cavity] or tumor can reduce chest expansion.)

Do you have any difficulty with body movement or pain in your joints?
(RATIONALE: These symptoms signal arthritis, which may occur with ulcerative colitis or Crohn's disease. Impaired mobility can lead to constipation.)

Have you noticed any swelling in your neck, underarms, or groin?
(RATIONALE: Enlarged lymph glands may cause swelling in those areas and may point to a GI infection or cancer.)

Have you had any problems with your mouth, throat, abdomen, or rectum that have lasted for a long time?
(RATIONALE: Many GI problems are chronic. Long-term GI problems, such as chronic ulcerative colitis or GI polyposis, may predispose a client to colorectal cancer.)

Have you had any nerve problems, such as weakness or numbness in your hands and fingers?
(RATIONALE: Many neurologic conditions, such as vascular accident, myasthenia gravis, and peripheral nerve damage, can also affect nervous innervation of the GI tract and alter GI function by slowing motility.)

Have you ever had surgery on your mouth, throat, abdomen, or rectum?
(RATIONALE: Surgery may cause adhesion formation, which can lead to strictures and altered GI function.)

Do you have any allergies, such as to milk products?
(RATIONALE: Allergic reactions to foods or medications may cause various GI symptoms.)

Do you use laxatives or enemas? If so, how often?
(RATIONALE: Laxatives and frequent enemas affect intestinal motility. Chronic use may cause constipation or diarrhea.)

Has anyone in your family ever had colorectal cancer or polyps?
(RATIONALE: A family history of either disorder increases the client's risk of developing colorectal cancer.)

Has anyone in your family ever had colitis?
(RATIONALE: A family history of colitis increases the client's risk for colitis.)

Pediatric client

When assessing a pediatric client, try to involve the child and the parent or guardian in the interview. For any child who can speak, encourage participation in the interview, and use age-appropriate words. To help assess a child thoroughly, ask the following questions (directed to the parent or guardian):

What is the color, consistency, and number of your newborn's stools?
(RATIONALE: During the first 5 to 6 days after birth, the stool normally changes from greenish black to greyish yellow, then to pasty yellow for the formula-fed infant and mushy yellow for the breast-fed infant. An infant typically passes 4 to 6 stools a day for the first 5 days, decreasing to 1 or 2 a day thereafter.)

What special words does your child use for having a bowel movement?
(RATIONALE: Learning the child's special words for elimination will help ease hospital adjustment.)

At what age was the child toilet trained? Did any problems occur?
(RATIONALE: Achievement of independent toileting is a developmental milestone indicating a level of physical maturity.)

Does the child seem to have more "accidental" bowel movements when ill?
(RATIONALE: Regression in bowel elimination habits is fairly common during illness and hospitalization.)

Are the child's underpants often stained with stool?
(RATIONALE: This may indicate encopresis, fecal incontinence caused by constipation with watery colonic contents bypassing the hard fecal masses.)

Do you suspect that the child sometimes deliberately holds back stool?
(RATIONALE: This may indicate the cause of constipation. Children sometimes use bowel function as a weapon in power struggles with parents.)

Do the child's stools ever appear large, bulky, and frothy and float in the toilet bowl? Are they especially malodorous?
(RATIONALE: This may indicate a malabsorptive state, such as celiac disease or cystic fibrosis.)

Does the infant have projectile vomiting (forceful vomiting that is propelled away from the body) but continually wants to eat?
(RATIONALE: Projectile vomiting may indicate pyloric stenosis or gastroesophageal reflux. An infant with such a disorder will be constantly hungry because he or she cannot retain food.)

Pregnant client

Do you ever experience nausea and vomiting? If so, does it occur at a specific time of day or throughout the day?
(RATIONALE: "Morning sickness" with early-morning nausea and vomiting—although afternoon or evening episodes also may occur—is common during the first trimester of pregnancy. However, continual nausea and vomiting throughout the day may indicate a more serious GI problem.)

How have your bowel habits changed since you became pregnant?
(RATIONALE: Constipation is common in pregnancy because of pressure on the bowel applied by the growing fetus.)

Do you ever experience abdominal pain?
(RATIONALE: Abdominal pain before the expected delivery date may indicate ectopic pregnancy, abruptio placentae, or uterine rupture. Conditions unrelated to pregnancy—for example, appendicitis—sometimes can occur.)

Do you ever experience heartburn?
(RATIONALE: Heartburn, caused by abnormal gastroesophageal sphincter activity from diaphragmatic pressure applied by the expanded uterus, commonly occurs during pregnancy.)

Elderly client

Do you ever lose control of your bowels?
(RATIONALE: Fecal incontinence in an elderly client may result from loss of sphincter tone or leakage of liquid stool around a fecal impaction.)

Do you experience constipation regularly? Does this represent a change in your normal bowel elimination habits?
(RATIONALE: Constipation is common in elderly clients, resulting from decreased intestinal motility with aging; however, sudden onset may herald colorectal cancer.)

Do you experience diarrhea after ingesting certain foods?
(RATIONALE: Diarrhea may result from a food intolerance, to which many elderly clients have increased susceptibility.)

Do you need assistance at home to go to the bathroom?
(RATIONALE: Decreased mobility or other problems associated with aging may interfere with the client's ability to use the bathroom effectively, possibly leading to constipation or incontinence.)

Health promotion and protection patterns

Do you smoke? If so, how much and for how many years?
(RATIONALE: Heavy smoking can aggravate an ulcer and may predispose the client to oral cancer.)

Do you drink alcohol? How much? How often? How long have you maintained this pattern?
(RATIONALE: Alcohol irritates the stomach lining and can precipitate hepatic and pancreatic disease.)

Do you drink coffee, tea, or cola, or use any other caffeine-containing products?

(RATIONALE: Caffeine irritates the stomach lining and increases intestinal motility.)

How do you care for your teeth and gums?
(RATIONALE: Poor dental hygiene habits can lead to gingivitis or other gum disease, and loss of teeth.)

How do you spend a typical day? Do you participate in any regular program of exercise?
(RATIONALE: Lack of regular activity and a sedentary life-style can contribute to constipation.)

What do you do for a living? How do you feel about your job?
(RATIONALE: The answers to these questions may identify unusual stressors or circumstances that could trigger GI problems. For example, an air-traffic controller or a single mother of teenagers may be predisposed to gastritis or diarrhea from the stress inherent in these situations. A sedentary job may predispose a person to constipation. Jobs that require varying shift rotations may cause a worker to skip meals or eat at odd hours, causing GI upset.)

Role and relationship patterns
Have you ever lived in or traveled to a foreign country? If so, where and when?
(RATIONALE: A client who has recently immigrated or spent time abroad may have a GI ailment endemic to the foreign country, such as intestinal parasites.)

In your family, who prepares the meals and who does the food shopping? Does the entire family normally eat together? Have these routines changed recently?
(RATIONALE: Illness can disrupt family roles and relationships, increasing stress and exacerbating GI symptoms.)

Have you recently lost a loved one, experienced a breakup of a relationship, or undergone a similar stressful event?
(RATIONALE: Depression, loss, and life changes can affect eating and elimination patterns and produce various GI symptoms.)

Assessment checklist

The nurse should ask herself or himself these questions before beginning the assessment:
☐ Have I gathered all necessary equipment?
☐ Have I washed and warmed my hands?
☐ Have I warmed the stethoscope's bell and diaphragm between my hands?
☐ Have I gathered specimen containers for stool samples?
☐ Do I have Hemoccult slides available to check the stool for occult blood?
☐ Have I reviewed laboratory data?
☐ Is the client's bladder empty?

PHYSICAL ASSESSMENT
The nurse uses the following equipment and techniques when performing a gastrointestinal system assesssment.
Equipment
- gloves
- stethoscope
- flashlight
- measuring tape
- felt-tip pen
- gown and drapes

Techniques
- inspection
- auscultation
- percussion
- palpation

Inspecting the abdomen
- Begin the abdominal assessment by inspecting the client's entire abdomen, noting overall contour and skin integrity, appearance of the umbilicus, and any visible pulsations.
- Assess abdominal contour from the foot of the bed and the client's side, stooping so that the abdomen is at eye level.
- Next, inspect the abdominal skin, which normally appears smooth and intact with varying amounts of hair.
- Observe the entire abdomen for movement from peristalsis or arterial pulsations.

• To detect any umbilical or incisional hernias, have the client raise his or her head and shoulders while remaining supine.
• Inspect the umbilicus for position, contour, and color.

Auscultating the abdomen

• After inspecting the client's abdomen, use a stethoscope to auscultate for bowel and vascular sounds. To auscultate bowel sounds, lightly press the stethoscope diaphragm on the abdominal skin in all four quadrants. Normal findings include soft, medium-pitched bowel sounds in all four quadrants every 5 to 15 seconds, and no borborygmi, hyperperistalsis, or hypoactive sounds.

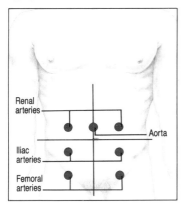

• Before reporting absent bowel sounds, be sure the client has an empty bladder; a full bladder may obscure the sounds.
• Gently pressing on the abdominal surface may initiate peristalsis and audible bowel sounds, as will having the client eat or drink something (if not contraindicated).
• Use the bell of the stethoscope to auscultate for vascular sounds. Normally, you should detect no vascular sounds.

Percussing the abdomen

• Abdominal percussion helps determine the size and location of abdominal organs and detect excessive accumulation of fluid and air in the abdomen.
• To perform this technique, percuss in all four quadrants, keeping approximate organ locations in mind as you progress. Normally,

you should detect tympany in all four quadrants and dullness over the liver and spleen. Normal percussion notes may range from tympany to dullness, depending on intestinal and bladder contents. In a pediatric client, percussion notes tend to be more tympanic.

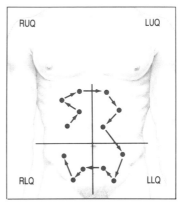

• Abdominal percussion or palpation is contraindicated in clients with suspected abdominal aortic aneurysm or abdominal organ transplants, and should be performed cautiously in clients with suspected appendicitis.

Palpating the abdomen

• Abdominal palpation provides useful clues about the character of the abdominal wall; the size, condition, and consistency of abdominal organs; the presence and nature of any abdominal masses; and the presence, degree, and location of any abdominal pain.
• To perform light palpation, gently press your fingertips about ½" to ¾" (1 to 2 cm) into the abdominal wall. The light touch helps relax the client. If the client finds the sensation disagreeable or ticklish, have the client place his or her hand atop yours and follow along. This usually relaxes the client and decreases involuntary muscle contractions in response to touch.
• To perform deep palpation, press the fingertips of both hands about 1½" (4 cm) into the abdominal wall. Move your hands in a slightly circular fashion, so that the abdominal wall moves over the underlying structures.

• Systematically palpate all four quadrants, assessing for organ location, masses, and areas of tenderness or increased muscular resistance. Normal findings include no masses or areas of tenderness or increased muscular resistance, and no organ enlargement.

• Ballottement involves the light, rapid bouncing or tapping of the fingertips against the abdominal wall. Use this technique to help you elicit abdominal muscle resistance or guarding that can be missed with deep palpation, or to detect the movement or bounce of a freely movable mass. Your fingers should also bounce at the underlying dense liver tissue in the upper right quadrant.

• If the client has ascites, you may need to use deep ballottement. To do so, push your fingertips deeply inward in a rapid motion, then quickly release the pressure, maintaining fingertip contact with the abdominal wall. You should feel the movement of an underlying organ or a movable mass toward your fingertips.

Advanced assessment skills: Liver assessment

• To percuss the client's liver, begin percussing the abdomen along the right midclavicular line, starting below the level of the umbilicus. Move upward until the percussion notes change from tympany to dullness, usually at or slightly below the costal margin. Mark the point of change with a felt-tip pen.

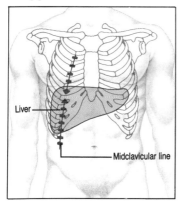

Liver —

Midclavicular line

• Next, percuss along the right midclavicular line starting above the nipple. Move downward until percussion notes change from normal lung resonance to dullness, usually at the 5th to 7th intercostal space. Again, mark the point of change with a felt-tip pen.

• Estimate liver size, which usually ranges from 2½" to 5" (6 to 12 cm), by measuring the distance between the two marks.

• If locating the inferior border of the liver through percussion is difficult or impossible, try a maneuver known as the "scratch test." To perform this test, lightly place the diaphragm of the stethoscope over the approximate location of the lower border of the liver. Auscultate while stroking the client's abdomen lightly with your right index finger (from well below the level of liver dullness) in the pattern used for locating the lower border of the liver through percussion. Start the stroke along the midclavicular line at the right iliac crest and move upward. Because the liver transmits sound waves better than the air-filled ascending colon, the scratching noise heard through the stethoscope becomes louder over the solid liver.

• To palpate the liver, place one hand on the client's back at the approximate height of the liver. Place your other hand below your mark of liver dullness on the right lateral abdomen. Point your fingers toward the right costal margin and press gently in and up as the client breathes in deeply. This maneuver may bring the liver edge down to a palpable position.

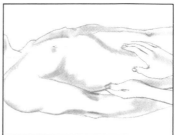

• If liver palpation is unsuccessful, try "hooking" the liver. To do so, stand on the client's right side at about shoulder level. Place your hands, side by side, below the

Common laboratory studies

For a client with GI signs and symptoms, various laboratory studies can provide valuable clues to the possible cause. This chart lists common studies along with normal values or findings. Remember that values differ among laboratories; check the normal value range for the specific laboratory.

TEST	NORMAL VALUES OR FINDINGS
Blood tests	
Alkaline phosphatase	1.5 to 4 Bodansky units/dl
Alpha-fetoprotein	No alpha-fetoprotein
Amylase and lipase	*Amylase:* 60 to 80 Somogyi units/dl *Lipase:* 32 to 80 units/liter
Bilirubin	*Direct:* 0.5 mg/dl or less *Indirect:* 1.1 mg/dl or less *Neonates:* 1 to 12 mg/dl (total)
Carcinoembryonic antigen (CEA)	5mg/dl
Cholesterol	120 to 220 mg/dl
Electrolytes	*Sodium* 135 to 145 mEq/liter
	Calcium 4.5 to 5.5 mEq/liter
	Chloride 100 to 108 mEq/liter
	Bicarbonate 22 to 26 mEq/liter
	Phosphate 1.8 to 2.6 mEq/liter
	Potassium 3.8 to 5.5 mEq/liter
	Magnesium 1.5 to 2.5 mEq/liter
Gamma glutamyl transpeptidase (GGT)	*Males:* 6 to 47 units/liter *Females under age 45:* 5 to 27 units/liter *Females over age 45:* 6 to 37 units/liter
pH (hydrogen ion concentration)	7.35 to 7.42
Phosphorus	3 to 4.5 mg/dl

Common laboratory studies continued

TEST	NORMAL VALUES OR FINDINGS
Total protein	6.6 to 7.9 g/dl
Serum glutamic-pyruvic transaminase (SGPT) and serum glutamic-oxaloacetic transaminase (SGOT)	*SGPT:* *Males:* 10 to 32 units/liter *Females:* 9 to 24 units/liter *SGOT:* 8 to 20 units/liter
Urine tests	
Bilirubin	No bilirubin
Urobilinogen	*Males:* 0.3 to 2.1 Ehrlich units/2 hr *Females:* 0.1 to 1.1 Ehrlich units/2 hr
Fecal tests	
Stool examination for ova and parasites	No parasites or ova in stool
Fecal occult blood test	2 to 2.5 ml/day
Stool culture	No pathogens

area of liver dullness. As the client inhales deeply, press your fingers in and upward, attempting to feel the liver with the fingertips of both hands.

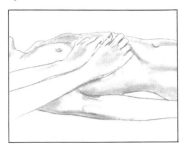

Advanced assessment skills: Rectal examination

• Rectal examination involves inspection and palpation. Usually, routine rectal examination is performed only for clients over age 40; however, it may also be performed for adult men with a urinary problem and for clients of any age with a history of bowel elimination changes or anal area discomfort.

• Client positioning for rectal examination depends on several factors: client mobility, age, or pregnancy, and the availability of an examination table or client's bed. Have an ambulatory client stand with the toes pointed inward and bend forward over the examining table. The knee-chest position, an excellent alternative position for the rectal examination for most clients confined to bed, often is not suitable for an ill, elderly, or pregnant client. Instead, position such a client in a left lateral Sims' position, with the knees drawn up and the buttocks near the edge of the bed or examination table.

• Begin the rectal examination with inspection. Spread the client's buttocks and inspect the skin around the anus and surrounding area. Inspect for breaks in the skin, fissures, discharge, inflammation, lesions, scars, rectal prolapse, skin tags, and external hemorrhoids.

• Ask the client to strain as though defecating. This maneuver can make visible internal hemorrhoids, polyps, rectal prolapse, and fissures.

Selected nursing diagnosis categories

The nurse may use these diagnosis categories to formulate nursing diagnoses for a client with a GI problem.
- Altered nutrition: Less than body requirements
- Altered nutrition: More than body requirements
- Bowel incontinence
- Constipation
- Diarrhea
- Fluid volume deficit
- Impaired skin integrity
- Impaired swallowing
- Sensory or perceptual alterations: Gustatory

- Next, palpate the external rectum. Put on a glove and apply lubricant to your index finger. As the client strains again, palpate for any anal outpouchings or bulges, nodules, or tenderness.
- Then, palpate the internal rectum. Before beginning, explain to the client that you will insert your gloved, lubricated finger a short distance into the rectum and that this maneuver will cause a feeling of pressure similar to that produced by the urge to defecate. Have the client breathe through the mouth and relax. When the anal sphincter is relaxed, gently insert your finger approximately 2½ to 4" (6 to 10 cm), angling it toward the umbilicus. (*Caution:* Do not force entry through a constricted sphincter. Wait with your fingertip resting lightly on the sphincter until it relaxes.)
- Once your finger is inserted, rotate systematically to palpate all aspects of the rectal wall for nodules, tenderness, irregularities, and fecal impaction.
- With your finger fully advanced, ask the client to bear down again; this may cause any lesions higher in the rectum to move down to a palpable level.
- To assess anal sphincter competency, ask the client to tighten the anal muscles around your finger. Finally, withdraw your finger and examine it for blood, mucus, or stool. If stool is present, note its color and test a sample for occult blood.

DOCUMENTATION

The SOAPIE method of documentation includes the following components: subjective (history) data, objective (physical) data, assessment, planning, implementation, and evaluation. The following example shows how to document nursing care for a client with altered bowel elimination.

Case history

Mrs. Maria Cortes, age 41, a married woman who works part-time as a sales clerk in a department store, was admitted to the hospital with a preliminary medical diagnosis of ulcerative colitis.

S　O　A　P　I　E

Client states, "I have a lot of cramps in my stomach and diarrhea," and "I feel so weak." Client says she sought medical attention after noticing blood in her stool and vomiting twice in one day. Client reports having 10 to 15 watery stools during the past 24 hours.

S　**O**　A　P　I　E

Client resting in bed with eyes closed, side rails up. Responds appropriately when roused. Pulse 112; sinus tachycardia noted on cardiac monitor; respirations 30 and regular; BP 100/66. Skin dry, skin turgor poor. Movement in all extremities; no tremors. Oral liquids taken in small amounts through straw. 1,000 ml 5% dextrose in ½ normal saline (5% D½ NS) infusing at 150 ml per hour via infusion pump to cephalic vein of left hand. No swelling or redness at infusion site. Bowel sounds hyperactive in all four quadrants, abdomen soft. One large diarrheal stool passed in bedpan: liquid, brown, no visible blood but Hemetest positive for occult blood. Perianal area superficially excoriated.

S　O　**A**　P　I　E

Fluid volume deficit related to bowel hypermotility. Client fatigued from numerous loose, watery stools.

S   O   A   **P**   I   E

Continue bed rest and fluid and electrolyte replacement. Monitor intake and output, serum electrolytes, and vital signs; provide skin care.

S   O   A   P   **I**   E

1,000 ml 5% D½ NS with 30 mEq KCl, 2 ml multivitamins started in cephalic vein of left hand using #20 Jelco. Perianal area cleansed, zinc oxide applied. Oral mucous membranes moistened.

S   O   A   P   I   **E**

Client weak, in bed with I.V. absorbing without difficulty. Liquid bowel movements continue.

SUGGESTED READINGS

Lockhart, J., and Hoelsken, R. (1993). Action stat! Abdominal hemorrhage. *Nursing93*, 23(3), 33.

Massoni, M. (1990). Nurse's GI handbook...gastrointestinal. *Nursing90*, 20(11), 65-80.

McConnell, E. (1991). Investigating abdominal pain. *Nursing91*, 21(11), 111-114.

O'Toole, M. (1990). Advanced assessment of the abdomen and gastrointestinal problems. *Nursing Clinics of North America*, 25(4), 771-776.

Rhodes, V. (1990). Nausea, vomiting, and retching. *Nursing Clinics of North America*, 25(4), 885-900.

Vonfrolio, L., and Bacon, K. (1991). Abdominal trauma. *RN*, 54(6), 30-36.

12

Urinary System

Certain urinary signs and symptoms—for example, hematuria, cloudy urine, incontinence, frequency, hesitancy, and urgency—should immediately indicate the need for a urinary system assessment. Other findings, such as abdominal pain and edema, also may warrant a complete urinary system assessment, even though their connection to this system may seem less obvious.

HEALTH HISTORY

Three groups of sample health history questions follow. Those on *health and illness patterns* help the nurse identify actual or potential urinary system problems; those on *health promotion and protection patterns* help the nurse determine how the client's life-style and behavior may affect urinary system functions; and those on *role and relationship patterns* help the nurse determine how the problem affects the client's body image and relationships with others.

Health and illness patterns

Do you ever have trouble starting or maintaining a urine stream?
(RATIONALE: Urinary hesitancy, or difficulty starting a urine stream, may result from a urethral stricture, such as from an enlarged prostate gland or from a partial obstruction from a renal calculus.)

Have you noticed a change in the size of your urine stream? If so, can you describe it?

(RATIONALE: Decreased stream size may indicate a partial urethral obstruction, such as from a renal calculus that has descended into the urethra or an enlarged prostate.)

Do you ever experience urinary urgency—the feeling that you must urinate immediately? If so, do you ever experience this without urinating?
(RATIONALE: Urinary urgency—with or without urination—suggests a bladder dysfunction or lower urinary tract infection. A client with urgency accompanied by urination may need to be near a bathroom or commode at all times.)

Does your bladder feel full after you urinate?
(RATIONALE: A full bladder sensation after voiding may indicate retention caused by bladder dysfunction or infection.)

Do you ever feel pain or a burning sensation when you urinate? If so, how often?
(RATIONALE: Pain or a burning sensation during urination may result from a lower urinary tract infection or obstruction.)

What color is your urine? Does it appear dark yellow and cloudy? Does it ever look red, brown, or black?
(RATIONALE: Urine normally appears amber or straw-colored. Abnormal urine colors, which range from dark yellow to black, may result from a urinary disorder, a change in

Anatomy review

The illustration below shows the anatomic structures of the urinary system.

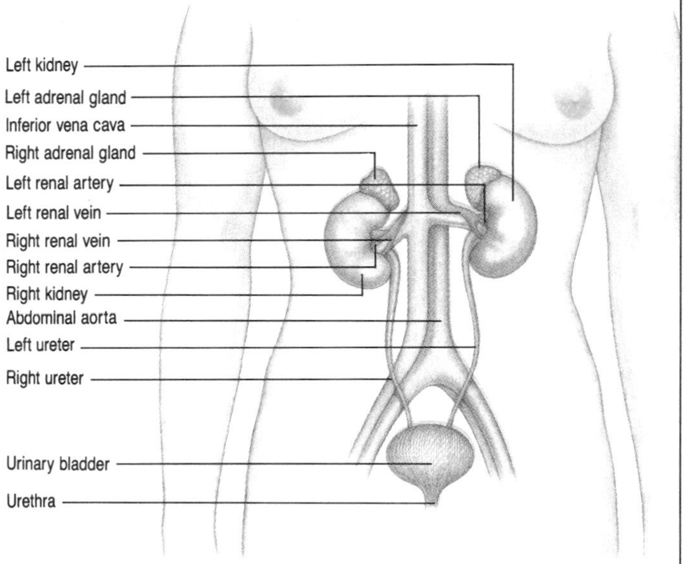

Left kidney
Left adrenal gland
Inferior vena cava
Right adrenal gland
Left renal artery
Left renal vein
Right renal vein
Right renal artery
Right kidney
Abdominal aorta
Left ureter
Right ureter
Urinary bladder
Urethra

fluid intake or diet, or administration of certain drugs.)

Do you ever have pain in your side that radiates around to your back or into your lower abdomen? If so, do position changes relieve the pain or make it worse?
(RATIONALE: Flank pain may indicate renal colic; lower abdominal pain may signal obstruction or infection. Pain relieved by lying down suggests inflammation from infection; pain unrelieved by position changes may mean renal colic.)

Do you ever have a urethral discharge? If so, how would you characterize its color and odor? How long have you had this discharge? How would you describe the
amount? Has the amount of the discharge increased or decreased?
(RATIONALE: Urethral discharge frequently accompanies a lower urinary tract infection or, in a male client, a sexually transmitted disease, such as gonorrhea. Discharge color, odor, and amount help identify the infection type.)

Have you ever had a kidney or bladder problem, such as a urinary tract infection? If so, describe the problem and tell when it first occurred.
(RATIONALE: A history of kidney or bladder problems increases the risk of recurrence or urinary system complications.)

Have you ever had syphilis, gonorrhea, or another sexually transmitted disease? If so, how long ago and how was it treated?
(RATIONALE: Sexually transmitted diseases can cause urinary and genital dysfunction.)

Has anyone in your family ever been treated for kidney problems?
(RATIONALE: Polycystic kidney disease and all types of hereditary nephritis are genetically transmitted.)

Has anyone in your family ever had kidney or bladder stones?
(RATIONALE: Kidney and bladder calculi have a familial tendency.)

Pediatric client

Ask the parent or guardian the following questions:
Does the child have a persistent diaper rash or excessive thirst?
(RATIONALE: Persistent diaper rash suggests a urine composition change, which may result from renal dysfunction; excessive thirst typically indicates that urine output exceeds fluid intake.)

Has the child experienced recent urinary changes, such as difficulty urinating or a urine stream change?
(RATIONALE: Difficulty urinating or a urine stream change suggests urinary obstruction.)

Does the child cry when urinating?
(RATIONALE: Crying during urination may indicate pain or a burning sensation, suggesting a lower urinary tract infection.)

If the child has not been toilet trained, how many diapers does the child wet each day? Has this number changed recently?
(RATIONALE: A change in the number of diapers wet daily may indicate a urine volume change. For example, urine volume may decrease with a fever and increased perspiration.)

Has the child's bladder control deteriorated recently?

(RATIONALE: Stress may cause a child's bladder control to regress. Enuresis [bed-wetting] results from an emotional disturbance, small bladder capacity, or a urinary tract infection.)

Does the child have a specific routine when urinating, for example, always urinating after a meal or before bed?
(RATIONALE: Determining the child's routine and attempting to maintain it can help prevent urine retention or loss of bladder control in a strange environment, such as a hospital.)

Pregnant client

Do you ever have pain during urination or in the kidney area? (Point out this area to the client.) *Have you ever been diagnosed with a urinary tract infection?*
(RATIONALE: Painful urination or pain in the kidney area may indicate a urinary tract infection—a common problem in the pregnant client because of her increased risk for urine retention and urinary tract infection.)

Elderly client

How much and what types of liquid do you drink in the evening?
(RATIONALE: A high fluid intake in the evening can exacerbate nocturia or incontinence. Intake of natural diuretics, such as tea, coffee, and beer, are especially likely to cause these problems.)

Do you ever lose control of your bladder? If so, does this occur suddenly or do you feel a warning, such as intense pressure?
(RATIONALE: Bladder muscle weakening commonly impairs bladder control in the elderly client. This problem can lead to more serious urinary dysfunction.)

Health promotion and protection patterns

Do you follow a special diet?
(RATIONALE: A diet that alters sodium intake or reduces fluid intake can affect urine output.)

Does the need to urinate awaken you at night? If so, how often? Does this happen

only when you drink large amounts of liquid in the evening?
(RATIONALE: Pathologic nocturia can result from bladder cancer, lower urinary tract infection, or renal disease, such as polycystic kidney disease or chronic interstitial nephritis. Nonpathologic nocturia can result from a high intake of fluids—especially coffee, tea, or beer—in the evening.)

What is your occupation?
(RATIONALE: Assembly-line workers, nurses, and others with limited on-the-job access to lavatory facilities may develop urinary stasis and subsequent infection. Other workers also have a high risk of urinary dysfunction. For example, jackhammer operators may develop renal ptosis [kidney drop] from operating drills with a constant pounding movement.)

How many times do you urinate daily? Have you noticed any change in frequency?
(RATIONALE: Voiding pattern changes can result from a local urinary disorder, such as a bladder infection, or a systemic disorder, such as diabetes mellitus.)

Have you noticed any increase or decrease in the amount of urine you void each time?
(RATIONALE: A urine volume change may result from renal dysfunction, a fluid intake change, or a systemic disorder, such as diabetes insipidus or diabetes mellitus.)

Role and relationship patterns

Can you carry out toileting independently?
(RATIONALE: Determining whether a client needs assistance with toileting can help you plan interventions that take this need into account. Such planning can reduce the risk of incontinence or urine retention.)

Have you noticed any local tenderness when you cleanse yourself after voiding? Do you ever have pain during sexual intercourse?
(RATIONALE: Bladder or urethral infection may cause perineal inflammation, leading to tenderness and dyspareunia [painful intercourse]. This, in turn, may impede the client's sexual behavior.)

PHYSICAL ASSESSMENT

The nurse uses the following equipment and techniques when performing a urinary system assessment.
Equipment
• stethoscope
• sphygmomanometer with inflatable cuff
• scale
• gown and drapes
• urine specimen cup
• gloves
Techniques
• inspection
• auscultation
• percussion
• palpation

Assessing related body structures

Before assessing the client's urinary system, evaluate various factors that may reflect renal function, including body weight, vital signs, and body position. Also assess the following factors and structures for changes that can occur with urinary system dysfunction:
• orientation—for changes related to toxin accumulation and electrolyte imbalance
• eyes—for retinal changes related to hypertension
• skin—for yellow-tan cast, pallor, dryness, poor turgor, ecchymoses, petechiae, uremic frost, or edema.

Inspecting the urethral meatus
• Drape the client to expose the urethral meatus. Note location of the meatus and any discharge, swelling, or lesions.
• In males, the meatus normally is centrally located at the end of the glans penis. In females, it is located midline. No discharge, swelling, or lesions should be noted.

Auscultating the renal arteries
• Auscultate with the bell of the stethoscope in the upper right and left quadrants.
• Normally, you should hear no bruits.

Assessment checklist

The nurse should ask herself or himself these questions before beginning the assessment:

☐ Have I gathered all equipment, including the urine specimen container?
☐ Has the client voided?
☐ Have I saved the urine specimen for laboratory analysis?
☐ Have I assessed the urine for color, amount, and odor?
☐ Has the client removed socks, stockings, or anti-embolism stockings so I can check for edema?

Percussing the urinary organs

The nurse can percuss the kidneys and bladder using the following techniques.

Kidney percussion

• With the client sitting upright, percuss each costovertebral angle (the angle over each kidney whose borders are formed by the lateral and downward curve of the lowest rib and the spinal column).

• To perform mediate percussion, place your left palm over the costovertebral angle, and gently strike it with your right fist.

• To perform blunt percussion, gently strike your fist over each costovertebral angle. During percussion, the client normally will feel a thudding sensation or pressure, but no tenderness.

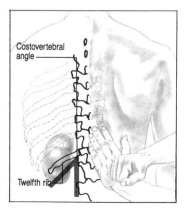

Bladder percussion

• Next, using mediate percussion, percuss the area over the bladder, beginning 2″ (5 cm) above the symphysis pubis.

• To detect differences in sound, percuss toward the base of the bladder.

• Percussion normally produces a tympanic sound. (Over a urine-filled bladder, it produces a dull sound.)

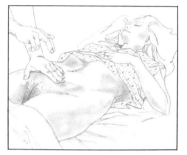

Palpating the urinary organs

In the normal adult, the kidneys usually cannot be palpated because of their location deep within the abdomen. However, they may be palpable in a thin client, an elderly client, or a client with reduced abdominal muscle mass. (Because the right kidney is slightly lower than the left, it may be easier to palpate.) Keep in mind that both kidneys descend with deep inhalation.

If palpable, the bladder normally feels firm and relatively smooth. However, keep in mind that an adult's bladder may not be palpable.

Before palpating the urinary organs, make sure the client has voided. Using bimanual technique, begin on the client's right side and proceed as follows.

Kidney palpation

• Help the client to a supine position, and expose the abdomen from the xiphoid process to the symphysis pubis.

• Standing at the client's right side, place your left hand under the back, midway between the lower costal margin and the iliac crest.

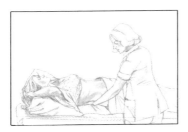

• Next, place your right hand on the client's abdomen, directly above your left hand. Angle this hand slightly toward the costal margin.

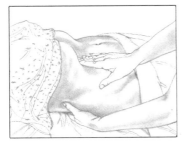

• To palpate the right lower edge of the right kidney, press your right fingertips about 1½" (4 cm) above the right iliac crest at the midinguinal line; press your left fingertips upward into the right costovertebral angle.
• Instruct the client to inhale deeply so that the lower portion of the right kidney can move down between your hands. If it does, note the shape and size of the kidney. Normally, it feels smooth, solid, and firm, yet elastic.

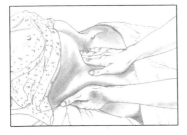

• Ask the client if palpation causes discomfort. (*Note:* Using excessive pressure to palpate the kidney may cause intense pain.)

• To assess the left kidney, move to the client's left side and position hands as described above, but with this change: place your right hand 2" (5 cm) above the left iliac crest.
• Then apply pressure with both hands as the client inhales. If the left kidney can be palpated, compare it to the right kidney; it should be the same size.

Bladder palpation

• Locate the edge of the bladder by pressing deeply in the midline about 1" to 2" (2.5 to 5 cm) above the symphysis pubis. As the bladder is palpated, note its size and location and check for lumps, masses, and tenderness.
• The bladder normally feels firm and relatively smooth. (Keep in mind that an adult's bladder may not be palpable.) During deep palpation, the client may report the urge to urinate—a normal response.

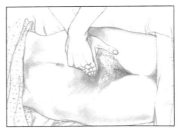

Advanced assessment skills: Kidney palpation

• The nurse can use the advanced palpation technique known as *capturing the kidney* if the lower edge of the kidney cannot be palpated. This technique resembles—but usually proves more successful than—bimanual palpation.
• To capture the right kidney, position your hands as for bimanual palpation. Place your left hand under the client, midway between the lower costal margin and the iliac crest.
• Then, place your right hand on the abdomen, directly above your left hand. Angle the right hand slightly toward the costal margin. Then instruct the client to inhale deeply.

Common laboratory studies

For a client with signs and symptoms of a urinary system disorder, various laboratory studies can provide valuable clues to the possible cause. This chart lists common laboratory studies along with normal values or findings. Remember that values differ among laboratories; check the normal value range for the specific laboratory.

TESTS	NORMAL VALUES OR FINDINGS
Blood tests	
Albumin	3.3 to 4.5 g/dl
Total protein	6.6 to 7.9 g/dl
Blood urea nitrogen (BUN)	8 to 20 mg/dl
Creatinine level	*Males:* 0.8 to 1.2 mg/dl *Females:* 0.6 to 0.9 mg/dl
Electrolytes	*Sodium* 135 to 145 mEq/liter
	Potassium 3.8 to 5.5 mEq/liter
	Chloride 100 to 108 mEq/liter
	Calcium 4.5 to 5.5 mEq/liter
	Phosphate 1.8 to 2.6 mEq/liter
	Magnesium 1.5 to 2.5 mEq/liter
Osmolality	280 to 295 mOsm/kg of water
Uric acid	*Males:* 4.3 to 8 mg/dl *Females:* 2.3 to 6 mg/dl
Urine tests	
Urinalysis	Straw color
	Slightly aromatic odor
	Clear appearance
	Specific gravity between 1.005 and 1.020, with slight variations from one specimen to the next
	pH between 4.5 and 8.0

Common laboratory studies continued

TESTS	NORMAL VALUES OR FINDINGS
Urinalysis continued	No protein
	No ketones
	No sugars
	0 to 3 red blood cells (RBCs)/high-power field
	0 to 4 white blood cells (WBCs)/high-power field
	Few epithelial cells
	No casts (except occasional hyaline casts)
	Some crystals
	No yeast cells
	No parasites

● At the peak of inhalation, press your hands together to capture the kidney. If the kidney can be palpated, note contour, size, lumps, masses, and tenderness.

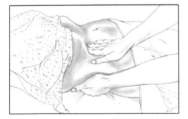

● Now, ask the client to exhale slowly as you release your hands. If the kidney was captured, it will slide back into place.

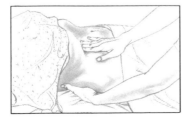

● To capture the left kidney, repeat this technique on the client's left side.

DOCUMENTATION

The SOAPIE method of documentation includes the following components: subjective (history) data, objective (physical) data, assessment, planning, implementation, and evaluation. The following example shows how to document nursing care for a client with burning on urination.

Case history

Ms. Susan Hudson, age 24, is a single Caucasian female who works as a legal secretary. She is visiting the clinic for relief of a burning sensation during urination, urinary frequency, and urinary urgency.

S   O   A   P   I   E

Client states, "I have a burning sensation when I urinate. I go to the bathroom a lot and feel pressure each time. I had a urinary tract infection 2 weeks ago with similar symptoms." Client states that she stopped taking the prescribed antibiotic after several

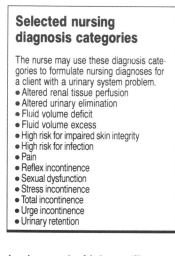

Selected nursing diagnosis categories

The nurse may use these diagnosis categories to formulate nursing diagnoses for a client with a urinary system problem.
- Altered renal tissue perfusion
- Altered urinary elimination
- Fluid volume deficit
- Fluid volume excess
- High risk for impaired skin integrity
- High risk for infection
- Pain
- Reflex incontinence
- Sexual dysfunction
- Stress incontinence
- Total incontinence
- Urge incontinence
- Urinary retention

S   O   A   P   I   **E**

Demonstrated how to clean the perineal area on a doll, and had client correctly return the demonstration. Had client explain medication regimen.

SUGGESTED READINGS

Abbott, D. (1992). Objective assessment ensures improved diagnosis: Principles and techniques of urodynamics. *Professional Nurse,* 7(11), 738-742.

Colley, W. (1991). The Colley model...assessment of bladder problems. *Nursing Times,* 87(7), 61-63.

Powers, I., and Williams, D. (1991). Urinary incontinence. *Advancing Clinical Care,* 6(2), 10-15.

Powers, I., and Williams, D. (1992). Urinary incontinence: Helping a patient regain control. *Nursing92,* 22(12), 46-47.

Toto, K. (1992). Acute renal failure: A question of location. *American Journal of Nursing,* 92(11), 44-57.

Wisby, M., et al. (1991). A nurse-managed health center offers early diagnosis of genitourinary problems: Assessing the male GU system. *Geriatric Nursing,* 12(1), 26-28.

days because she felt better. (She cannot remember the drug's name or the dose but states that she took it four times a day.) She reports that this is the fifth time in the last year that the problem has occurred. She admits to wiping herself back to front.

S   **O**   A   P   I   E

Blood pressure 120/80; temperature 99° F.; pulse 75 regular; respirations 18 regular. Abdominal and suprapubic tenderness elicited on palpation. Urine appears cloudy and smells foul. No hematuria noted.

S   O   **A**   P   I   E

Knowledge deficit related to lack of information about personal hygiene.

S   O   A   **P**   I   E

Teach client about proper personal hygiene. Teach client about medication regimen.

S   O   A   P   **I**   E

Instructed client about personal hygiene techniques that reduce the risk of urinary tract infection. Gave client a printed booklet to take home on proper feminine hygiene. Instructed client on importance of completing medication regimen.

13

Female Reproductive System

In the past, women were discouraged from discussing reproductive system problems, privately or publicly. Recently, however, women's health care issues have emerged as important discussion topics. Reproductive concerns such as contraception, infertility, and premenstrual syndrome (PMS) are commonly discussed in clinics and women's support groups. Because of their knowledge, nurses are particularly qualified to provide health care services and instruction related to these concerns.

HEALTH HISTORY

Obtain health history data in a comfortable environment that protects the client's privacy. Conduct the interview at an unhurried pace; otherwise the client may overlook important details. Ideally, the client should remain seated and dressed until the physical assessment. This ensures client comfort and confidence.

Three groups of sample questions follow. Those on *health and illness patterns* help the nurse identify actual or potential reproductive system problems; those on *health promotion and protection patterns* help the nurse deter-mine how the client's life-style and behavior affect reproductive functions; and those on *role and relationships patterns* help the nurse assess how the client's sexual or reproductive problem affects her life-style and relationships with others.

Health and illness patterns

When was the first day of your last menstrual period (LMP)?
(RATIONALE: Knowing when the last true menses occurred is necessary to evaluate such conditions as pregnancy or abnormal bleeding episodes.)

Was that period normal compared with your previous periods?
(RATIONALE: Determine what is usual for the client and how the menstrual period has changed. Some pregnant women continue to have what appear to be menses, but with different characteristics. The client could interpret a change, such as spotting [small amounts of bloody discharge from the vagina], as a period. However, spotting could indicate an ectopic pregnancy, a cervical infection, or a problem with hormonal support of the endometrium.)

Anatomy review

The illustrations below show the anatomic structures of the female genitalia.

View of external genitalia in lithotomy position

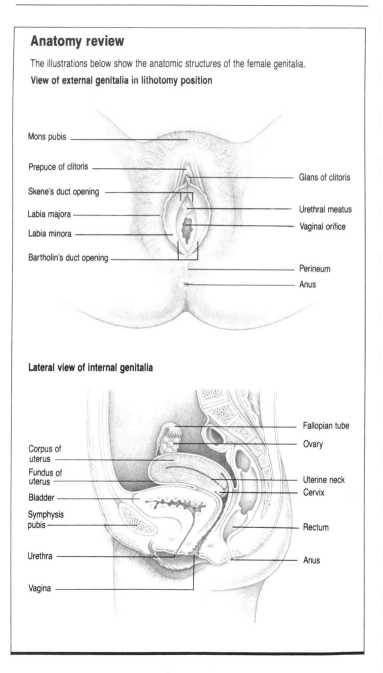

Mons pubis

Prepuce of clitoris

Skene's duct opening

Labia majora

Labia minora

Bartholin's duct opening

Glans of clitoris

Urethral meatus

Vaginal orifice

Perineum

Anus

Lateral view of internal genitalia

Corpus of uterus

Fundus of uterus

Bladder

Symphysis pubis

Urethra

Vagina

Fallopian tube

Ovary

Uterine neck

Cervix

Rectum

Anus

When was the first day of your previous menstrual period (PMP)?
(RATIONALE: The answer to this question may reveal a pattern of irregularity. A change in menstrual flow from PMP to LMP may signal pregnancy or another condition, such as anovulation.)

How often do your periods occur?
(RATIONALE: The cycle length, from day 1 of one menses to day 1 of the next, should be more than 21 and fewer than 35 days. Deviations could indicate ovulatory problems, fibroid tumors, or a malignant process.)

How long do your periods normally last?
(RATIONALE: The usual duration is 3 to 7 days, varying for each woman from cycle to cycle. Extremely long or short periods may signal an abnormality, such as anovulation or anorexia nervosa.)

How would you describe your menstrual flow? How many pads or tampons do you use on each day of your period?
(RATIONALE: How many heavy flow days, the heaviest flow day, and whether blood clots are expelled are important factors that help provide insight into the client's normal pattern. Heavy flow and clots that constitute a new pattern could indicate uterine fibroids. Women who use oral contraceptives or an intrauterine device [IUD] report wide variations in the menstrual flow.)

Are you currently using an oral contraceptive? If so, what do you use? How long have you used it?
(RATIONALE: Many oral contraceptives can cause adverse reactions, such as headaches, chest pain, or breast tenderness. An elderly client need not be questioned about current contraceptive use. However, a climacteric client may be questioned because conception is possible until the client completes menopause.)

If you do not use oral contraceptives, what method of contraception do you use? How long have you used it? If it is a device, is it in good condition?

(RATIONALE: Discussion of contraceptive methods and proper usage could reveal a knowledge deficit. Troublesome adverse reactions to any method should be explored.)

Do you have any signs or symptoms of infection, such as vaginal discharge, itching, sores, painful intercourse, fever, chills, or swelling?
(RATIONALE: Such signs and symptoms could result from a sexually transmitted disease [STD], candidiasis (*Monilia* infection), vaginitis, or toxic shock syndrome.)

Does your sexual partner have any signs or symptoms of infection, such as genital sores or penile discharge?
(RATIONALE: Such symptoms may result from STD. If the client's sexual partner has infection symptoms and is untreated, instruct the client to insist her partner undergo diagnostic testing [to prevent spreading STD].)

Are you sexually active? If so, when was the last time you had intercourse?
(RATIONALE: Answers to these questions help assess some reproductive system disorders, such as infections, and also provide clues for the physical assessment.)

Do you ever bleed between periods? If so, how much and for how long?
(RATIONALE: Bleeding between menstrual periods can indicate problems, such as hormonal imbalance or cancer.)

Do you ever have vaginal bleeding after intercourse?
(RATIONALE: Postcoital bleeding can indicate a vaginal infection with *Trichomonas* or other organisms.)

Have you had any uncomfortable signs and symptoms before or during your periods?
(RATIONALE: Uncomfortable signs and symptoms before the period, such as irritability, headache, abdominal bloating, breast tenderness, and constipation, can indicate PMS. Dysmenorrhea [discomfort or pain during menstruation] is common for some women. A change in pattern may be significant.)

Has anyone ever told you that something is wrong with your womb or other female organs?
(RATIONALE: The answer to this question provides information about previous problems as well as the client's readiness or reluctance to discuss them.)

Have you ever had a sexually transmitted disease or other genital or reproductive system infection?
(RATIONALE: Repetitive infections may indicate several problems. For example, a woman who continues to have candidal infections may have diabetes mellitus. Constant STD reinfections may mean an untreated partner or multiple partners. Pelvic inflammatory disease from such organisms as *Chlamydia trachomatis* and *Neisseria gonorrhoeae* can cause sterility.)

Have you had surgery for a reproductive system problem?
(RATIONALE: Tubal ligation, dilatation and curettage, and hysterectomy are common gynecologic surgical procedures.)

Have you ever been pregnant?
(RATIONALE: Specific data about the prenatal, labor, delivery, and postpartum periods; complications; neonatal weight; outcome; problems; treatments; and sequelae, if any, are important—particularly in women of childbearing age.)

Have you ever had problems conceiving?
(RATIONALE: Lack of pregnancy after more than 1 year of regular coitus without contraception may indicate a fertility problem and the need for referral to a gynecologist or a fertility specialist, if the couple desires. The couple trying unsuccessfully to conceive may be experiencing stress and anxiety and may welcome a counseling referral.)

Has anyone in your family ever had any reproductive problems?
(RATIONALE: Spontaneous abortion, menstrual difficulties, multiple births, congenital anomalies, or difficult pregnancies can have a familial tendency.)

Has any immediate member of your family had gynecologic surgery?
(RATIONALE: The client's answer could indicate a familial history of endometriosis, fibroid tumors, or ovarian or cervical cancer.)

Adolescent client

At what age did you first notice hair on your pubic area? When did you first notice your breasts growing?
(RATIONALE: In females, the appearance of secondary sex characteristics is the most accurate physical maturity indicator. (Pubic hair growth usually begins between ages 8 and 14.)

Have you noticed any moistness on your underpants?
(RATIONALE: Infection as well as increasing estrogen and androgen production from the ovaries result in increased vaginal secretions. To deal with body changes, the adolescent client must understand them. Any signs of infection should be evaluated and frank, open explanations provided.)

Have you noticed any blood on your underpants?
(RATIONALE: Although ovarian estrogen production may be potent enough to trigger the first menstrual flow, ovulation may not occur for some time. Adolescent girls commonly complain of irregular menses, which are caused by anovulation. Usually, no medical therapy is indicated unless heavy bleeding [which may cause anemia] occurs.)

When did you begin having menstrual periods?
(RATIONALE: The mean onset of menarche is age 12.8; the normal age range, 9.1 to 17.7. By age 14, if no menses occur and no secondary sex characteristics appear, the adolescent should be evaluated medically; no menses by age 16, regardless of secondary sex characteristics, also warrants medical evaluation.)

How old were you when you first had sex? Do you ever have pain with sex?
(RATIONALE: Many adolescents are sexually active. Asking the questions in this manner

assumes sexual activity and is nonthreatening.)

Climacteric client
Do you experience hot flushes or flashes? If so, how bothersome are they?
(RATIONALE: Menopausal experiences are subjective. Hot flashes or flushes may bother one woman and not another.)

Do you experience vaginal dryness, pain, or itching during sexual intercourse?
(RATIONALE: Such symptoms are caused by decreased estrogen levels that lead to decreased vaginal secretions.)

Are you experiencing menstrual irregularities?
(RATIONALE: Reassure the client that climacteric menstrual irregularities are common, but refer a client with excessive or frequent bleeding to a physician.)

Do you practice contraception?
(RATIONALE: The woman may become pregnant during the climacteric if she does not practice contraception because she thinks that she can no longer conceive.)

Are you having any problems or changes you attribute to menopause? What are they? Could anything else be causing these problems or changes?
(RATIONALE: These questions help the client differentiate between the signs and symptoms related to menopause and those related to stress caused by other life changes.)

How do you feel about approaching menopause (or menopause if it has occurred)?
(RATIONALE: This question allows the client to vent feelings about menopause and life changes occurring during that time. Listen actively.)

Are you receiving hormone therapy for menopause?
(RATIONALE: Some women need medical assistance during menopause—for example, estrogen replacement therapy, which can decrease symptoms but increases the risk of uterine cancer.)

If you have completed menopause, have you had any bleeding?
(RATIONALE: Any bleeding in a postmenopausal woman, except that associated with estrogen-progesterone replacement therapy, is abnormal and a possible sign of endometrial carcinoma.)

Health promotion and protection patterns
When was your last Pap test?
(RATIONALE: A Pap test can detect precancerous and cancerous cell changes in the cervix. It may also detect human papillomavirus [which causes venereal warts], *Chlamydia trachomatis*, and herpes simplex, which may not produce symptoms but may cause abnormal cellular changes.)

Are you currently having any problems that you feel are related to your reproductive system or any other problems that we have not talked about?
(RATIONALE: These questions offer the client a chance to air any concerns.)

Have you any questions about your reproductive organs or sexual activity?
(RATIONALE: The client's questions may be significant to her health. The elderly client, for example, may want to discuss her sexual activity. The adolescent client may have questions that she is reluctant to ask.)

Role and relationship patterns
Have you noticed any changes in your sexual interest, frequency of intercourse, or sexual functioning?
(RATIONALE: Changes in libido [psychic energy or instinctual drive associated with sexual desire or pleasure] or sexual function could indicate pain, infection, hormonal changes, disease [for example, diabetes mellitus], changes in mental status [for example, depression], or altered role and relationship patterns.)

Are you experiencing any sexual problems?
(RATIONALE: Physical problems in the reproductive system can alter sexual relationships. The client's answer may lead not only to exploring possible changes in her sexual rela-

tions, but also to assessing whether a physical problem is contributing to the changes.)

PHYSICAL ASSESSMENT

The nurse uses the following equipment and techniques when performing female reproductive system assessment.

Equipment
- gloves
- speculum
- lubricant
- spatula
- swabs
- endocervical brush
- glass slides and covers
- cytologic fixative
- culture bottles or plates
- light source
- mirror

Techniques
- inspection
- palpation

Inspecting and palpating the pubic area

- Position the client supine with the pubic area uncovered, and begin the assessment by determining sexual maturity. Inspect pubic hair for amount and pattern, which should be appropriate for the client's age.
- Then, using a gloved index finger and thumb, gently spread the labia majora and look for the following: labia majora and labia minora, clitoris, vaginal introitus, and discharge, which is odorless and nonirritating to the mucosa.
- The external genitalia should be pink and moist with no varicosities, lesions, organisms, edema, or abnormal discharge.
- Palpate the Skene's and Bartholin's glands, noting any swelling, tenderness, or discharge.

Advanced assessment skills: Using the speculum

- To avoid startling the client, touch her thigh before touching her genitalia, and explain the procedure. Then gently spread the labia majora with the left hand, insert the right index finger into the vagina about 4 to 5 cm (1½″ to 2″), turn the finger pad

upward, and milk the urethra and Skene's glands very gently by exerting upward pressure on either side of the urethra and then directly over it.

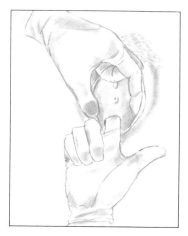

- Rotate the index finger downward and, using the thumb and index finger, palpate the areas of Bartholin's glands (at the 5 and 7 o'clock positions) in the vaginal walls at the introitus. The areas should feel smooth with no swelling, masses, or tenderness.

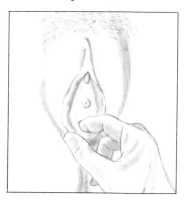

- Place the index and middle fingers on either side of the vaginal opening and spread the fingers to separate the opening. To check pelvic support, ask the client to bear down. Some slight muscle bulging is normal. Assess vaginal tone by having the client tighten her vaginal muscles around your two fingers. Tone should be greater in women who have not borne children vaginally. Next, palpate the perineum between the index finger and thumb. The tissue should feel smooth and thick in nulliparous women and thicker and rigid in multiparous women.

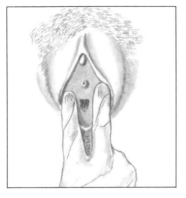

• Place the index and middle fingers of one hand inside the vaginal orifice to spread it apart about 2.5 cm (1″). Exert downward pressure with the fingers while introducing the closed speculum with the opposite hand over the spread fingers at about a 45-degree angle. This maneuver bypasses the sensitive urethra adjacent to the anterior vaginal wall. Hold the blades closed with the index and middle fingers of the introducing hand, and insert the speculum at about a 45-degree angle. Make sure not to pinch or pull skin or hair.

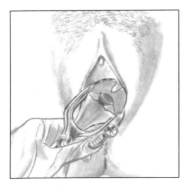

Assessment checklist

The nurse should ask herself or himself these questions before beginning the assessment:
☐ Have I gathered all the necessary equipment?
☐ Have I washed and warmed my hands?
☐ Is the room warm?
☐ Have I gathered culture materials?
☐ Have I checked that I have enough fixative and lubricant for the examination?
☐ Have I checked the bulb in the light?
☐ Have I reviewed the workings of the examination table?
☐ Do I have a mirror available?
☐ Have I reviewed relevant laboratory data?

• Once the blades pass the introitus, rotate the speculum to a horizontal plane and remove the fingers, exerting downward pressure. Maintain pressure in a downward and posterior manner on the blades until the instrument is completely inserted.

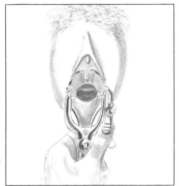

• Open the speculum blades and look for the cervix. If you cannot see it, reposition the speculum more anteriorly, posteriorly, or laterally until the complete cervix appears. The speculum may have to be removed, the cervix located digitally, and the speculum reinserted. Tell the client when the speculum will be moved or reinserted.

To fix the blade of the metal speculum in open position, tighten the thumbscrew. During speculum repositioning maneuvers, remind the client to relax. The cervix will be more posterior with the anteverted or anteflexed uterus and more anterior with the retroverted or retroflexed uterus.

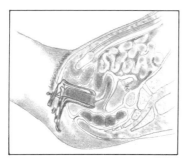

The cervix should be shiny pink. However, it may be pale if the client is anemic or menopausal. Pregnancy gives it a bluish purple cast (Chadwick's sign). The cervix, with a diameter of about 2 to 3 cm (¾″ to 1¼″), projects about 1 to 3 cm (¼″ to 1¼″) into the vagina. The cervix position correlates with the position of the uterus; it should be midline.

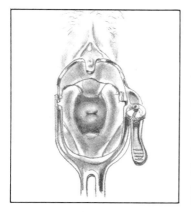

● After inspecting the cervix, obtain an endocervical specimen by inserting a cotton-tipped swab, an endocervical brush, or the longer serrated end of a spatula about 0.5 cm into the cervical os and rotating the instrument 360 degrees clockwise. Then

smear the specimen onto a glass slide with a smooth, painting motion; too much pressure can destroy the cells. Then spray the slide with cytologic fixative. (See *Obtaining specimens for culture.*)

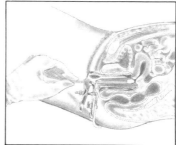

● Retrieve a specimen from the ectocervix (the outer layer of the cervix) with the softly curved end of the spatula. Some health care facility protocols permit collecting both the ectocervical and endocervical smears simultaneously on the same slide (one on each end). Regardless, the procedure is the same: Place the curved end of the spatula in the os, apply pressure while turning it 360 degrees, transfer the scrapings to a slide, and spray the slide with fixative.

If the client has no cervix, as after a complete hysterectomy, scrape the vaginal cuff and obtain a vaginal pool specimen with a cotton-tipped applicator from the posterior vaginal area. If the client has dry mucosa, the applicator tip can be moistened with normal saline solution. Prepare the slide specimen as described previously; label the slide to indicate where the specimen came from.

A vaginal wall specimen may be needed to evaluate the maturation index (estrogen and progesterone influence on the cells). Take this specimen by scraping the blunt end of a spatula along the lateral middle third of the vaginal wall.

Transfer specimens from all cervical areas to the slide and spray with cytologic fixative. (*Note:* If the specimen is too thick, it may be inadequate for microscopic examination.)

Obtaining specimens for culture

This chart describes the sites and equipment used to obtain specimens for culture studies that may accompany assessment of the female reproductive system.

ORGANISMS	SPECIMEN SITE	EQUIPMENT
Neisseria gonorrhoeae	Endocervix, anus, or oropharynx	• Cotton-tipped swab • Thayer-Martin medium culture plate or bottle
Chlamydia trachomatis	Endocervix	• Special swab (provided with test medium) • Special medium slide • Acetone
Candida albicans, Trichomonas vaginalis, or *Haemophilus vaginalis*	Vaginal secretions from posterior vaginal pool	• Cotton-tipped applicator • Normal saline solution • Potassium hydroxide (KOH) • Glass slides and coverslips

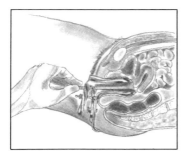

• After collecting all the specimens, unlock the speculum thumbscrew and begin to withdraw the speculum. Slowly rotating the blades in a moderately open fashion, inspect the vaginal wall for abnormalities, such as lesions, discharge, swelling, abnormal color, and the presence or absence of rugae. Women with adequate estrogen levels have pink, moist, rugose vaginal walls.

• Finally, close the speculum blades just before the distal ends reach the area adjacent to the urethral meatus and the introitus (to avoid trauma to the area), making sure that no mucosa, skin, or hair remains between the closed blades before withdrawing them. Place the speculum into a soaking solution or container or discard it if it is disposable.

Advanced assessment skills: Bimanual palpation

• After inspecting the cervix and obtaining a Papanicolaou smear and any other specimens, bimanually palpate the internal genitalia as follows. Use your dominant hand internally for the most comfortable approach, but try your other hand if this seems awkward.

• Put on clean gloves and apply lubricant. Lubricant comes in a tube or foil packet and may be squeezed onto a disposable gauze or paper square for easy use. Never touch the tube end with your gloved fingers; instead, allow the lubricant to drop freely onto the fingers. Discard the packet after one use.

After lubricating the index and middle fingers of your gloved hand, introduce them into the vagina using downward and posterior pressure. With your thumb abducted and your other two fingers flexed, palpate every aspect of the vaginal wall with the palmar surfaces of your fingers, rotating them as necessary. Rugae, a normal finding, feel like small ridges running concentrically around the vaginal wall. Note any nodules, tenderness, or other abnormalities. Women with small vaginal openings may need to be examined with one finger.

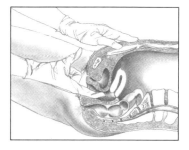

• Insert your fingers deeper until the cervix is located with the palmar surface of the fingers. Grasp the cervix gently between your fingers and feel the surface. Also run your fingers around the circumference. Gently moving the cervix from side to side 1 to 2 cm (½″ to ¾″; this should not hurt the client), assess the size, shape, position, consistency, regularity of contour, mobility, and sensitivity of the cervical surface. It should feel firm, smooth, mobile, and non-tender when moved and touched. The cervix of an older woman is smaller and is usually recessed, as in a prepubertal girl; a pregnant woman's cervix is usually softened and enlarged. The os should admit your index finger about 1 cm (¼″) or less, unless the woman is pregnant. The cervix, usually in the midline, should point posteriorly, anteriorly, or midplane.

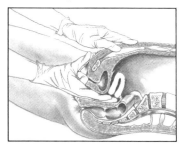

• Position your hands for examination of the uterus. Place your external hand on the abdomen between the umbilicus and symphysis pubis. Then, inserting the first and second fingers of your examining hand into the vagina and pressing the bent digits of the fingers remaining outside the vagina

against the perineum, reach under and behind the cervix and lift the uterus toward the abdomen and toward your external hand, which is applying pressure toward the internal fingers. Keep the wrist straight to keep your internal hand and forearm in a straight line. Most examination tables have a step at the examiner's end, allowing the examiner to step up and elevate one knee. Then, stabilize the elbow of the examining hand on the elevated knee, or on the hip if no step or stool is available.

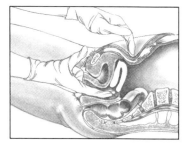

• After inserting your examining hand into the vagina, examine the uterus for position, size, shape, consistency, tenderness, mobility, and surface regularity. If your internal fingers can move underneath and behind the cervix without encountering an obstacle in the cul-de-sac (a deep recess formed by the peritoneum as it covers the lower posterior wall of the uterus and upper portion of the vagina), the uterus is probably anteflexed, anteverted, or midplane. If you encounter an obstacle (the body of the uterus), the uterus is posteriorly positioned, either retroflexed or retroverted. (Flexion indicates that the uterus is bent upon itself; version refers to a deflection of the long axis of the uterus from the long axis of the body, either anteriorly or posteriorly. Midplane position means the long axis of the uterus is parallel to the long axis of the body.) The position of the cervix may be a clue to the uterine position. A cervix pointing anteriorly indicates a retroverted uterus; a cervix pointing posteriorly indicates an anteverted uterus. Also note whether the uterus lies midline or deviates to the left or right of the pelvis.

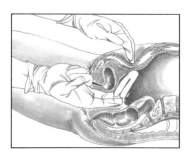

• Determine whether the uterus is normal sized, enlarged, or immature. If it is enlarged, the size is estimated in weeks of gestation. The normal nonpregnant uterus is small and fits comfortably beneath the symphysis pubis in the pelvis; it is not palpable by abdominal examination. The uterus of a postmenopausal woman is usually smaller than before menopause.

Normally, the uterus is pear-shaped and symmetrical. Note any deviations; for example, a protruding mass on the fundal surface.

Normally, the muscular composition of the uterus makes it feel firm. Although the uterus is not particularly tender on palpation (unless the woman is menstruating), some tenderness normally may occur. The ligaments suspending the uterus in the pelvis allow the uterus to be slightly mobile on the anterior to posterior plane. Limited mobility may indicate a pathologic condition, such as carcinoma, infection, or scarring.

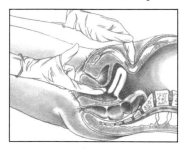

• Assess the right and left adnexal areas (ovaries and fallopian tubes). Place your internal fingers deeply inward and upward toward the external hand on the right lower abdominal quadrant and lift your internal fingers as the external hand is swept down and inward toward the symphysis pubis. This maneuver allows the ovary and any masses to slip between the fingers of your two hands; it should be repeated on the left side.

If palpable, the ovaries are mobile, oval, somewhat flattened, firm, smooth organs shaped like 3 x 2 x 1 cm (1¼" x ¾" x ¼") almonds. They may be sensitive to palpation. The ovaries of a postmenopausal woman or prepubertal girl should not be palpable. Normal fallopian tubes are usually not palpable or sensitive. The round ligaments may be palpable as cordlike apparatuses in the adnexa.

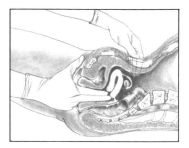

• After completing the bimanual assessment, prepare for rectovaginal palpation. The rectovaginal assessment is useful for examining women with small vaginal openings that permit only one finger to be introduced. The finger used rectally can lift organs anteriorly that cannot be reached by the finger used vaginally.

Change the glove of your internal hand to prevent transfer of vaginal organisms into the rectum. Be careful not to touch the anal area with the index finger that will be introduced into the vagina. Changing gloves also prevents a positive occult blood test result of rectal contents (caused by introducing vaginal or cervical blood into the rectum with a contaminated glove). An inadvertently contaminated index finger must be newly gloved before the assessment proceeds.

• First, explain the procedure to the client. Then, after lubricating the index and middle fingers of your gloved examining hand, ask the client to bear down, as if to have a bowel movement (she should be assured she will not), and carefully insert your middle finger into the rectum. Inspect for hemorrhoids or other painful areas and avoid these lesions when inserting your finger. Next, as you insert your index finger into the vagina, tell the client to stop bearing down and to relax using the techniques taught earlier. Use the finger in the vagina to find the cervix and keep it from being confused with a mass by the finger in the rectum.

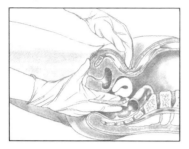

- Sweep the rectum within the reach of your examining finger. No masses or nodules should be felt. A high percentage of rectal growths can be felt by the examining hand. The rectovaginal assessment provides a more complete evaluation of the posterior side of the uterus.

The posteriorly positioned uterus must be examined rectally to examine its surface characteristics. The anteriorly positioned or midplane uterus is also assessed posteriorly when the rectovaginal assessment is performed. Reevaluation of the adnexa and the cul-de-sac may reveal masses or nodules not palpated during the bimanual assessment.
- After withdrawing your gloved finger from the client's rectum, check it for stool color and note any blood. When the examination is complete, clean the client with tissue in a front-to-back motion to remove excess lubricant. Help her to a sitting position. Wash your hands and advise the client to wash her hands if she has touched her genitals.

DOCUMENTATION

The SOAPIE method of documentation includes the following components: subjective (history) data, objective (physical) data, as-

Selected nursing diagnosis categories

The nurse may use these diagnosis categories to formulate nursing diagnoses for a client with a reproductive system problem.
- Altered family processes
- Altered growth and development
- Altered parenting
- Anticipatory grieving
- Anxiety
- Body image disturbance
- Pain
- Rape-trauma syndrome
- Rape-trauma syndrome: Compound reaction
- Rape-trauma syndrome: Silent reaction
- Sexual dysfunction
- Stress incontinence

sessment, planning, implementation, and evaluation. The following example shows how to document nursing care for a client with irregular periods.

Case history

Shelly Jordan is a 13-year-old Black female eighth grader. Her mother brought her to the clinic. She complains of "funny periods" since the onset of menses 6 months ago. She states her periods come every 12 to 36 days and last from 1 to 10 days. She also reports extreme fatigue.

S O A P I E

Client states, "My periods have not been regular since they started 6 months ago. They come every 12 to 36 days and last from 1 to 10 days. I'm really tired, have missed a lot of school, and I'm afraid something is wrong with me."

S **O** A P I E

Bimanual palpation of internal pelvic organs reveals no tenderness, pain, or masses. Inspection with speculum reveals pink cervix with no abnormal discharge. Dietary recall reveals diet low in iron and vitamin C. Crying and clinging to mother. HCT 32%; Hb 10.8 g; RBC indices indicate iron-deficiency anemia.

S   O   **A**   P   I   E

Altered nutrition: less than body requirements, related to poor dietary habits. Client
very fearful, needs mother's support. Menses irregular with heavy flow.

S   O   A   **P**   I   E

Instruct the client about nutritional needs and
supplemental iron use, including potential adverse reactions. Using anatomic models and a
booklet for the client to take home and read,
teach client about female reproductive system
and menstrual cycle. Show client how to keep
menstrual-cycle calendar.

S   O   A   P   **I**   E

Client taught that iron supplements should
be taken ½ hour after meals and also taught
potential adverse reactions. Client taught
about anatomy of female reproductive system, including the menstrual cycle and normal maturational changes.

S   O   A   P   I   **E**

Client discussed supplemental iron use and
explained importance of eating properly. She
discussed female reproductive organs and
menstrual cycle in quiet, embarrassed manner.

SUGGESTED READINGS

Cohen, S., Kenner, C., and Hollingsworth,
   A. (1991). *Maternal, Neonatal, and
   Women's Health Nursing.* Springhouse,
   PA: Springhouse Corp.
Swehla, M. (1990). Identifying and vali-
   dating nursing diagnoses in a gynecologic
   ambulatory-care setting. *JOGNN,* 19(5),
   439-447.
Willms, J., and Newman, L. (1990). The
   pelvic examination in primary practice:
   Making it easier for your patients...and
   for you. *Consultant,* 30(10), 61-64.
Yoder, L. (1990). The epidemiology of
   ovarian cancer: A review. *Oncology
   Nursing Forum,* 17(3), 411-415.

14

Male Reproductive System

Assessing the male reproductive system, although potentially uncomfortable for the nurse and client, is an essential part of a complete health assessment. Careful assessment may uncover actual or potential problems or concerns that the client usually would not volunteer willingly. Such information may be crucial. Many common disorders of the male reproductive system carry potentially serious psychological or physiologic consequences. For example, sexual or reproductive dysfunction, such as impotence or infertility, can dramatically affect the client's quality of life. Also, sexually transmitted diseases—the most common communicable diseases in the United States—can produce devastating complications unless detected and treated early.

HEALTH HISTORY

Interviewing a male client about his reproductive system requires sensitivity and tact, tempered with a professional approach. The initial goal should be to establish a rapport with the client so that he will relax and confide in you. An uncomfortable client may withhold valuable information.

Three groups of sample questions follow. Those on *health and illness patterns* help the nurse identify actual or potential reproductive

system problems; those on *health promotion and protection patterns* help the nurse determine how the client's life-style and behavior affect sexual and reproductive function; and those on *role and relationship patterns* help the nurse evalate the client's sexual practices and relationships with others.

Health and illness patterns

Have you noticed any changes in the color of the skin on your penis or scrotum?
(RATIONALE: Reddened penile skin may indicate an inflammation; reddened scrotal skin could result from orchitis—inflammation of the testes. Dark blue to black discoloration may point to gangrene. Altered skin integrity may occur in sexually transmitted diseases, inflammatory disorders, and cancer. Small skin lumps on the scrotum may be sebaceous cysts.)

If you are uncircumcised, can you retract and replace the foreskin easily?
(RATIONALE: Inability to retract the prepuce [foreskin] from the glans penis [phimosis] sometimes occurs in uncircumcised men. Inability of the retracted prepuce to return to its normal position over the glans penis [paraphimosis] could, if untreated, impair local circulation and lead to edema and even gangrene of the glans penis.)

Have you noticed the appearance of a sore, lump, or ulcer on your penis?

Anatomy review

The illustration below shows the anatomic structures of the male reproductive system.

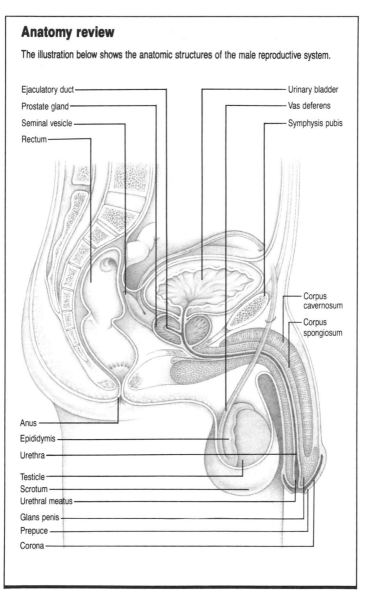

Ejaculatory duct

Prostate gland

Seminal vesicle

Rectum

Urinary bladder

Vas deferens

Symphysis pubis

Corpus cavernosum

Corpus spongiosum

Anus

Epididymis

Urethra

Testicle

Scrotum

Urethral meatus

Glans penis

Prepuce

Corona

(RATIONALE: Such findings may point to a sexually transmitted disease, an inflammatory disorder, or cancer.)

Have you noticed any discharge or bleeding from the urethral opening?
(RATIONALE: Copious amounts of thick, yellowish discharge may indicate gonorrhea. Thin, watery discharge may point to nonspecific urethritis or prostatitis. Bloody discharge may indicate infection or cancer in the urinary or reproductive tract.)

Have you noticed any swelling in your scrotum?
(RATIONALE: Scrotal swelling may point to inguinal hernia, hematocele, epididymitis, or testicular tumor.)

Are you experiencing any pain in the penis, testes, or scrotal sac? If so, where? Does the pain radiate? If so, to where? What measures aggravate or relieve the pain? When does it occur?
(RATIONALE: Dull, aching pain in the scrotal sac may indicate inguinal hernia. Sudden onset of extremely sharp pain may point to testicular torsion. Sharp pain of more gradual onset usually indicates infection, such as orchitis or epididymitis.)

Have you felt a lump, painful sore, or tenderness in the groin?
(RATIONALE: These findings may point to a tumor or an infection.)

Do you get up during the night to urinate? Do you have urinary frequency, hesistancy, or dribbling or pain in the area between your rectum and penis, hips, or lower back?
(RATIONALE: These signs and symptoms are especially significant in men over age 50; they may point to a prostate problem, such as benign prostatic hypertrophy or prostatic cancer.)

Do you have any difficulty achieving and maintaining an erection during sexual activity? If so, do you have erections at other times, such as on awakening?
(RATIONALE: The ability to achieve an erection is an important diagnostic clue in evaluating the cause of impotence.)

Do you have any difficulty with ejaculation?
(RATIONALE: Problems with ejaculation— such as premature, retarded [delayed] , or retrograde [backward] ejaculation—may provide clues to the underlying cause of impotence or other sexual problems.)

Do you ever experience pain from erection or ejaculation?
(RATIONALE: Painful erection or ejaculation may point to inflammation in the genitourinary tract.)

Have you fathered any children? If so, how many and what are their ages? Have you ever had a problem with infertility? Is it a current concern?
(RATIONALE: If infertility is a problem, further exploration will be required. This is best done by a professional who specializes in this field.)

Have you ever been diagnosed as having a sexually transmitted disease or any other infection in the genitourinary tract? If so, what was the specific problem? How long did it last? What treatment was provided? Did any associated complications develop?
(RATIONALE: Depending on its nature and course, infection can cause infertility and other reproductive system abnormalities.)

Do you have a history of undescended testes or an endocrine disorder, such as hypogonadism?
(RATIONALE: These conditions may cause infertility.)

Has anyone in your family had infertility problems?
(RATIONALE: Infertility often has a familial tendency.)

Has anyone in your family had a hernia?
(RATIONALE: Hernias also tend to occur in families.)

Pediatric client
When assessing a male child, try to involve both the child and the parent or guardian in the interview. Obviously, the parent or guardian will answer for an infant or very young child. Questions to ask include:

Did the child's mother use any hormones during pregnancy?
(RATIONALE: Some hormones taken during pregnancy can have an adverse effect on the development of a male child's reproductive system.)

If the child is uncircumcised, what hygienic measures do you use?
(RATIONALE: Poor hygiene increases the risk of infection under the prepuce.)

Do you notice any scrotal swelling when the child cries or has a bowel movement?
(RATIONALE: This finding may point to an inguinal hernia.)

Did the child exhibit any genitourinary abnormalities at birth? If so, what treatment was received?
(RATIONALE: If uncorrected, congenital defects such as hypospadias and epispadias can lead to further problems.)

Adolescent client
Do you have pubic hair? If so, at what age did it appear?
(RATIONALE: Normally, pubic hair appears between ages 12 and 14, usually indicating normal sexual development.)

How would you describe your sexual activity?
(RATIONALE: This question gives the adolescent client the opportunity to ask questions and express concerns about sexual function. It also allows the nurse to share information and clear up any misconceptions the client may have.)

If you are sexually active, do you use condoms for intercourse?
(RATIONALE: This question elicits information on the adolescent client's knowledge of contraception and prevention of sexually transmitted diseases. It also gives the nurse a chance to teach the client about the proper use of prophylactics for these purposes.)

Elderly client
Have you experienced any change in your frequency of or desire for sex?
(RATIONALE: Depression, loss of partner, or physical illness may cause these changes.)

Have you noticed any changes in your sexual performance?
(RATIONALE: Such physiologic changes as slower and less-firm erections, longer time required to reach orgasm, and decreased ejaculatory volume normally occur with age or may result from use of certain drugs or from physical illness.)

Health promotion and protection patterns
Do you examine your testes periodically? Have you been taught the proper procedure?
(RATIONALE: Testicular cancer, the most common form of cancer in males between ages 15 and 30, is treated most successfully after early detection.)

If you are sexually active, do you have more than one partner?
(RATIONALE: Having multiple sex partners increases the risk of acquiring a sexually transmitted disease.)

Do you take any precautions to prevent contracting a sexually transmitted disease or acquired immunodeficiency syndrome (AIDS)? If so, what do you do?
(RATIONALE: Take this opportunity to discuss measures for preventing these disorders, such as use of condoms during intercourse and avoiding exchange of body fluids during any sexual activity.)

Are you now or have you been exposed to radiation or toxic chemicals?
(RATIONALE: Such exposure may increase the client's risk of developing infertility or testicular cancer.)

Do you engage in sports or in any activity that requires heavy lifting or straining? If so, do you wear any protective or supportive devices, such as a jock strap, protective cup, or truss?
(RATIONALE: Any activity involving heavy lifting or abdominal straining can increase the risk of hernia formation. Certain sports activities—for example, playing the catcher's position in a baseball or softball game—can predispose the client to genital trauma.)

Role and relationship patterns

Do you have a supportive relationship with another person?
(RATIONALE: Problems with family or other relationships can produce stress, which in turn can cause sexual dysfunction.)

Are your sexual practices heterosexual, homosexual, or bisexual?
(RATIONALE: The answer to this question provides information about the client's possible risk level for certain sexually transmitted diseases and forewarns of certain sexual practices that can injure the anal sphincter, which may be noted during the physical assessment.)

If you are experiencing sexual difficulty, is it affecting your emotional and social relationships?
(RATIONALE: Feelings of emotional or social isolation can increase stress, which in turn can exacerbate sexual dysfunction.)

PHYSICAL ASSESSMENT

The nurse uses the following equipment and techniques when performing male reproductive system assessment.
Equipment
- gloves
- water-soluble lubricant
- flashlight
Techniques
- inspection
- palpation

Inspecting the genitals and inguinal area

Physical assessment of the male reproductive system begins with inspection of the genitals and inguinal area. Be sure to put on gloves before starting.

Penis inspection
- Inspection of the penis should start with an evaluation of the color and integrity of the penile skin. Over the shaft, the skin should appear loose and wrinkled; over the glans penis, taut and smooth.

- The skin should be pink to light brown in Caucasians and light to dark brown in Blacks, and free of scars, lesions, ulcers, or breaks of any kind.
- If the client is uncircumcised, ask him to retract his prepuce to allow inspection of the glans penis. The client should be able to retract the prepuce with ease, and then easily replace it over the glans.
- The urethral meatus, a slitlike opening, should be located at the tip of the glans.

Scrotum inspection
- Inspection of the scrotum begins with evaluation of the amount, distribution, color, and texture of pubic hair. Pubic hair should cover the symphysis pubis and scrotum.
- Next, inspect the scrotal skin for obvious lesions, ulcerations, induration, or reddened areas, and evaluate the sac for size and symmetry. The scrotal skin should be coarse and more deeply pigmented than the body skin. Both testicles should hang freely in the scrotum; the left testicle usually hangs slightly lower than the right.

Inguinal area inspection
- Inspect the inguinal area for obvious bulges—a sign of hernias.
- Then ask the client to bear down as if passing a stool as you inspect again. (Bearing down increases intra-abdominal pressure, which pushes any herniation downward and makes it more easily visible.)

Palpating the genitals and inguinal area

After inspection, palpate the penis and scrotum for structural abnormalities; then palpate the inguinal area for hernias.

Penis palpation
- Gently grasp the shaft of the penis between the thumb and first two fingers.
- Palpate along its entire length, noting any indurated, tender, or lumpy areas.

Scrotum palpation
- Using the thumb and first two fingers, palpate the scrotal skin by feeling its rough, wrinkled surface for nodules, lesions, or ulcers.

• Palpate the testes; they should feel like separate, smooth, freely movable, oval masses low in the scrotal sac.
• Palpate the epididymis by grasping each testicle at the posterolateral surface between the thumb and forefinger. The epididymis should feel like a ridge of tissue lying vertically on the testicular surface.

Inguinal area palpation
• To palpate a client's inguinal area for hernias, first place the index and middle finger of each hand over each external inguinal ring and ask the client to bear down or cough to increase intra-abdominal pressure momentarily.

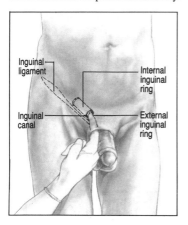

• Then, with the client relaxed, proceed as follows: Gently insert the middle or index finger (if the client is an adult) or the little finger (if the client is a young child) into the scrotal sac and follow the spermatic cord upward to the external inguinal ring, to an opening just above and lateral to the pubic tubercle known as Hesselbach's triangle. Holding the finger at this spot, ask the client to bear down or cough again. A hernia will palpate as a mass or bulge.
• To palpate for a femoral hernia, place the right hand on the client's thigh with the index finger over the femoral artery. The femoral canal is then under the ring finger in an adult client and between the index and

ring finger in a child. A hernia here will palpate as a soft bulge or mass.

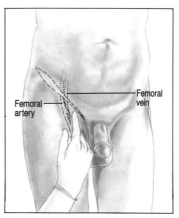

Advanced assessment skills: Palpating the prostate gland
• Because palpation of the prostate usually is uncomfortable and may embarrass the client, the nurse should begin by explaining the procedure and reassuring the client that the procedure should not be painful.
• Have the client urinate to empty the bladder and reduce discomfort during the examination.

Common laboratory studies

For a male client with signs and symptoms of a reproductive system problem, various laboratory studies can provide clues to the cause. This chart lists common laboratory studies along with normal values or findings. Remember that values differ among laboratories; check the normal value range for the specific laboratory.

TEST	NORMAL VALUES OR FINDINGS
Semen tests	
Semen analysis	60 to 150 million/ml
Blood tests	
Serum alpha-fetoprotein	< 30 ng/ml
Venereal disease research laboratory (VDRL) test	Nonreactive
Serum acid phosphatase	0 to 1.1 Bodansky unit/ml; 1 to 4 king Am strong units/ml; 0.13 to 0.63 Bessey-Lowery-Brock units/ml
Prostatic specific antigen (PSA)	0 to 2.7 ng/ml (under age 40); 0 to 4.0 ng/ml (age 40 and over)
Urine tests	
Divided urine test	Absence of bacteria
Culture and sensitivity	Absence of infectious microorganisms

• Ask the client to stand at the end of the examination table, with his elbows flexed and his upper body resting on the table. If the client cannot assume this position because he is unable to stand, have him lie on his left side with his right knee and hip flexed or with both knees drawn up toward his chest.
• Wear a glove on your examining hand and apply water-soluble lubricant to the gloved index finger. Inspect the skin of the perineal, anal, and posterior scrotal surfaces. The skin should appear smooth and unbroken, with no protruding masses.
• Introduce the gloved, lubricated index finger into the rectum, pad down. Instruct the client to relax to ease passage of the finger through the anal sphincter.
• Using the pad of the index finger, palpate the prostate on the anterior rectal wall, lo-

cated just past the anorectal ring. The prostate should feel smooth and rubbery. Normal size varies, but usually is about the size of a walnut. The prostate should not protrude into the rectal lumen. The proximal portions

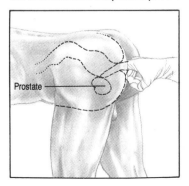

Prostate

of the seminal vesicles sometimes may be palpated above the superolateral to midpoint section of the gland as corrugated structures.

DOCUMENTATION

The SOAPIE method of documentation includes the following components: subjective (history) data, objective (physical) data, assessment, planning, implementation, and evaluation. The following example shows how to document nursing care for a client with a penile lesion.

CASE HISTORY

Mr. Tom Sloan, age 20, is a single college student who has come to the university health care clinic because of a sore on his penis.

S   O   A   P   I   E

Client states, "I have a sore on my penis. I don't have any trouble urinating, but I'm afraid the sore is a sign of syphilis."

S   **O**   A   P   I   E

Anxious client with oval ulcer on top of penile shaft. Ulcer is indurated with raised edges; clear exudate. Enlarged inguinal lymph nodes bilaterally on palpation, 1 cm in diameter, firm, freely movable. Laboratory report is positive for syphilis.

S   O   **A**   P   I   E

Anxiety related to penile ulcer. Client is upset with himself and worried about what others will think.

S   O   A   **P**   I   E

Teach client about disease to reduce anxiety. Teach the importance of condom use. Ascertain which other students were involved.

S   O   A   P   **I**   E

Client provided with film and written literature on syphilis and use of condoms. Discussed with client the need to treat other involved parties.

S   O   A   P   I   **E**

Client verbalizes correct information con-

Selected nursing diagnosis categories

The nurse may use these diagnosis categories to formulate nursing diagnoses for a client with a reproductive system problem.
- Altered growth and development
- Altered parenting
- Altered role performance
- Altered urinary elimination
- Anxiety
- Body image disturbance
- High risk for infection
- Impaired physical mobility
- Pain
- Rape-trauma syndrome
- Sexual dysfunction
- Total incontinence
- Urinary retention

---

cerning syphilis and use of condoms. Reluctant to provide information on other participants.

SUGGESTED READINGS

Bonnar, I., and Gordon, M. (1991). Testicular self-examination. *Occupational Health*, 43(2), 52-56.

Bonnar, I., and Gordon, M. (1991). Testicular self-examination, part 2. *Occupational Health*, 43(3), 87-88.

Willis, D. (1992). Taming the overgrown prostate. *American Journal of Nursing*, 92(2), 34-42.

Willson, P. (1991). Testicular, prostate, and penile cancers in primary care settings: The importance of early detection. *Nurse Practitioner*, 16(11), 18-26.

Wozniak-Petrofsky, J. (1991). BPH: Treating older men's most common problem. *RN*, 54(7), 32-38.

15

Nervous System

The nurse may encounter signs and symptoms of nervous system disorders in clients of any age. Cerebrovascular accidents (CVAs, or strokes)—the third most common cause of death in the United States—produce varying degrees of neurologic dysfunction, mostly in elderly clients. Young adults are more likely to suffer traumatic injuries to the nervous system, especially the spinal cord and brain. Degenerative neurologic disorders, such as Huntington's chorea or multiple sclerosis, cause a progressive deterioration of the nervous system and can occur at any age. Nervous system infections (meningitis, encephalitis, and brain abscess) and cancer (brain and spinal cord tumors) also affect clients in different age groups.

HEALTH HISTORY

To begin an accurate neurologic assessment, the nurse asks questions that focus on the health history. Ask questions in a systematic manner, proceeding from head to toe to avoid omitting information. Progress from general to specific questions, from non-threatening to more threatening ones.

Three groups of sample questions follow. Those on *health and illness patterns* help the nurse identify actual or potential neurologic-related health problems; those on *health promotion and protection patterns* help the nurse determine how the client's life-style and behavior affect neurologic function; and those on *role and relationship patterns* help the nurse determine how a neurologic problem affects the client's self-image and relationships with family members and others.

Health and illness patterns

To assess the client's health and illness patterns related to the nervous system, investigate the client's current, past, and family health status as well as any pertinent developmental considerations.

Do you have headaches? If so, how would you describe them?
(RATIONALE: The pattern and characteristics of a headache can help identify its etiology. For example, vascular [migraine or cluster] headaches recur, frequently following a pattern. Early morning headaches that are present upon awakening and disappear after arising may be an early warning sign of a brain tumor in an adult.)

Have you ever had a head injury? If so, when? How would you describe what happened? Do you have any lasting effects?
(RATIONALE: Even minor head injuries can produce long-term effects. In an elderly client, a minor head injury can cause a subdural hematoma that may take weeks or months to produce symptoms. Post-concussion syndrome causes various symptoms, such as insomnia, headache, or depression, which can persist up to a year after the injury.)

Anatomy review

The illustration below shows the anatomic structures of the central nervous system.

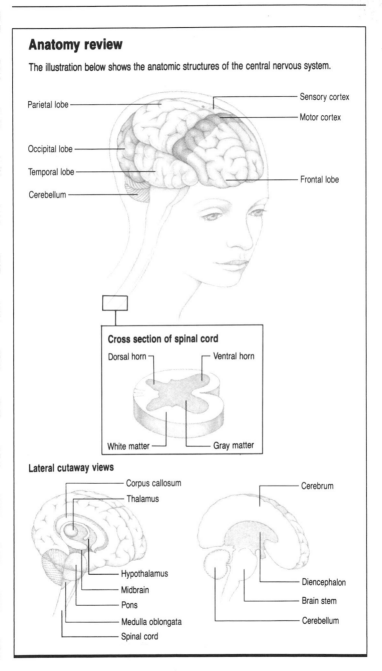

Parietal lobe

Occipital lobe

Temporal lobe

Cerebellum

Sensory cortex

Motor cortex

Frontal lobe

Cross section of spinal cord

Dorsal horn

Ventral horn

White matter

Gray matter

Lateral cutaway views

Corpus callosum

Thalamus

Hypothalamus

Midbrain

Pons

Medulla oblongata

Spinal cord

Cerebrum

Diencephalon

Brain stem

Cerebellum

Peripheral nervous system

The peripheral nervous system is composed of the cranial nerves, spinal nerves, and the autonomic nervous system—which has two major divisions: the sympathetic (thoracolumbar) nervous system and the parasympathetic (craniosacral) nervous system.

Cranial nerves

The 12 pairs of cranial nerves (CNs) transmit motor or sensory messages, or both, primarily between the brain or brain stem and the head and neck. All cranial nerves, except for the olfactory and optic nerves, exit from the mid-brain, pons, or medulla oblongata of the brain stem. The chart and illustration show the origin of each cranial nerve.

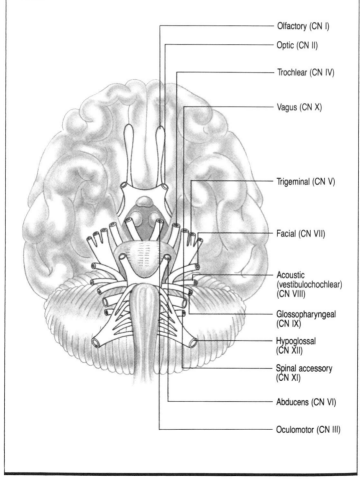

Olfactory (CN I)

Optic (CN II)

Trochlear (CN IV)

Vagus (CN X)

Trigeminal (CN V)

Facial (CN VII)

Acoustic (vestibulochochlear) (CN VIII)

Glossopharyngeal (CN IX)

Hypoglossal (CN XII)

Spinal accessory (CN XI)

Abducens (CN VI)

Oculomotor (CN III)

Have you noticed a change in your ability to remember things? If so, how would you describe this change?
(RATIONALE: Impaired recent memory is an early sign of cerebral degeneration, such as accompanies Alzheimer's disease. High stress levels and fatigue can also impair memory.)

Do you experience blurred vision, double vision, or any other visual disturbances, such as blind spots?
(RATIONALE: Blurred or double vision can indicate disorders of cranial nerves III, IV, and VI. Blind spots suggest a localized retinal injury or damage to the optic tracts in the brain caused by a CVA or trauma. Transient blind spots or the loss of vision in one eye may signal transient cerebral ischemia and an impending stroke. Transient blind spots accompanied by flashing lights [scotomata] precede a classic migraine.)

Have you noticed any change in your sense of smell or taste? If so, how would you describe this change?
(RATIONALE: A loss of the sense of smell [olfaction] called anosmia frequently follows a facial fracture or head injury. Occasionally, impaired olfaction can indicate a brain tumor or lesion; unusual smells can accompany temporal lobe seizures. Disorders of cranial nerve VII or IX can affect the sense of taste. A decreased sense of taste always accompanies an impaired sense of smell.)

Do you have any difficulty swallowing? If so, how would you describe it?
(RATIONALE: A dysfunction of cranial nerves IX, X, and XII can produce impaired swallowing and other bulbar symptoms in such disorders as myasthenia gravis and amyotrophic lateral sclerosis [ALS]. Poor neuromuscular control from CVA or Parkinson's disease also can impair swallowing.)

Do you have difficulty speaking or expressing the words you are thinking?
(RATIONALE: Difficulty understanding or using language indicates a language dysfunction [aphasia] from an injury to the cerebral cortex.)

Have you recently noticed any change in strength? Have you recently noticed a change in your muscle coordination?
(RATIONALE: Degenerative neurologic disorders, such as ALS, produce progressive muscle weakness and wasting. Disturbed coordination implies a disease of the cerebellum, basal ganglia, or extrapyramidal tracts.)

Do you have tremors or muscle spasms in your hands, arms, or legs?
(RATIONALE: A positive answer may indicate a disorder of the cerebellum or basal ganglia.)

Do you have problems with your balance?
(RATIONALE: Poor balance implies a cerebellar disorder or impairment of the vestibular portion of cranial nerve VIII. A client with such a problem requires assistance when walking and other safety precautions.)

Do you have dizzy spells? If so, how would you describe them?
(RATIONALE: Dizziness accompanies many neurologic disorders, and its characteristics vary. Vertigo, which is a sensation of spinning or whirling, differs from simple dizziness, which is a sensation of unsteadiness or disequilibrium accompanied by lightheadedness, giddiness, or feeling faint.)

Have you ever had a seizure? If so, please describe it and indicate under what circumstances it occurred.
(RATIONALE: Besides identifying individuals at risk for seizures, the answer to this question helps differentiate between a client with a seizure disorder [recurrent seizures] and one who experiences an isolated seizure because of a metabolic disturbance.)

Have any of your immediate family members (mother, father, or siblings) had high blood pressure or a stroke?
(RATIONALE: Hypertension in the family can predispose the client to CVA.)

Pediatric client

When interviewing the parents of an infant or young child, include the following questions:

Was the baby full term at birth or born prematurely? If premature, how early was the baby born?

(RATIONALE: The nervous system of a premature infant is not as developed as that of a full-term infant at birth; therefore, age-related developmental milestones will not be accurate for the premature infant.)

Was the labor and delivery difficult?

(RATIONALE: Difficult labor and delivery can cause neurologic birth injuries, such as cerebral palsy, paralysis, or paresis.)

How did the baby look right after the delivery?

(RATIONALE: A limp, gray, or mottled appearance suggests anoxia, which could produce neurologic sequelae.)

During the first month after birth, did the baby have any problems with sucking or swallowing, or any other problems, such as high bilirubin levels or a positive phenylketonuria test?

(RATIONALE: Metabolic disorders can affect nervous system functioning.)

Has the child reached developmental milestones at the expected age? Has the child lost any functions that were previously mastered?

(RATIONALE: Delayed neuromuscular development implies an underlying neurologic disorder. Remember that premature infants are less developed neurologically and therefore are behind the expected age-related developmental milestones for age. Loss of previously mastered skills could indicate an underlying neurologic disorder.)

Elderly client

How would you describe your walking pattern? Has it changed? Have you developed tremors?

(RATIONALE: Gait changes or tremors could signify Parkinson's disease or another degenerative neurologic disorder.)

Have you noticed any change in your memory or thinking abilities, vision, hearing, or sense of smell or taste?

(RATIONALE: A change in any of these may indicate cerebral or cranial nerve changes, which may interfere with the client's lifestyle, health maintenance, and safety.)

Health promotion and protection patterns

Do you have difficulty following conversations or television programs? Do you have difficulty concentrating on activities that you once found enjoyable, such as reading or watching movies?

(RATIONALE: Difficulty following conversations or decreased attention span may be early signs of cognitive or hearing impairment. Depression can also cause a loss of interest in previous pastimes.)

Are you exposed to any toxins or chemicals, such as insecticides, petroleum distillates, or lead, in your home or on the job?

(RATIONALE: Exposure to toxins can cause neurologic signs and symptoms.)

On the job, do you perform any strenuous or repetitive activities? Do you sit, stand, or walk while performing your job?

(RATIONALE: Repetitive motions, such as on an assembly line, can cause peripheral nerve injuries from overuse. Strenuous activities or heavy lifting increases the risk of intervertebral disc injuries; prolonged sitting or standing can cause neuromuscular stiffness or discomfort.)

Role and relationship patterns

How has your disability affected you? Has it made you feel differently about yourself?

(RATIONALE: Nervous system disorders that produce obvious deficits, such as paralysis, paresis, or impaired gait or coordination, or that impair the client's memory, facility with language, or other cognitive skills, can adversely affect the client's self-image.)

Can you fulfill your usual family responsibilities? If not, who has assumed them?

(RATIONALE: Neurologic impairment may prevent the client from fulfilling certain roles that would then have to be assumed by another family member.)

How has your illness or disability affected members of your family emotionally and financially?
(RATIONALE: Nervous system disorders can devastate the family emotionally. Chronic or degenerative processes often require prolonged treatment, hospitalization, or special equipment, which can drain a family financially.)

PHYSICAL ASSESSMENT

Because the nervous system is so extensive, a complete neurologic assessment is complicated and time-consuming; it can take several hours to complete. A complete neurologic assessment provides information about five broad categories of neurologic function:

• cerebral function (including level of consciousness [LOC], mental status, and language)
• cranial nerves
• motor system and cerebellar functions
• sensory system
• reflexes.

Except when working as a nurse practitioner, the nurse probably will not perform a complete neurologic assessment. Instead, the nurse usually will perform a neurologic screening assessment. This type of assessment evaluates some of the key indicators of neurologic function and helps identify areas of dysfunction. A neurologic screening assessment usually includes:

• evaluation of LOC (including a brief mental status examination and evaluation of verbal responsiveness)
• selected cranial nerve (CN) assessment (usually CN II, III, IV, and VI)
• motor screening (strength, movement, and gait)
• sensory screening (tactile and pain sensations in extremities).

If the neurologic screening assessment identifies areas of neurologic dysfunction, the nurse must evaluate those areas in more

Assessment checklist

The nurse should ask herself or himself these questions before beginning the assessment:
☐ Have I gathered all the necessary equipment?
☐ Have I washed my hands?
☐ Have I provided a safe environment for the client?
☐ Does the client require any special assistance, such as a cane, a walker, or braces? If so, have I provided for it?
☐ Have I reviewed all relevant laboratory data?

detail. For this reason, the nurse must be familiar with the neurologic screening assessment as well as with the components of a complete neurologic assessment.

Finally, the nurse should be able to perform a very brief neurologic assessment, called a *neuro check*. This assessment is used to make rapid, repeated evaluations of several key indicators of nervous system status: LOC, pupil size and response, verbal responsiveness, extremity strength and movement, and vital signs. After establishing a baseline, regularly reevaluating these key indicators reveals trends in a client's neurologic functioning and helps detect transient changes that can be warning signs of problems.

Assessing cerebral function

Basic assessment of cerebral function includes LOC, communication, and, briefly, mental status.

Level of consciousness

Evaluation of LOC includes assessing level of arousal and orientation.

• Begin by quietly observing the client's behavior. Is the client awake, dozing, or asleep? Moving about or motionless?
• If the client is dozing or sleeping, attempt arousal by providing an appropriate auditory, tactile, or painful stimulus, in that sequence. Always start with a minimal stimulus, increasing its intensity as necessary.

Glasgow Coma Scale

Originally designed as part of a tool for predicting survival and recovery after a head injury, the Glasgow Coma Scale is now used to assess a client's level of consciousness (LOC). This scale minimizes the subjectivity historically associated with LOC evaluations by testing and scoring three faculties: eye response, motor response, and verbal response. Each response receives a point value. An assessment totaling 15 points indicates that the client is alert, completely oriented to person, place, and time, and can follow simple commands. In a comatose client, the score will total 7 or less. A score of 3, the lowest possible score, indicates deep coma and a poor prognosis.

Many facilities display the Glasgow Coma Scale on neurologic flowsheets to show changes in the client's LOC over time.

FACULTY MEASURED	RESPONSE ELICITED	SCORE
Eye response	• Opens spontaneously	4
	• Opens to verbal command	3
	• Opens to pain	2
	• No response	1
Motor response	• Reacts to verbal command	6
	• Reacts to painful stimuli	
	—Identifying localized pain	5
	—Flexing and withdrawing	4
	—Assuming flexor posture	3
	—Assuming extensor posture	2
	• No response	1
Verbal response	• Oriented and converses	5
	• Disoriented but converses	4
	• Uses inappropriate words	3
	• Makes incomprehensible sounds	2
	• No response	1

• Use painful stimuli only to assess an unconscious client or one with a markedly decreased LOC who is unresponsive to other stimuli. Techniques to test response to painful stimuli include application of firm pressure over a nailbed with a blunt hard object, such as a pen, or a firm pinch of the Achilles tendon between your thumb and index finger.

• After assessing the client's level of arousal, compare the findings with those of previous assessments. Note any trends, such as lethargy following several hours of drowsiness in a client who is usually awake.

• When assessing the client's orientation to person, place, and time, ask questions that require the client to provide information, rather than a yes or no answer.

• To minimize the subjectivity of LOC assessment and to establish a greater degree of reliability, many health care facilities use the Glasgow Coma Scale. (For details, see *Glasgow Coma Scale.*)

Communication

• Note the quantity of what the client says. Does the client speak in complete sentences? In phrases? In single words? Is communication spontaneous? Or does the client rarely speak?

• Note the quality of the client's speech. Is it unusually loud or soft? Does the client articulate clearly, or are words difficult to understand?

• Are the client's verbal responses appropriate? Does the client choose the correct words to express thoughts, or appear to have problems finding or articulating words?
• Can the client understand and follow commands?

Mental status

• Consider conducting a mental status screening when the client's responses seem unreliable or indicate a possible disturbance of memory or cognitive processes.
• Ask the following questions: What is your name? (This screens orientation to person.) What is today's date? (This screens orientation to time.) What year is it? (This screens orientation to time.) Where are you now? (This screens orientation to place.) How old are you? (This screens memory.) Where were you born? (This screens remote memory.) What did you have for breakfast? (This screens recent memory.) Who is the U.S. president? (This screens general knowledge.) Can you count backwards from 20 to 1? (This screens attention and calculation skills.) Why are you here? (This screens judgment.)

Advanced assessment skills: Cerebral function

Advanced assessment of cerebral function includes assessment of communication by a formal language skills evaluation and a complete mental status assessment. A speech pathologist usually performs the language skills evaluation; a physician or specially trained nurse conducts the complete mental status assessment.

Assessing cranial nerve function

Cranial nerve assessment provides valuable information about the condition of the central nervous system (CNS), particularly the brain stem. Because of their anatomic locations, some cranial nerves are more vulnerable than others to the effects of increasing intracranial pressure. That is why a neurologic screening assessment of the cranial nerves focuses on these key nerves: the optic (II), oculomotor (III), trochlear (IV), and abducens (VI). Evaluate the other

nerves only if the client's history or symptoms indicate a potential cranial nerve disorder or when a complete nervous system assessment must be performed. However, because disorders can affect any of the cranial nerves, become familiar with methods for testing each nerve. (For a description of assessment techniques and normal findings, see *Cranial nerve assessment,* pages 190 to 192.)

Assessing motor system and cerebellar function

A complex neurologic assessment of the motor system includes evaluation of motor functions (muscle size, tone, strength, and movement), cerebellar functions (balance and coordination), and gait. (For a description of how to assess muscle tone, see Chapter 16, Musculoskeletal System.)

Motor function

• Evaluate muscle strength (including size and symmetry) of the arms and legs, movement of arms and legs, and gait for all clients.
• Assess arm strength by asking the client to push you away as you apply resistance. If this test suggests mild weakness in one arm, confirm your suspicions by evaluating for downward drift and pronation of the arm.
• Assess the client's movement in response to a command. Instruct the client who is very weak to open and close each fist, or to move each arm without raising it off the bed or examination table.
• Assess leg movement, first asking the client to move each leg and foot. If the client fails to move the leg on command, observe for spontaneous movement.

Cerebellar function

The nurse can evaluate the client's cerebellar function by assessing balance and coordination. To assess balance, have the client perform tandem-gait (heel-to-toe) walking, the Romberg test, and heel and toe walking. To assess coordination, evaluate the client's ability to perform rapid alternating movements, point-to-point localization, and the leg coordination test.

(Text continues on page 192.)

Cranial nerve assessment

The nurse's techniques for cranial nerve assessment vary according to the nerve being tested. The chart below describes these techniques and identifies normal findings.

ASSESSMENT TECHNIQUE	NORMAL FINDINGS
Olfactory (CN I)	
After checking the patency of the client's nostrils, have the client close both eyes. Then occlude one nostril, and hold a familiar, pungent-smelling substance, such as coffee, tobacco, soap, or peppermint, under the client's nose and ask its identity. Repeat this technique with the other nostril.	The client should be able to detect and identify the smell correctly. If the client reports detecting the smell but cannot name it, offer a choice, such as "Do you smell lemon, coffee, or peppermint?"
Optic (CN II) and oculomotor (CN III)	
To assess the optic nerve, check visual acuity, visual fields, and the retinal structures. To assess the oculomotor nerve, check pupil size, pupil shape, and pupillary response to light. (For a description of how to perform these assessments, see Chapter 7, Eyes and Ears.)	The pupils should be equal, round, and reactive to light. When assessing pupil size, be especially alert for any trends. For example, watch for a gradual increase in the size of one pupil or the appearance of unequal pupils in a client whose pupils were previously equal.
Oculomotor (CN III), trochlear (CN IV), and abducens (CN VI)	
To test the coordinated function of these three nerves, assess them simultaneously by evaluating the client's extraocular eye movement. (For a description of how to perform these assessments, see Chapter 7, Eyes and Ears.)	The eyes should move smoothly and in a coordinated manner through all six directions of eye movement. Observe each eye for rapid oscillation (nystagmus), movement not in unison with that of the other eye (dysconjugate movement), or inability to move in certain directions (ophthalmoplegia). Also note any complaint of double vision (diplopia).
Trigeminal (CN V)	
To assess the sensory portion of the trigeminal nerve, gently touch the right, then the left side of the client's forehead with a cotton ball while the client's eyes are closed. Instruct the client to state the moment the cotton touches the area. Compare the client's response on both sides. Repeat the technique on the right and left cheek and on the right and left jaw. Next, repeat the entire procedure using a sharp object. (If an abnormality appears, also test for temperature sensation by touching the client's skin with test tubes filled with hot and cold water and asking the client to identify the temperature.)	The client with a normal trigeminal nerve should report feeling both light touch and sharp stimuli in all three areas (forehead, check, and jaw) on both sides of the face.

Cranial nerve assessment continued

ASSESSMENT TECHNIQUE	NORMAL FINDINGS
To assess the motor portion of the trigeminal nerve, ask the client to clench the jaws. Palpate the temporal and masseter muscles bilaterally, checking for symmetry. Try to open the client's clenched jaws. Next, watch the client's opening and closing mouth for asymmetry. Then assess the corneal reflex. (See Chapter 7, Eyes and Ears.)	The jaws should clench symmetrically and remain closed against resistance. The lids of both eyes should close when a wisp of cotton is lightly stroked across a cornea.

Facial (CN VII)

To test the motor portion of the facial nerve, ask the client to wrinkle the forehead, raise and lower the eyebrows, smile to show teeth, and puff out the cheeks. Also, with the client's eyes tightly closed, attempt to open the eyelids. Observe closely for symmetry. To test the sensory portion of the facial nerve, which supplies taste sensation to the anterior two-thirds of the tongue, apply in succession (using a cotton swab or dropper and having the client rinse the mouth between applications) salt solution, sugar solution, vinegar or lemon, and quinine or bitters to one side of the anterior tongue. Ask the client to identify each application as sweet, salty, sour, or bitter. Repeat on the other side of the tongue. Taste sensations to the posterior third of the tongue are supplied by the glossopharyngeal nerve and usually are tested at the same time.	Normal facial movements are symmetrical. So are normal taste sensations.

Acoustic (CN VIII)

To assess the acoustic portion of this nerve, test the client's hearing acuity. (See Chapter 7, Eyes and Ears.)	The client should be able to hear a whispered voice or a watch tick.

Glossopharyngeal (CN IX) and vagus (CN X)

To assess these nerves, first listen to the client's voice for indications of hoarseness or nasality. Then watch the client's soft palate when the client says "ah." Next, test the gag reflex.	The client's voice should sound strong and clear. The soft palate and the uvula should rise when the client says "ah," and the uvula should remain midline. The palatine arches should remain symmetrical during movement and at rest. The gag reflex should be intact. If the gag reflex appears decreased or the pharynx moves asymmetrically, evaluate each side of the posterior wall of the pharynx.

continued

Cranial nerve assessment continued

ASSESSMENT TECHNIQUE	NORMAL FINDINGS
Spinal accessory (CN XI)	
To assess, press down on the client's shoulders while the client attempts to shrug against this resistance. Note shoulder strength and symmetry while inspecting and palpating the trapezius muscle. Then, apply resistance to the client's turned head while the client attempts to return to a midline position. Note neck strength while inspecting and palpating the sternocleidomastoid muscle. Repeat for the opposite side.	Normally, both shoulders should be able to overcome the resistance equally well. The neck should overcome resistance in both directions.
Hypoglossal (CN XII)	
To assess, observe the client's protruded tongue for any deviation from midline, atrophy, or fasciculations (very fine muscle flickerings indicative of lower motor neuron disease). Next, ask the client to move the tongue rapidly from side to side with the mouth open, curl the tongue up toward the nose, and then curl the tongue down toward the chin. Then use a tongue depressor or folded gauze pad to apply resistance to the client's protruded tongue, and ask the client to try to push the depressor to one side. Repeat on the other side and note tongue strength. Listen to the client's speech for the sounds *d, l, n,* and *t,* which require use of the tongue. If general speech suggests a problem, have the client repeat a phrase or series of words containing these sounds.	Normally, the tongue should be midline and the client should be able to move it right to left equally. The client should be able to move the tongue up and down. Pressure exerted by the tongue on the tongue depressor should be equal on either side. Speech should be clear.

• To perform the Romberg test, have the client stand with feet together, arms at sides, and without support. Observe the client's ability to maintain balance with both eyes open and then with them closed. Normally, a small amount of swaying occurs when the eyes are closed. Note any abnormal problems with balance. Impaired coordination and balance (ataxia) is the classic sign of cerebellar disease.

• To assess heel and toe walking, first ask the client to walk on the heels. Then have the client walk on the toes. Observe balance, coordination, and ankle strength during both procedures. Note any deviation from the normal ability to walk steadily on the heels and toes.

• To assess tandem gait (heel-to-toe) walking, ask the client to walk heel-to-toe in a straight line, as shown. Observe for normal coordination and balance. If the client leans or falls to one side, note the direction. When performing heel-to-toe walking, the client will tend to lean or fall toward the side of the lesion. If the lesion is midline, the client cannot perform heel and toe walking and displays a wide-based, ataxic gait. (See illustration on next page.)

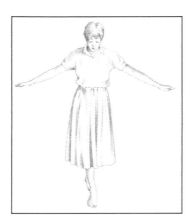

• To assess rapid alternating movements, begin with the arms. Have the seated client pat one thigh with one hand as rapidly as possible. Test the other arm, noting speed and rhythm.

Next, have the client place an open palm on one thigh and then turn the hand over, touching the thigh with the top of the hand, as shown. Have the client repeat this pronation and supination of the hand as rapidly as possible. Note the speed and the degree of ease or difficulty in performing the maneuver.

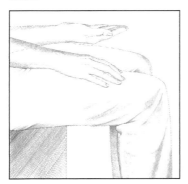

Have the client use the thumb of one hand to touch each finger of the same hand in rapid sequence. Repeat with the other hand. The nondominant hand will perform rapid alternating movement tasks more slowly than the dominant hand.

To assess the legs, have the client rapidly tap the floor with the ball of one foot. Test each leg separately. Note any slowness or awkwardness in performing rapid alternating movements.

• To assess point-to-point localization, have the client stand or sit with arms extended and then touch the nose. Have the client perform the test first with both eyes open, and then with them closed.

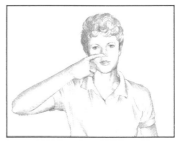

Next, hold one index finger in front of the client and ask the client to touch it with his or her index finger. Repeat the maneuver at various positions, as shown. Evaluate the client's ability to adjust.

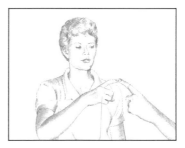

• To assess leg coordination, have the client lie supine and place one heel on the shin of the opposite leg just below the knee. Then have the client slowly slide the heel along the shin toward the ankle. Repeat with the other leg. Note the client's ability to position each heel on the shin accurately as well as the ease, speed, and accuracy with which the client can move the heel down the shin.

Assessing sensory system function

Basic neurologic screening usually consists of evaluating light-touch sensation in all extremities and comparing both arms and legs for symmetry of sensation.

• Before beginning the sensory system screening, ask the client about any areas of numbness or unusual sensations. Such areas require special attention.

• To perform the assessment, have the client sit with eyes closed. Ask the client to say "yes" or "now" when you lightly touch the client's forearm with a cotton wisp. Allow time for the client's response, and then lightly touch the same area on the client's other arm.

• Compare sensations on both sides of the client's body in the upper arm, back of the hand, thigh, lower leg, and top of the foot. Occasionally skip an area to test the reliabilty of the client's responses. However, be sure to check the skipped area for sensory response before concluding the assessment.

• Be alert for complaints of numbness, tingling, or unusual sensations that accompany the tactile stimulus. Also note the degree of stimulation required to evoke a response. A light, brief touch should be sufficient.

Advanced assessment skills: Sensory system

The nurse can evaluate the client's sensory function further by assessing for superficial pain, temperature sensation, response to vibration, and sense of position (proprioception). Further, the nurse can assess the client's ability to recognize objects by the sense of touch (stereognosis), number identification, two-point discrimination, point localization, and extinction. All sensory testing must be performed with the client's eyes closed.

• To assess for superficial pain, lightly touch—but do not puncture—the client's skin using a sharp object, such as a sterile hypodermic needle. Occasionally alternate sharp and blunt ends.

Ask the client to identify the sensation as sharp or dull. Test and compare the distal and proximal portions of all extremities. If the client displays abnormal pain sensation, test for temperature sensation.

• To assess temperature sensation, fill two test tubes with water, one hot and the other cold. Alternately touch the client's skin with the hot and cold test tubes, asking the client to differentiate between them. Test and compare distal and proximal portions of all extremities.

• To assess response to vibration, tap a low-pitched tuning fork (preferably 128 cycles per second) on the heel of your hand and then place the base of the tuning fork firmly on an interphalangeal joint (any of the client's fingers or the great toe).

Ask the client to describe the sensation, differentiating between pressure and vibration, and then to state when the feeling stops. Proceed from distal to proximal areas.

• To assess proprioception, grasp the sides of the client's great toe between your thumb and forefinger. Move the toe upward or downward, asking the client to describe the position. Repeat on the other foot, and then perform the same technique on the client's fingers.

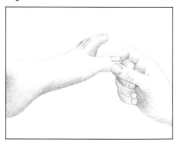

If the client exhibits impaired proprioception, proceed to the next joint on the extremity and repeat the procedure. On the leg, progress from the ankle to the knee; on the arm, from the wrist to the elbow.

• To assess for stereognosis, place a familiar object, such as a key, pencil, or paper clip, in the client's hand and ask the client to identify the object by feel—which the client should be able to do. A particularly sensitive test of stereognosis involves having the client identify the "heads" and "tails" sides of a coin.

• To assess number identification, trace a large number on the client's palm, using a blunt object, such as the blunt end of pen or pencil, as shown. The client should be able to identify the number.

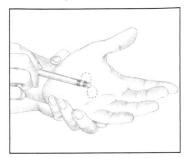

• To assess two-point discrimination, alternately touch one or two sharp objects to the client's skin, as shown. First assess whether the client can feel one or two points; then assess the smallest distance between the two points at which the client can still discriminate the presence of two points. Acuity varies in different body areas. On the finger pads, an area rich in tactile sensory receptors, the average distance necessary for two-point discrimination is less than 5 mm.

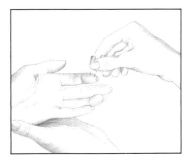

• To assess extinction, touch two corresponding parts on the client (such as the forearms just above the wrist) simultaneously, as shown. Ask the client to describe the location of the touch. The client should sense the touch in both locations.

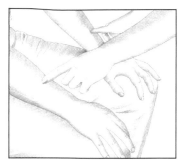

Advanced assessment skills: Reflexes

Reflex assessment helps evaluate the intactness of the specific cervical (C), thoracic (T), lumbar (L), or sacral (S) spinal segments shown in parentheses below.

Assessment of deep tendon reflexes includes evaluation of the biceps, triceps, brachioradialis, quadriceps, and Achilles reflexes. Assessment of the superficial reflexes includes evaluation of the pharyngeal, abdominal, and cremasteric reflexes as well as the anal and bulbocavernous reflexes. (Assess the last two reflexes, known as the perineal reflexes, only in clients with suspected sacral spinal cord or sacral spine nerve disorders.) Pathologic reflexes include the grasp, sucking, snout, and Babinski reflexes. Although healthy adults do not display these reflexes, the nurse may assess them to detect signs of CNS damage.

Deep tendon reflexes

• To assess the biceps reflex (C5, C6), have the client partially flex one arm at the elbow with the palm facing down. Place your thumb or finger over the biceps tendon. Then tap lightly over your finger with the reflex hammer. An impulse from the tapping should travel to the biceps tendon and cause brisk elbow flexion that is visible and palpable.
• To assess the triceps reflex (C7, C8), have the client partially flex one arm at the elbow with the palm facing the body. Support the arm and pull it slightly across the client's chest. Using a direct blow with the reflex hammer, tap the triceps tendon at its insertion (about 1" to 2" [2.5 to 5 cm] above the elbow on the olecranon process of the ulnar bone).

Common laboratory studies

For a client with neurologic signs and symptoms, various laboratory studies can provide the nurse with valuable clues to the possible cause. This chart lists commonly ordered laboratory studies along with their normal values or findings. Remember that values differ among laboratories, and check the normal value range for the specific laboratory.

TEST	NORMAL VALUES OR FINDINGS
Blood tests	
Electrolytes	*Sodium:* 135 to 145 mEq/liter
	Potassium: 3.8 to 5.5 mEq/liter
	Calcium: 4.5 to 5.5 mEq/liter
	Magnesium: 1.5 to 2.5 mEq/liter
Cerebrospinal fluid tests	
Cerebrospinal fluid (CSF) analysis	*Color:* Clear, colorless
	Glucose: 50 to 80 mg/dl (or ⅔ of blood glucose)
	Protein: 15 to 45 mg/dl
	Gamma globulin: 3% to 12% of total protein
	Blood cells: No red blood cells 0 to 5 white blood cells

Normally, this action causes brisk extension of the client's elbow.

• To assess the brachioradialis (supinator) reflex (C5, C6), position the client with one arm flexed at the elbow, palm down, and resting in the lap, or, if the client is lying down, against the abdomen. Then tap the styloid process of the radius with the reflex hammer, about 1″ to 2″ above the wrist. Normally, this action causes flexion of the client's elbow, supination of the forearm, and flexion of the fingers and hand.

• To assess the quadriceps (knee-jerk or patellar) reflex (L2, L3, L4), seat the client with one knee flexed and the lower leg dangling over the side of the examination table, or place the client in the supine position. (For the supine client, place your hand under the knee, slightly raising and flexing it.) Then tap the patellar tendon with the reflex

hammer. The client's knee should extend and the quadriceps should contract.

• To assess the Achilles (ankle-jerk) reflex (S1, S2), first position the client with the knee bent and the ankle dorsiflexed. (The best position is with the client seated and the legs dangling over the side of the examination table.) Then tap the Achilles tendon, which should cause plantar flexion followed by muscle relaxation.

Superficial reflexes

• To assess the pharyngeal (gag) reflex (CN IX, CN X), have the client open the mouth wide. Then touch the posterior wall of the pharynx with a tongue depressor. The normal response to this action is gagging.

• To assess the upper abdominal reflex (T8, T9, T10), use a fingernail or the tip of the handle of the reflex hammer to stroke one

Selected nursing diagnosis categories

The nurse can use these diagnosis categories to formulate nursing diagnoses for a client with a neurologic problem.
- Altered nutrition: Less than body requirements
- Altered role performance
- Altered thought processes
- Altered urinary elimination
- Bathing or hygiene self-care deficit
- Bowel incontinence
- Dressing/grooming self-care deficit
- High risk for altered body temperature
- High risk for injury
- Hyperthermia
- Impaired verbal communication
- Impaired home maintenance management
- Impaired physical mobility
- Impaired skin integrity
- Impaired swallowing
- Ineffective breathing pattern
- Ineffective family coping: Compromised
- Ineffective individual coping
- Powerlessness
- Sensory or perceptual alteration
- Toileting self-care deficit
- Total incontinence

side, and then the opposite side, of the client's abdomen above the umbilicus. To assess the lower abdominal reflex (T10, T11, T12), repeat on the lower abdomen. Normally, the abdominal muscles contract and the umbilicus deviates toward the stimulated side.
- To assess the cremasteric reflex (L1, L2) on a male client, use a tongue depressor to scratch the inner aspect of each thigh gently. This should cause elevation of the testicles.
- To assess the anal reflex (S3, S4, S5), gently scratch the skin at the side of the anus with a blunt instrument, such as a tongue depressor or gloved finger. Look for puckering of the anus, a normal response.
- To assess the bulbocavernous reflex (S3, S4) on a male client, apply direct pressure over the bulbocavernous muscle behind the scrotum and gently pinch the foreskin or glans. This action should cause contraction of the bulbocavernous muscle.

Pathologic reflexes
- To assess the grasp reflex, stimulate the palm of the client's hand with your fingers. (*Note:* Because a lack of inhibition by the brain can cause the client to squeeze very tightly, avoid finger injury or pain by crossing your middle and index fingers before placing them in the client's palm.) In a positive grasp reflex, the client's hand will grasp yours upon stimulation, indicating frontal lobe damage, bilateral thalamic degeneration, or cerebral degeneration or atrophy.
- To assess the sucking reflex, stimulate the client's lips with a mouth swab. A sucking movement on stimulation can indicate cerebral degeneration.
- To assess the snout reflex, gently percuss the oral area with your fingers. This action may make the client's lips pucker, indicating cerebral degeneration or late-stage dementia.
- To assess the plantar reflex (L5, S1), stroke the lateral aspect of the sole of the client's foot. Toe flexion is the normal response. A positive Babinski's sign occurs when the toes dorsiflex and fan out, indicating upper motor neuron disease.

Assessing vital signs
The CNS, primarily by way of the brain stem and autonomic nervous system, controls the body's vital functions: heart rate and rhythm; respiratory rate, depth, and pattern; blood pressure; and body temperature. However, because these vital control centers lie deep within the cerebral hemispheres and in the brain stem, changes in vital signs – temperature, pulse, respiration, and blood pressure – are not usually early indicators of CNS deterioration. Furthermore, the significance of vital sign changes must be evaluated by considering each sign individually as well as in relation to each other.

DOCUMENTATION

The SOAPIE method of documentation includes the following components: subjective (history) data, objective (physical) data, assessment, planning, implementation, and evaluation. The following example shows how to document nursing care for a client with a neurologic problem.

Case history
Joseph Collins, age 73, comes to the clinic because his right arm feels "heavy and clumsy" and, unlike previous episodes, this sensation has not gone away.

S   O   A   P   I   E

Client states that right arm is "heavy and clumsy." Reports having "spells" of being unable to move right hand or arm, feels numb and tingling. Having difficulty finding appropriate words. Episodes started 8 months ago, now occur every other day and last 10 minutes. Client has had hypertension "for 40 years." Stopped taking prescribed antihypertensive medication last year because he was "feeling good." Father died of a stroke at age 82.

S   **O**   A   P   I   E

T 98.8° F.; P 78, regular; R 22, even and unlabored; BP 182/96. Alert and oriented. Remote and recent memory intact. Speech slightly slurred. Pupils round, equal, and reactive to light. Motor: right-handed. Moves all extremities on command without difficulty. Upper and lower extremities strong bilaterally; right grasp slightly weaker than left. Right arm drifts. Sensory: light touch, pain, temperature sensation absent in right hand and forearm; intact in left arm and both legs.

S   O   **A**   P   I   E

Knowledge deficit related to warning signs of stroke and importance of adhering to antihypertensive regimen. Correlates hypertension medications with feeling bad and having headaches.

S   O   A   **P**   I   E

Teach client importance of following antihypertensive regimen and warning signals of TIAs. Encourage client to keep appointments.

S   O   A   P   **I**   E

Taught client about antihypertensive regimen and importance of adherence. Explained TIAs and associated warning signs that should be reported. Gave client printed material for reinforcement. Discussed importance of regular checkups to monitor blood pressure and TIAs.

S   O   A   P   I   **E**

Client repeats some information and states that he will make a follow-up appointment.

SUGGESTED READINGS

Barker, E., et al. (1992). Cranial nerve assessment. *RN*, 55(5), 62-69.

Jackson, S. (1992). Action Stat! Assessing a head injury. *Nursing92*, 22(9), 49.

Kaufman, J. (1990). Nurse's guide to assessing the 12 cranial nerves. *Nursing90*, 20(6), 56-58.

Lower, J. (1992). Rapid neuro assessment. *American Journal of Nursing*, 92(6), 38-48.

Sullivan, J. (1990). Neurologic assessment. *Nursing Clinics of North America*, 25(4), 795-809.

16

Musculoskeletal System

Assessing the musculoskeletal system entails examination of muscles, bones, and joints. Because the central nervous system (CNS) coordinates muscle and bone function, the examiner must understand how the two systems interrelate. (For information about the CNS, see Chapter 15, Nervous System.)

Usually, the musculoskeletal system assessment is a small fraction of the overall physical assessment, especially for the client who has other complaints. However, where the general assessment reveals an abnormality or the symptom history suggests musculoskeletal involvement, a complete assessment of the system is necessary.

HEALTH HISTORY

Obtaining a thorough and accurate client health history is crucial to the nurse's assessment of the musculoskeletal system.

Three groups of sample questions follow. Those on *health and illness patterns* help the nurse identify actual or potential musculoskeletal-related health problems; those on *health promotion and protection patterns* help the nurse determine how the client's life-style and behavior affects musculoskeletal function; and those on *role and relationship patterns* help the nurse determine how the problem affects the client's self-image and life-style.

Health and illness patterns

Are you having any pain? Can you point to the area where you feel pain?
(RATIONALE: The client's response will validate your understanding of the client's verbal description.)

How would you describe the pain—for instance, aching, burning, stabbing, or throbbing?
(RATIONALE: Frequently, the client's description provides clues to identify the tissue affected; for example, "sore or aching" points to muscle pain; "throbbing," to bone pain.)

When you have this pain, do you also have pain in any other location?
(RATIONALE: An affirmative response requires further assessment to check for referred pain. For example, pain felt in the leg may result from lumbosacral nerve root irritation.)

When did this pain begin? What were you doing at the time it began?
(RATIONALE: These questions establish whether onset was gradual or sudden. Certain activities increase the potential for injury and pain; for example, lifting heavy or awkward loads can strain ligaments and vertebral disks, causing acute, immediate pain.)

(Text continues on page 202.)

Anatomy review

The illustrations below show the anatomic structures of the musculoskeletal system.

Muscle system

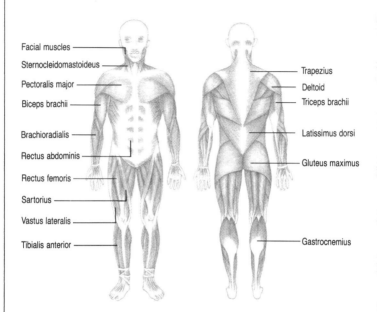

Facial muscles
Sternocleidomastoideus
Pectoralis major
Biceps brachii
Brachioradialis
Rectus abdominis
Rectus femoris
Sartorius
Vastus lateralis
Tibialis anterior

Trapezius
Deltoid
Triceps brachii
Latissimus dorsi
Gluteus maximus
Gastrocnemius

Muscle structure

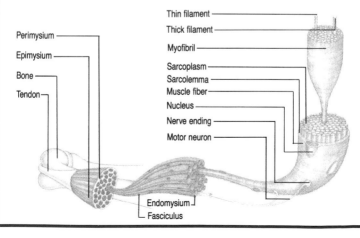

Perimysium
Epimysium
Bone
Tendon

Thin filament
Thick filament
Myofibril
Sarcoplasm
Sarcolemma
Muscle fiber
Nucleus
Nerve ending
Motor neuron

Endomysium
Fasciculus

Skeletal system

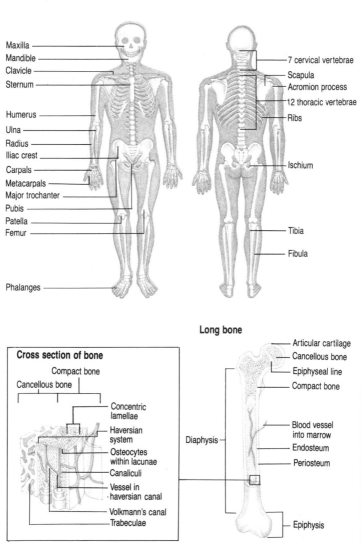

Long bone

Cross section of bone

What activities seem to decrease or eliminate the pain?
(RATIONALE: Resting and elevating the affected body part usually decrease pain.)

What activities seem to increase the pain?
(RATIONALE: Weight bearing usually increases pain if the client has a degenerative disease of the hip, knee, or vertebrae.)

Do you have any other unusual sensations, such as tingling, with the pain?
(RATIONALE: Paresthesias—sensations of tingling, burning, or prickling—can accompany compression of nerves or blood vessels serving a body area.)

Will you describe your weakness? When did you first notice muscle weakness? Did the weakness begin in the same muscles where you now notice it?
(RATIONALE: Muscle weakness associated with certain diseases migrates, traveling from muscle to muscle or to groups of muscles. Knowing the symptom patterns and when they occur helps identify the disease process, if any, responsible for weakness.)

When did you first notice swelling? Did you injure this area? Is the area tender? Does the overlying skin ever look red or feel hot?
(RATIONALE: These findings may indicate infection or recent trauma to the area.)

What have you tried to reduce the swelling? Have you tried heat or ice applications?
(RATIONALE: The client's response may help identify remedies that can be continued or may uncover inappropriate client actions.)

When did the stiffness begin? Has stiffness increased since it began? Do you feel stiff only upon awakening or all the time?
(RATIONALE: Some diseases have remission and exacerbation periods. Others, such as osteoarthritis, cause stiffness upon awakening that decreases with activity.)

Is pain associated with the stiffness, or do you sometimes hear a grating sound or feel a grating sensation?

(RATIONALE: Pain, stiffness, and a crackling noise [crepitus] indicate rough, irregular articular cartilage, as found in osteoarthritis.)

How have you tried to reduce stiffness?
(RATIONALE: The stiffness of rheumatoid arthritis usually decreases if the client exercises the affected joints.)

Have you ever had any injury to a bone, muscle, ligament, cartilage, joint, or tendon? If so, what was the injury and how and when did it occur? How was it treated? Have you experienced any aftereffects?
(RATIONALE: The client's answers provide useful guides to physical assessment activities, particularly evaluating muscle strength and joint range of motion.)

Have you had surgery or treatment involving bone, muscle, joint, ligament, tendon, or cartilage? What was the outcome?
(RATIONALE: The answers to these questions can guide physical assessment.)

Have you had bone X-rays? What was X-rayed and when? What was found?
(RATIONALE: X-ray studies show bone and joint integrity as well as previous injuries.)

Have you had joint fluid removal or a biopsy performed?
(RATIONALE: Synovial fluid analysis and tissue biopsy usually provide important diagnostic information.)

Has anyone in your family had osteoporosis, gout, arthritis, or tuberculosis?
(RATIONALE: A family history of certain diseases or a history of infectious tuberculosis increases the possibility that the client may have or be at risk for these conditions.)

Pediatric client

A complete musculoskeletal assessment of a child should include the following questions (directed to a parent or guardian):

Was labor and delivery difficult?
(RATIONALE: Birth injuries may include fractures or nerve damage. A neonate's difficult

breathing at birth may cause hypoxia leading to decreased muscle tone.)

At what age did your child first hold up his (or her) head, sit, crawl, and walk?
(RATIONALE: The answers to these questions help determine whether the child is achieving appropriate developmental milestones or if a musculoskeletal problem prevents normal development.)

Have you noted any lack of coordination? Can your child move about normally? Would you describe your child's strength as normal for his (or her) age?
(RATIONALE: Poor coordination may point to a serious musculoskeletal problem, such as cerebral palsy, or may indicate something less serious, such as a vision problem. Muscle weakness may signify muscular dystrophy.)

Has your child ever broken a bone? If so, which one and when? Did any complications occur during the healing?
(RATIONALE: The answers to these questions help guide subsequent physical assessment.)

Female client
At what age did you begin menstruating? If you have undergone menopause, at what age did it occur? Are you taking estrogen?
(RATIONALE: Late menarche and early menopause allow fewer years for exposure to estrogen levels that provide for bone mass, placing a woman at risk for osteoporosis.)

Pregnant client
Are you having back pains or spasms?
(RATIONALE: Often, the forward abdominal tilt during pregnancy strains the lower back.)

Are you experiencing weakness, pain, or tingling in one or both hands?
(RATIONALE: A pregnant client is at increased risk for carpal tunnel syndrome — compression neuropathy of the median nerve in the wrist — from the hand and wrist edema that occurs during the last trimester of pregnancy.)

Elderly client
Have you broken any bones recently? If so, how?
(RATIONALE: Bones lose density with age. The vertebrae, hips, and wrists are particularly susceptible to fractures in an elderly client. Some fractures result from trauma; others result from a pathologic [nontraumatic] cause.)

Have you noticed any change in agility, speed of movement, or endurance?
(RATIONALE: Decreased agility, reaction time, and endurance occur normally with aging.)

Do you exercise regularly? If not, why not?
(RATIONALE: Regular exercise slows the musculoskeletal deterioration attributed to aging. Encourage the client to engage in regular exercise appropriate to ability.)

Health promotion and protection patterns
How much alcohol do you drink daily? How much coffee, tea, or other caffeine-containing beverages?
(RATIONALE: High alcohol or caffeine consumption may increase the risk of osteoporosis.)

Do you follow an exercise schedule? If so, describe it. How has your current problem affected your usual exercise routine?
(RATIONALE: Routine exercise helps maintain strength, muscle tone, bone density, and flexibility.)

Have any of your usual activities, such as dressing, grooming, climbing stairs, or rising from a chair, become difficult or impossible for you to do?
(RATIONALE: The client's response helps establish the degree of weakness and assesses its impact on daily living.)

Are you now using or do you think you would be helped by an assistive device, such as a cane, walker, or brace?
(RATIONALE: The answer shows how the client feels about an assistive device and its effects on daily life.)

Do you supplement your diet with vitamins, calcium, protein, or other products? If so, what kinds and in what amounts?
(RATIONALE: Although controversy surrounds using dietary supplements, an affirmative answer indicates an interest in nutritional status. The amount and type of supplements the client takes are important to know because they could be helpful or detrimental.)

What is your current weight? Is this your normal weight?
(RATIONALE: Obesity adds stress to weight-bearing joints, such as the knees, putting the client at greater risk for certain musculoskeletal disorders, such as osteoarthritis.)

Does your current problem affect your ability to prepare food and to eat? For instance, do you have difficulty opening cans or cutting meat?
(RATIONALE: Finger stiffness that accompanies osteoarthritis or rheumatoid arthritis can interfere with such tasks, possibly compromising the client's nutritional status.)

Has this problem adversely affected your hobbies, leisure pursuits, and social life?
(RATIONALE: An affirmative answer indicates the need to help identify new activities within the client's capabilities.)

Do weather changes seem to affect the problem in any way; for example, does pain increase in cold or damp weather?
(RATIONALE: A low temperature with increased humidity tends to exacerbate muscle pain in inflammatory conditions and joint pain in osteoarthritis.)

Role and relationship patterns
Do you feel any stress because of your current problem?
(RATIONALE: Certain musculoskeletal problems can interfere with life-style and self-image. For example, finger flexion associated with Dupuytren's contracture [progressive thickening and tightening of subcutaneous tissue of the palm] severely limits a client's dexterity. Pronounced scoliosis [lateral curvature of the spine] can cause self-consciousness and low self-es-

teem in a child or adolescent. A large tophaceous deposit [urate crystals] in the first metatarsal joint and gout pain can make footwear feel unbearable.)

What effect, if any, does this problem have on your sexual relationship?
(RATIONALE: Chronic back pain or other musculoskeletal problems can interfere with sexual desire and performance.)

PHYSICAL ASSESSMENT
The nurse uses the following equipment and techniques when assessing the musculoskeletal system.
Equipment
• tape measure
• goniometer
Techniques
• inspection
• palpation

Inspecting and palpating muscles
• Although inspection and palpation are performed separately in many assessments, they are performed simultaneously during the musculoskeletal assessment. Muscle assessment includes evaluating muscle tone, mass, and strength.
• Palpate the muscles gently, never forcing movement when the client reports pain or when you feel resistance. Watch the client's face and body language for signs of discomfort; a client may suffer silently.
• Assess muscle tone—the consistency or tension in the resting muscle—by palpating a muscle at rest and during passive range of motion (ROM).
• Palpate a muscle at rest from the muscle attachment at the bone to the edge of the muscle. Normally, a relaxed muscle should feel soft, pliable, and nontender; a contracted muscle, firm.
• Assessment of muscle mass usually involves measuring the circumference of the thigh, the calf, and the upper arm. When measuring, establish landmarks to ensure measurement at the same location on each extremity.

• When measuring the upper midarm circumferences to assess muscle size, be sure to ask the client which side is dominant (that is, whether the client is right- or left-handed). Expect symmetry of size; greater than a ½″ (1-cm) circumferential difference between opposite thighs, calves, and upper arms is considered abnormal unless the increased muscle size results from specific physical activities.

• To evaluate muscle strength, have the client perform active range-of-motion movements as you apply resistance. Note the strength that the client exerts against resistance. If the muscle group is weak, lessen the resistance to permit a more accurate assessment. Record findings according to a five-point scale. (For information on how to test and grade muscle strength, see "Assessing muscle strength and joint range of motion," pages 207 to 213.)

Inspecting and palpating joints and bones

• Assessment of the joints and bones includes measuring the client's height and the length of the extremities (arms and legs) and evaluating joint and bone characteristics and joint ROM.

• During joint assessment, never force joint movement if you feel resistance or if the client complains of pain.

• Measure the height of the client as well as the length of the extremities for comparison.

• To measure the extremities, place the client in the supine position on a flat surface with the arms and legs fully extended and the shoulders and hips adducted. Measure each arm from the acromion process to the tip of the middle finger. Measure each leg from the anterior superior iliac spine to the medial malleolus with the tape crossing at the medial side of the knee. More than ½″ (1 cm) disparity in the length between each limb is abnormal.

• Inspect the cervical spine from three viewpoints: from behind, from the side, and facing the client. The client may sit or stand.

• Observe the alignment of the head with the body. The nose should be in line with the midsternum and extend beyond the shoulders

---

Assessment checklist

The nurse should ask herself or himself these questions before beginning the assessment:

☐ Have I gathered all the necessary equipment?

☐ Have I washed my hands?

☐ Have I provided seating in case the client tires?

☐ Does the client require any special assistance (cane, walker, or brace)? If so, have I provided for it?

☐ Have I reviewed all relevant laboratory data?

---

when viewed from the side. The head should align with the shoulders. Normally, the seventh cervical and first thoracic vertebrae are more prominent than the others.

• Inspect and palpate the length of the clavicles, including the sternoclavicular and acromioclavicular joints. Normal findings include firm, smooth, and continuous bone.

• To inspect and palpate the scapulae, sit directly behind the client, who sits with shoulders thrust backward. Normally, the scapulae are located over thoracic ribs 2 through 7. Check for an equal distance from the medial scapular edges to the midspinal line.

• After assessing the scapulae, inspect and palpate the anterior, posterior, and lateral surfaces of the ribs. Normal findings include firm, smooth, continuous bones.

• Palpate the moving joints for crepitus. Inspect the skin overlying the shoulder joint for erythema, masses, or swelling.

• Palpate the acromioclavicular joint and the area over the greater humeral tuberosity. Shoulder joint palpation begins with the client's arm at the side. Ask the client to move the arm across the chest (adduction). Then, place your thumb on the anterior portion of the client's shoulder joint and your fingers on the posterior portion of the joint. Ask the client to move the arm backward. Palpate the shoulder joint as the client's arm moves backward.

Grading muscle strength

When evaluating muscle strength, use the scale below. Column 1 describes the possible muscle response and the significance of the response. Column 2 shows how to grade the response.

A rating of less than 3 on the scale indicates significant muscular dysfunction or disability. Total lack of contractility (the flaccid muscle) accompanies paralysis, which is a complete loss of voluntary movement. Slight contractility (the hypotonic muscle) accompanies paresis.These conditions are secondary to neurologic dysfunction.

MUSCLE RESPONSE AND SIGNIFICANCE	GRADE RATING
No visible or palpable contraction felt • Paralysis	0
Slightly palpable contraction felt • Paresis, severe weakness	1
Passive range of motion (ROM) maneuvers when gravity is removed • Paresis, moderate weakness	2
Active ROM against gravity alone or against light resistance • Mild weakness	3 to 4
Active ROM against full resistance • Normal	5

• Next, stand behind the client. With your fingertips placed over the greater humeral tuberosity, instruct the client to rotate the shoulder internally by moving the arm behind the back. Besides palpating the bony structures of the shoulder joint, you can also palpate a portion of the musculotendinous rotator cuff in this way.

• Inspect joint contour and the skin over each elbow. Palpate the joint at rest and during movement.

• Inspect the wrists for masses, erythema, skeletal deformities, and swelling. Palpate the wrist at rest and during movement by gently grasping it between your thumb and fingers.

• On each hand, inspect the fingers and thumb for nodules, erythema, spacing, length, and skeletal deformities. Palpate fingers and thumb at rest and during movement for crepitus, heat (inflammation), and pain.

• Besides evaluating the curvatures of the thoracic and lumbar spine during the postural assessment, palpate the length of the spine for tenderness and vertebral alignment. To check for tenderness, percuss each spinous process (directly over the vertebral column) with the ulnar side of your fist.

• Normal spinal assessment findings include the client's ability to perform movements with a full ROM, while maintaining balance, smoothness, and coordination.

• Inspect and palpate over the bony prominences: iliac crests, symphysis pubis, anterior spine, ischial tuberosities, and greater trochanters. Palpate the hip at rest and during movement.

• Inspect the knees with the client seated. Palpate the knees at rest and during movement. Inspect and palpate the popliteal spaces (behind the knee joint). Knee movements should be smooth.

• Inspect and palpate the ankles and feet at rest and during movement.

• The client may be sitting or lying supine for toe assessment. Inspect all toe surfaces. Palpate toes at rest and during movement.

Assessing muscle strength and joint range of motion

Assessment of joint ROM tests the integrity of joint function; assessment of muscle strength against resistance tests function of the muscles surrounding the joint. To assess joint ROM, the nurse asks the client to move specific joints through the normal ROM. If the client is unable to do so, the nurse can move the client's joints through passive ROM. To assess muscle strength, the nurse applies pressure to a specific point at or near the muscles surrounding a joint. The client should also be able to apply strong resistance (grades) to pressure applied against movement. If two sides are being assessed (the right and left knee, for example), strength should be symmetrical.

Cervical spine and neck
Below is a posterior view of the upper spine.

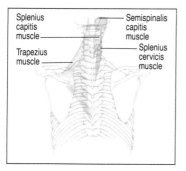

Splenius capitis muscle

Trapezius muscle

Semispinalis capitis muscle

Splenius cervicis muscle

Muscle strength. To assess flexion of the cervical spine, place your hand on the client's forehead, applying pressure. Ask the client to bend the head forward and touch the chin to the chest.

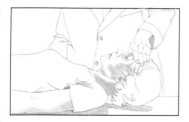

To assess rotation of the cervical spine, ask the client to push laterally against your hand positioned firmly against the left side of the face to prevent movement. At the same time, palpate the sternocleidomastoid muscle on the opposite side. Repeat the procedure on the right side.

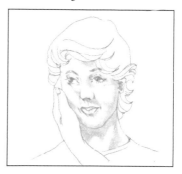

To assess extension of the cervical spine, apply pressure with your hand on the client's occipital bone. Ask the client to bend the head backward as far as possible.

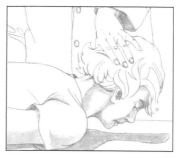

Range of motion. Ask the client to flex the neck (attempt to touch the chin to the chest), then extend the neck (bend the head backward). Next, ask the client to bend laterally, touching the ears to the shoulders. Then ask the client to rotate the head from side to side.

Shoulder

Below is an anterior view of the right shoulder.

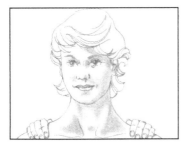

Clavicle
Supraspinatus muscle
Biceps brachii tendon
Biceps
Deltoid

Muscle strength. The trapezius muscles (of the shoulder and upper back) are best tested simultaneously. Ask the client to shrug the shoulders freely, then again as you press down on them.

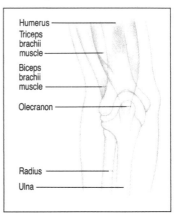

Range of motion. Observe and measure ROM as the client demonstrates forward flexion with the arms straight in front and backward extension with the arms straight and extended backward.

To assess abduction, ask the client to raise the arm out to the side with the arm straight; to assess adduction, ask the client to move the arm to midline with the arm straight.

To assess internal rotation, ask the client to abduct the arm with the elbow bent and the fingers pointed downward by placing the hands behind the small of the back.

To assess external rotation, ask the client to abduct the arm with the elbow bent and the fingers pointed upward by placing the hands behind the head.

Upper arm and elbow

Below is a posterior view of the left arm.

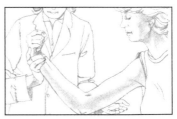

Humerus
Triceps brachii muscle
Biceps brachii muscle
Olecranon
Radius
Ulna

Muscle strength. To test tricep strength, try to flex the client's arm while the client tries to extend it.

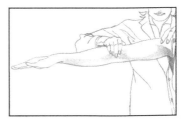

To test deltoid strength, push down on the client's arm (abducted to 90 degrees) while the client resists.

To assess bicep strength, attempt to pull the client's flexed arm into extension while the client resists.

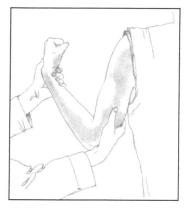

Range of motion. Ask the client to sit or stand. Then, assess flexion by having the client bend the arm and attempt to touch the shoulder. To assess extension, ask the client to straighten the arm.

Assess pronation by holding the client's elbow in a flexed position while the client rotates the arm until the palm faces the floor. Assess supination by holding the client's elbow in a flexed position while the client rotates the arm until the palm faces upward.

Wrist and hand

Below is a lateral view of the left hand and wrist.

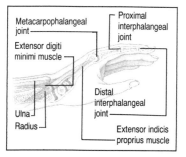

Muscle strength. Test muscle strength and movement of both hands simultaneously by having the client squeeze the first two fingers of your hand, make a fist, resist your efforts to straighten the client's flexed wrist, and resist your efforts to flex the client's straightened wrist. (Normally, the dominant hand is slightly stronger.)

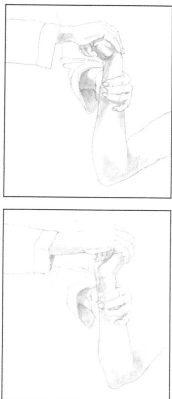

Range of motion. To assess flexion, ask the client to bend the wrist downward; assess extension by having the client straighten the wrist. To assess hyperextension or dorsiflexion, ask the client to bend the wrist upward.

Assess ulnar deviation by asking the client to move the hand toward the ulnar side; assess radial deviation by asking the client to move the hand toward the radial side.

To assess the metacarpophalangeal joints, ask the client to hyperextend (dorsiflex), extend (straighten), and flex (make a fist) the fingers. Also ask the client to straighten the fingers, then spread them and bring them together. Abduction should be 20 degrees between fingers; in adduction, the fingers should touch.

To assess palmar adduction, ask the client to bring the thumb to the index finger; assess palmar abduction by asking the client to move the thumb away from the palm. Also assess opposition by having the client touch the thumb to each fingertip.

Thoracic and lumbar spine

Below is a posterior view of the spine and pelvis.

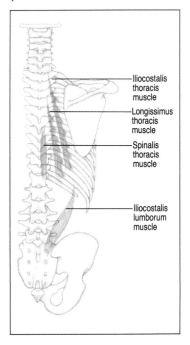

Iliocostalis thoracis muscle

Longissimus thoracis muscle

Spinalis thoracis muscle

Iliocostalis lumborum muscle

Range of motion. With the client standing, observe and evaluate spinal ROM as the client demonstrates hyperextension by bending backward from the waist and flexion by bending to touch the floor with the knees slightly bent.

Next, assess rotation by first stabilizing the client's pelvis, then asking the client to rotate the upper body from side to side. Finally, ask the client to bend to each side.

Hip and pelvis

Below is a posterior view of the right hip and thigh.

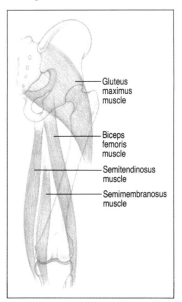

Gluteus maximus muscle

Biceps femoris muscle

Semitendinosus muscle

Semimembranosus muscle

Muscle strength. With the client lying (prone and, later, supine), then sitting, evaluate muscle strength and palpate muscles as you carry out the following tests.

To assess hip extensors, ask the prone client to hyperextend the leg backward (toward the ceiling) as you try to push the leg downward.

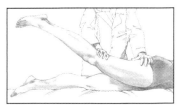

To assess hip abductors, ask the supine client to move the straightened leg away from midline as you attempt to push the client's leg toward midline.

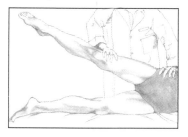

To assess hip flexors, ask the client to sit and raise the knee to the chest as you apply downward pressure proximal to the knee.

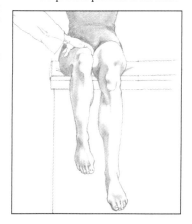

To assess hip adductors, ask the supine client to move the leg toward midline as you try to pull the leg away from midline.

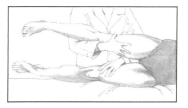

Range of motion. With the client prone or standing, observe and evaluate ROM as the client demonstrates flexion by bending the knee to the chest with the back straight. *Caution:* Do not perform this movement on a client who has undergone total hip replacement without the surgeon's permission because the motion can cause the prosthesis to dislocate.

Next, evaluate extension by asking the client to straighten the knee and hyperextension by asking the client to extend the leg backward with the knee straight. *Note:* This motion can be performed with the client prone or standing.

To assess abduction, have the client move the straightened leg away from midline; assess adduction by having the client move the straightened leg toward midline. *Caution:* This motion can displace a hip prosthesis.

Finally, assess internal and external rotation by asking the client to turn the foot inward and outward, respectively.

Knee

Below is an anterior view of the right knee.

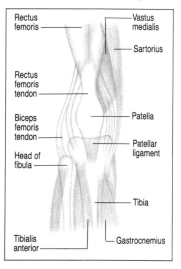

Muscle strength. To assess knee extensors, ask the client to sit or lie supine and extend the leg as you attempt to flex it.

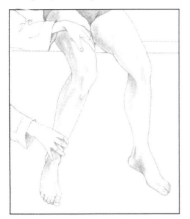

To assess knee flexors, ask the client to sit or lie supine while you try to extend the client's leg as the client flexes the knee.

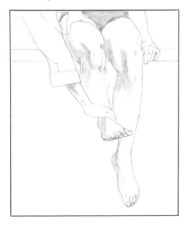

Range of motion. With the client sitting or standing, observe and measure ROM as the client demonstrates extension by straightening the leg at the knee and flexion by bending the leg at the knee and bringing the foot up to touch the buttock.

Ankle and foot

Below is an anterior view of the right ankle and foot.

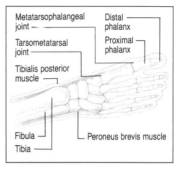

Muscle strength. To assess dorsiflexion of the ankle joint, place your hand on the dorsal surface of the client's foot and apply pressure. Ask the client to bend the foot up against your resistance.

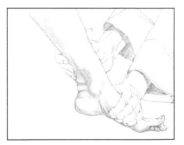

To assess plantar flexion, apply pressure with your hand to the plantar surface of the client's foot as the client attempts to bend the foot down.

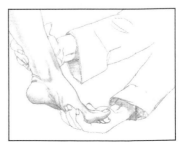

To assess inversion, apply pressure with your hand to the medial surface of the client's first metatarsal bone as the client attempts to move the toes inward. To assess eversion, place your hand on the lateral surface of the fifth metatarsal bone and apply pressure as the client attempts to move the toes outward.

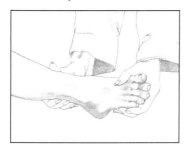

Range of motion. Ask the client who is sitting, lying, or standing to demonstrate plantar flexion by bending the foot downward and dorsiflexion by bending the foot upward.

Then ask the client to invert the foot by pointing the toes and turning the foot inward and to evert the foot by pointing the toes and turning the foot outward.

To assess forefoot adduction and abduction, stabilize the client's heel while the client turns the forefoot inward and outward, respectively.

Toes
Below is an anterior view of the left foot.

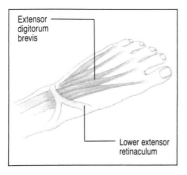

Muscle strength. To assess flexion, apply pressure with your finger to the plantar surface of the client's toes as the client attempts to bend the toes downward.

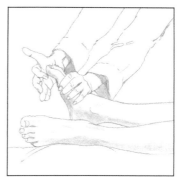

To assess extension, apply pressure with your finger to the dorsal surface of the client's toes as the client attempts to point the toes upward.

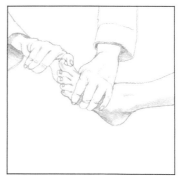

Range of motion. To assess the metatarsophalangeal joints, ask the client to extend (straighten) and flex (curl) the toes. Then, ask the client to hyperextend the toes by straightening and pointing them upward.

Common laboratory studies

For a client with musculoskeletal signs and symptoms, various laboratory studies can provide the nurse with valuable clues to the possible cause. This chart lists commonly ordered laboratory studies along with their normal values or findings. Remember that values differ among laboratories, and check the normal value range for the specific laboratory.

TEST	NORMAL VALUES OR FINDINGS
Blood tests	
Alanine aminotransferase (ALT), formerly SGPT	*Males:* 10 to 32 units/liter *Females:* 9 to 24 units/liter *Infants:* twice the adult values
Aspartate aminotransferase (AST), formerly SGOT	*Adults:* 8 to 20 units/liter *Infants:* four times the adult values
Creatine phosphokinase (CPK) enzyme with isoenzyme (CPK-MM)	*CPK males:* 23 to 99 units/liter *CPK females:* 15 to 57 units/liter *CPK-MM:* 5 to 70 IU/liter
Rheumatoid factor (RF)	Nonreactive test with titer value less than 1:20
Alkaline phosphatase	*Males:* 90 to 239 units/liter *Females under age 45:* 76 to 196 units/liter *Females over age 45:* 87 to 250 units/liter
Calcium	4.5 to 5.5 mEq/liter
Urine tests	
Uric acid	250 to 750 mg/24 hours
Bence Jones protein	Absence of Bence Jones protein in urine

DOCUMENTATION

The SOAPIE method of documentation includes the following components: subjective (history) data, objective (physical) data, assessment, planning, implementation, and evaluation. The following example shows how to document nursing care for a client with rheumatoid arthritis who needs pain management.

Case history

Mrs. Linda Jackson, age 40, was referred to the clinic for pain management related to moderately advanced rheumatoid arthri-

tis. She recently resigned her job as a third grade teacher when arthritis limited her ability to function. Her reason for coming to the clinic at this time is pain management.

S   O   A   P   I   E

Client states, "My pain and stiffness are much worse in the morning." Client also reports limited use of hands and "pain in both feet," which increases on weight bearing. Client reports that arthritis was diagnosed at age 32 and is progressively more "crippling" and "intolerable."

S **O** A P I E

Distal phalangeal hyperextension, proximal phalangeal flexion, and ulnar deviation of fingers noted. Joints are swollen, slightly red, warm to the touch, and painful when palpated. Atrophy of hand muscles noted. Grip poor; client cannot form a tight fist. Muscle strength rating is 2. ROM markedly reduced: flexion of distal interphalangeal joints, 20 degrees; flexion of proximal interphalangeal joints, 40 degrees. Findings are symmetrical.

Metatarsophalangeal joints are swollen and painful with joint movement. Marked reduction of ROM bilaterally: flexion of first metatarsophalangeal joints, 10 degrees; flexion of distal interphalangeal joints, 20 degrees; flexion of proximal interphalangeal joints, 10 degrees; flexion of metatarsophalangeal joints, 5 degrees; hyperextension of metatarsophalangeal joints, 5 degrees.

Other less-involved joints include wrists, elbows, knees, and ankles.

X-rays show joint space narrowing and marked bilateral erosion of finger and toe articular joint cartilages. WBC slightly elevated (12,500/mm³). ESR elevated (30 mm/hour).

S O **A** P I E

Pain in hand and foot joints related to inflammatory changes.

S O A **P** I E

Help client control and relieve pain.

S O A P **I** E

Assessed pain. Developed an appropriate pain medication schedule. Taught client to apply heat and cold to joints. Encouraged regular ROM exercise.

S O A P I **E**

Emphasize importance of medication and exercise schedule.

Selected nursing diagnosis categories

The nurse can use these diagnosis categories to formulate nursing diagnoses for a client with a musculoskeletal problem.
- Activity intolerance
- Altered growth and development
- Altered sexuality patterns
- Bathing or hygiene self-care deficit
- Dressing or grooming self-care deficit
- High risk for injury
- Impaired physical mobility
- Pain
- Sleep pattern disturbance

SUGGESTED READINGS

Bailey, M., and Michalski, J. (1992). Close-up on clavicle fracture. *Nursing92*, 22(8), 41.

Bailey, M., and Michalski, J. (1992). Close-up on scapula fracture. *Nursing92*, 22(12), 64.

Dykes, P. (1993). Minding the five P's of neurovascular assessment. *American Journal of Nursing*, 93(6), 38-39.

Hayden, J. (1992). Triage of hand injuries. *Emergency Medicine*, 24(15), 91-102.

Nussman, D., and Poole, R. (1991). Rescue and recovery in traumatic hip dislocation. *American Journal of Nursing*, 91(11), 34-38.

17

Immune System and Blood

The main purpose of the immune system is to defend the body from assault by microorganisms. Blood, the body's major transportation fluid, performs a vital function by maintaining homeostasis (natural, physiologic equilibrium of the body's internal environment). Through its lymphatic channels, the immune system also performs a transport function.

Unlike other body systems, the immune system and blood are not composed of simple organ groups. The immune system consists of billions of circulating cells and specialized structures, such as lymph nodes, that are located throughout the body. The blood includes fluid (plasma) and formed elements (blood cells and platelets) that circulate throughout the body. The spleen assists the blood and immune system by serving as a reservoir for blood and producing blood cells. The spleen also aids in defense against microorganisms. Because of their diffuse nature, the immune system and the blood can affect, and be affected by, every other body system; for this reason, assessing the immune system and blood is complex. Sometimes, immune or blood disorders produce characteristic signs or symptoms, such as the butterfly rash of systemic lupus erythematosus (SLE). Usually, though, they cause vague symptoms, such as fatigue or dyspnea (shortness of breath), that initially seem related to other body systems.

The nurse should consider assessing the immune system and blood whenever a client reports such symptoms as frequent or recurring infections, slow wound healing, or blood clotting problems.

HEALTH HISTORY

Focus the health history on detecting the most common signs and symptoms of immune and blood disorders: abnormal bleeding, lymphadenopathy (hypertrophy of lymphoid tissue, often called swollen glands), fatigue, weakness, fever, and joint pain. Focus on blood and immune system concerns, but maintain a holistic approach by inquiring about the status of other systems and about health-related concerns. Blood and immune problems may result from problems in other systems, may cause problems in other systems, or may impair other aspects of the client's life.

Three groups of sample questions follow. Those on *health and illness patterns* help the nurse identify actual or potential immune- or blood-related health problems; those on *health promotion and protection patterns* help the nurse determine how the client's life-style and behavior may affect the immune system or blood; and those on *role and relationship patterns* help the nurse determine how an immune- or blood-related problem affects the client's life-style and relationships with others.

Anatomy review

The illustration below shows the anatomic structures of the immune system.

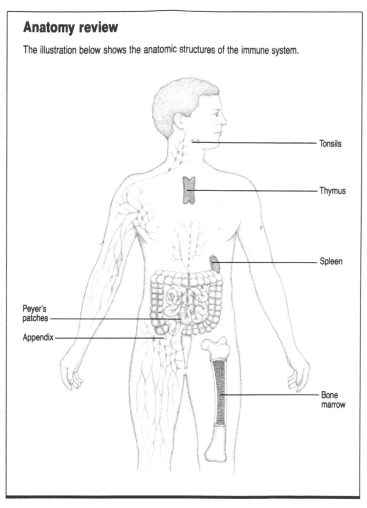

Tonsils

Thymus

Spleen

Peyer's patches

Appendix

Bone marrow

Health and illness patterns

How have you been feeling lately? Have you noticed any changes in your usual health? If so, please tell me more about them.
(RATIONALE: Because immune and blood disorder symptoms may be vague, open-ended questions usually elicit more information than a checklist might. The client may discuss seemingly insignificant health deviations when comparing current and past health status. Draw the client out about dif-

ficult-to-pinpoint, vague complaints. The more specific the information, the better the probability of identifying interrelationships among the client's discomforts.)

Have you noticed any unusual bleeding— for example, frequent nosebleeds or bruises that you don't remember getting?

(Text continues on page 220.)

Hematopoiesis: Development of blood and immune cells

Hematopoiesis produces all of the body's blood cells, including those for immunologic defense. The process occurs in the bone marrow, where multipotential stem cells give rise to five distinct cell types known as unipotential stem cells. Each unipotential cell can differen-

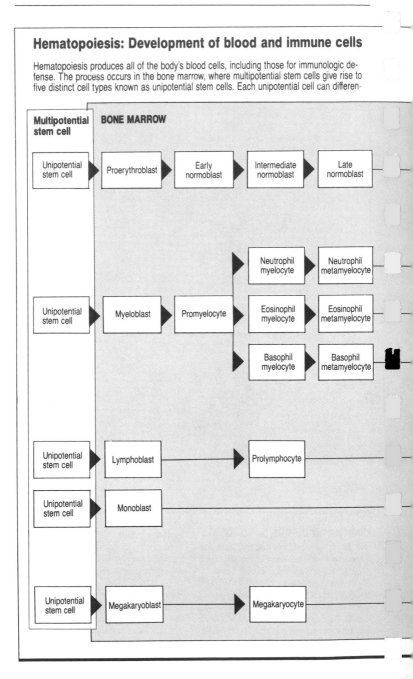

tiate (diversify) into one of the following: an erythrocyte, a granulocyte (neutrophil, eosinophil, or basophil), an agranulocyte (lymphocyte or monocyte), or a thrombocyte, as shown in the chart below.

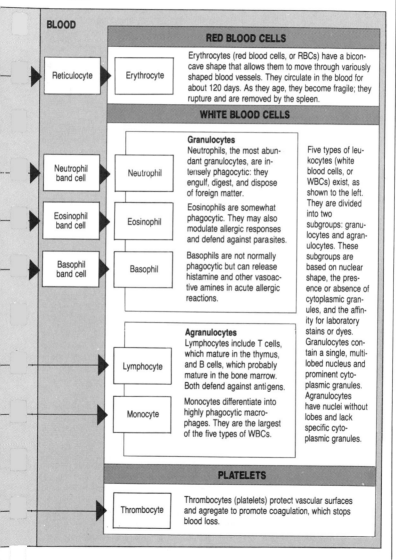

BLOOD

RED BLOOD CELLS

Reticulocyte → Erythrocyte

Erythrocytes (red blood cells, or RBCs) have a biconcave shape that allows them to move through variously shaped blood vessels. They circulate in the blood for about 120 days. As they age, they become fragile; they rupture and are removed by the spleen.

WHITE BLOOD CELLS

Granulocytes
Neutrophils, the most abundant granulocytes, are intensely phagocytic: they engulf, digest, and dispose of foreign matter.

Eosinophils are somewhat phagocytic. They may also modulate allergic responses and defend against parasites.

Basophils are not normally phagocytic but can release histamine and other vasoactive amines in acute allergic reactions.

Neutrophil band cell → Neutrophil
Eosinophil band cell → Eosinophil
Basophil band cell → Basophil

Five types of leukocytes (white blood cells, or WBCs) exist, as shown to the left. They are divided into two subgroups: granulocytes and agranulocytes. These subgroups are based on nuclear shape, the presence or absence of cytoplasmic granules, and the affinity for laboratory stains or dyes. Granulocytes contain a single, multilobed nucleus and prominent cytoplasmic granules. Agranulocytes have nuclei without lobes and lack specific cytoplasmic granules.

Agranulocytes
Lymphocytes include T cells, which mature in the thymus, and B cells, which probably mature in the bone marrow. Both defend against antigens.

Monocytes differentiate into highly phagocytic macrophages. They are the largest of the five types of WBCs.

Lymphocyte
Monocyte

PLATELETS

Thrombocyte

Thrombocytes (platelets) protect vascular surfaces and aggregate to promote coagulation, which stops blood loss.

(RATIONALE: With low platelet counts or clotting factor deficiencies, a client's unusual bleeding or unexplained ecchymoses can occur secondary to minimal trauma. The extremities are most prone to such injuries, but no body part is exempt.)

Have you ever bled for a long time after accidentally cutting yourself?
(RATIONALE: Prolonged bleeding may indicate a platelet or clotting mechanism deficiency, which can occur with certain immune disorders. If it occurs regularly, it can lead to anemia.)

Have you noticed any bleeding from your gums?
(RATIONALE: Because oral mucosal tissues are highly vascular [and visible], the client may note bleeding from these tissues before noting abnormal bleeding in other areas. Gingivae may bleed after the client masticates coarse foods or roughage, or after daily oral hygiene; they may bleed vigorously after dental hygiene or repair.)

Have you noticed any rash or skin discolorations? If so, on which part of your body?
(RATIONALE: Petechiae, pinpoint accumulations of blood in the skin or mucous membranes, may appear to the client as a rashlike discoloration. Petechiae occur when small vessels leak under pressure and platelet numbers are insufficient to stop the bleeding. They are likely to appear where clothing constricts circulation, such as at the waist and wrists.)

Have you noticed any swelling in your neck, armpits, or groin? If so, are the swollen areas sore, hard, or red? Do they appear on one or both sides?
(RATIONALE: Lymphadenopathy may signal inflammation, infection, or elevated lymphocyte production associated with certain leukemias. Primary lymphatic tumors usually are not painful; tender, red, swollen lymph nodes may occur in Hodgkin's disease.)

Do you ever feel tired? If so, are you tired all the time or only after exertion? Do you
need frequent naps, or do you sleep an unusually long time at night?
(RATIONALE: Fatigue is a prominent symptom of many hematologic disorders. The change may be subtle [the client requires a bit more sleep at night] or dramatic [the client can no longer climb a flight of stairs comfortably or requires a longer time to do so]. The client may complain of *always* feeling tired.)

Do you ever feel weak? If so, are you weak all the time or only at certain times? Does weakness ever interfere with your ability to perform your usual daily tasks, such as cooking or driving a car?
(RATIONALE: Although weakness is different from fatigue, these symptoms often occur together in a client with immune or blood disorders. Exertional fatigue and weakness suggest moderate anemia; constant or extreme fatigue and weakness, severe anemia or neuropathy from an autoimmune disorder. *Note:* Instead of reporting weakness, the client may complain of heavy extremities, "as if my ankles and wrists had weights around them.")

Have you had a fever recently? If so, how high was it? Was it constant or intermittent? Did it follow any particular pattern?
(RATIONALE: A fever that recurs every few days (for example, Pel-Ebstein fever) may indicate Hodgkin's disease; a temperature that rises and falls within 24 hours suggests an infection. Frequently recurring fevers may signal immune system impairment or rapid blood cell proliferation.)

Do you ever have joint pain? If so, which joints are affected? Do swelling, redness, or warmth accompany the pain? Do your bones ache?
(RATIONALE: Pain in the knees, wrists, or hands may indicate an autoimmune process or hemarthrosis [blood in a joint] from a blood disorder. Pain accompanied by swelling, redness, or warmth typically suggests inflammation, which may be relieved by heat application or salicylates. Aching bones may result from the pressure of expanding bone marrow [from blood cell proliferation and subsequent crowding].)

Have you noticed any change in your skin's texture, color, or other characteristics?
(RATIONALE: Hard, thickened skin may indicate scleroderma; dry skin, Hashimoto's disease; sallow skin, SLE.)

Have you noticed any sores that heal slowly?
(RATIONALE: With too few white blood cells [WBCs] to control infection and promote healing, a client may have delayed wound healing from compromised hematopoietic or immune functions.)

Are you bothered by a persistent or recurrent cough or cold? Do you cough up sputum? Do you feel chest pain when you cough, breathe deeply, or laugh?
(RATIONALE: Immunodeficiency increases the risk of persistent or recurrent respiratory infections, especially pneumonia. Sputum color and consistency may suggest the underlying disorder. For example, greenish sputum suggests bacterial infection; rust-colored sputum suggests pneumococcal pneumonia. Pleuritic pain [a sharp, knife-like pain that increases with coughing, deep breathing, or laughing] commonly occurs with pneumonia.)

Have you vomited recently? If so, how would you describe the vomitus?
(RATIONALE: Hematemesis [vomiting blood] may produce bright red, brown, or black vomitus that is the color and consistency of coffee grounds. This sign may be caused by thrombocytopenia or a clotting factor disorder.)

Have you noticed any blood in your bowel movements or have you had any black, tarry bowel movements? Do you experience any discomfort when defecating?
(RATIONALE: Hematochezia [passing bloody stools] can cause bright red, blood-streaked, or dark-colored stools. It may be caused by thrombocytopenia or a clotting factor deficiency. It may also result from tears in the rectal mucosa caused by straining or hemorrhoidal irritation. In either case, the rectal mucosa is predisposed to infection in the client with an immune or blood disorder because macrophages that normally inhabit the area are absent.)

Have you noticed any change in how your urine looks or in your urination pattern?
(RATIONALE: The urine may appear pink or grossly bloody from bladder capillary hemorrhages in a client who has a coagulation disorder. It may appear cloudy and malodorous in a client who has an external genitalia inflammation caused by a WBC deficiency, immunodeficiency, or a urinary tract infection. Such a client may also experience changes in usual urinary patterns, such as nocturia [urination at night], dysuria [painful urination], urinary frequency, urinary urgency, or urinary incontinence.)

Do you have any difficulty walking, or do you experience a pins-and-needles sensation?
(RATIONALE: These neurologic effects may result from pernicious anemia.)

Have you recently suffered from emotional instability, headaches, irritability, or depression?
(RATIONALE: These effects commonly occur with SLE and other chronic immune disorders.)

Did you have sore throats frequently in the past?
(RATIONALE: Frequent sore throats suggest poor immune response to infecting organisms.)

Do you recall being seriously ill as a child or having a long illness requiring frequent visits to a physician?
(RATIONALE: Information about childhood illnesses can provide clues to immune or blood disorders. For example, Hodgkin's lymphoma, sarcoma, and acute lymphocytic leukemia, which occur mostly in childhood and adolescence, require aggressive bone marrow suppression therapy with drugs or radiation. Some chemotherapeutic agents, known as alkylating agents, may induce bone marrow dysfunction or leukemia.)

Do you have any allergies? If so, what causes them and which symptoms are most bothersome?
(RATIONALE: Multiple allergies to foods, drugs, insects, or environmental pollutants are common. A description of the allergic reaction symptoms helps differentiate between a food intolerance or an adverse drug reaction and a true allergic reaction that indicates an immune system dysfunction.)

Have you ever had asthma?
(RATIONALE: A history of asthma may indicate immunopathology.)

Do you have an immune disease, such as acquired immunodeficiency syndrome (AIDS)? Have you tested positive for human immunodeficiency virus (HIV)?
(RATIONALE: An immune disease history may mean the client is predisposed to other diseases because the immune system does not function properly.)

Have you had any other disorders or health problems?
(RATIONALE: Hepatitis or tuberculosis promote bone marrow failure. Liver failure or cirrhosis can disrupt normal production of prothrombin and fibrinogen needed for blood coagulation. A history of peptic ulcer with excessive bleeding may suggest anemia.)

Have you ever had surgery? If so, what kind and when? What follow-up care did you receive?
(RATIONALE: Surgery can exert a negative effect on the immune system and blood. For example, gastric surgery can contribute to malabsorption of nutrients and vitamins needed for blood formation. A splenectomy places the client at increased risk for disseminated infection.)

Have you had an organ transplant?
(RATIONALE: Organ transplants usually require prolonged treatment with immunosuppressant agents to prevent organ rejection. Such therapy compromises the immune system, predisposing the client to numerous disorders, such as infections and lymphoreticular cancers.)

Have you ever had a blood transfusion? If so, when? How many units did you receive?
(RATIONALE: Blood products can transmit infectious agents, such as hepatitis virus [non-A, non-B, and B], cytomegalovirus, plasmodia that cause malaria, and the Epstein-Barr virus. Donor blood has been screened for hepatitis B for many years. Donor blood is now screened for HIV, which causes AIDS, but before March 1985, it was not routinely tested and could have transmitted this virus.)

Have you ever been rejected as a blood donor?
(RATIONALE: A blood donation refusal may stem from chronic anemia or a history of hepatitis or jaundice from an unknown cause.)

How would you describe the health of your blood relatives? How old are your living relatives? How old were those who died? What caused their deaths? Do or did any of them have immune, blood, or other problems of the kinds we have discussed?
(RATIONALE: Several blood and immune disorders are transmitted genetically, such as hemophilia, sickle cell anemia, and hemolytic anemia. To determine the client's risk for developing such disorders, trace the occurrence of these disorders on a family genogram.)

Pediatric client
Involve the child who is old enough in the interview. For an infant or young child, direct your questions to the parent or guardian.
Is the infant breast-fed or bottle-fed? If the infant is bottle-fed, what type of formula do you use?
(RATIONALE: Breast-feeding introduces immunoglobulins into the infant's GI tract, conferring some immunity. If the infant is bottle-fed, the formula should be iron-fortified to prevent anemia.)

Does your child ever seem pale or lethargic? Does the child sleep too much? Has the child been gaining weight at a normal rate?
(RATIONALE: Pallor, lethargy, fatigue, and failure to gain weight are common signs of anemia.)

Did the mother have any obstetric bleeding complications? Was parental blood Rh compatible?
(RATIONALE: Obstetric bleeding complications or Rh incompatibility of the parents may lead to clotting disorders in the child.)

Does the child have frequent or continuous severe infections?
(RATIONALE: Constant severe infections may suggest thymic deficiency or bone marrow dysfunction.)

Does the child have any allergies? If so, to what? Does anyone else in the family have allergies?
(RATIONALE: Children are more susceptible to allergies than adults, but a family history of infections and allergic or autoimmune disorders may suggest a pattern of immunodeficiencies.)

Which immunizations has the child received?
(RATIONALE: Immunizations can prevent many common communicable diseases. However, immunization timing is important. Every effort should be made to follow the recommended immunization schedule.)

Elderly client
Do you have any difficulty using your hands?
(RATIONALE: Weakness and numbness in the hands and impaired fine finger movement may suggest a blood disorder, such as anemia. Joint pain in the hands and other areas may indicate an autoimmune disorder, such as rheumatoid arthritis.)

Do you ever have headaches, faintness, vertigo, ringing in the ears, or confusion?
(RATIONALE: These symptoms are especially probable in an elderly client with anemia.)

Have you ever had arthritis, osteomyelitis, or tuberculosis?
(RATIONALE: These disorders can predispose the client to anemia related to chronic illness.)

Health promotion and protection patterns

What is your typical daily diet? What types and amounts of food do you eat at each meal? What do you eat between meals?
(RATIONALE: Certain foods, such as beef, liver, milk, and kidney beans, contain iron, vitamin B_{12}, and folic acid—the nutrients required for red blood cell [RBC] development. A diet lacking these foods may lead to anemia. Inadequate caloric and protein intake alter the immune response by compromising antibody formation, antigen recognition and processing, and phagocytosis. When this happens, the client runs a higher risk of developing infections.)

Do you drink alcoholic beverages? If so, what kind, how much, and how often do you drink?
(RATIONALE: Alcohol, especially when combined with decreased food intake, may cause folic acid-deficiency anemia.)

How would you rate your stress level? In the past 2 years, have you experienced death of a loved one, a job change, divorce, marriage, or other major change?
(RATIONALE: Persistently high levels of stress can reduce the client's resistance to infection. Researchers are exploring the possible connection between high stress and immune system suppression.)

Have you ever used intravenous (I.V.) drugs? If so, which ones and under what conditions?
(RATIONALE: All I.V. drugs compromise intact skin, one of the body's first defenses against invasion by microorganisms. However, illegal I.V. drugs are most likely to be unsanitary, which promotes transmission of such infectious agents as HIV or hepatitis virus.)

Have you ever been in military service? If so, when and where did you serve?
(RATIONALE: A client who served in Vietnam in the 1960s may have been exposed to such dioxin-containing defoliants as Agent Orange. These agents may be oncogenic and are linked to the development of leukemia and lymphoma.)

What type of work do you do? In what kind of environment do you work?
(RATIONALE: On the job, many workers are exposed to substances that increase the risk of blood and immune disorders.)

Role and relationship patterns

Are you sexually active? If so, are you involved in a monogamous relationship?
(RATIONALE: A client who has multiple sexual partners may acquire or transmit infectious organisms, such as HIV. Barrier contraceptives, such as condoms, are effective in reducing this risk.)

Have you noticed any change in your usual pattern of sexual functioning? If so, can you describe this change?
(RATIONALE: Any chronic illness or pain can profoundly affect sexual performance and satisfaction. For example, anemia may cause such severe cellular hypoxia and fatigue that the client has loss of sexual desire or difficulty with erection or ejaculation.)

What is your sexual preference? Do you or have you engaged in anal intercourse?
(RATIONALE: The AIDS virus can be transmitted by intimate sexual contact, especially that associated with the rectal mucosal trauma that occurs during anal intercourse.)

PHYSICAL ASSESSMENT

To assess the client's immune system and blood, the nurse evaluates factors that reflect changes (for example, vital signs); related body structure status (for example, the skin and respiratory system); and, of course, the lymph nodes (the only accessible immune system organs). Often nonspecific, the initial complaints and findings may involve several body systems.

The nurse uses the following equipment and techniques when assessing the immune system and blood.

Equipment
- flashlight
- ruler
- nonstretchable tape measure
- gown and drapes

Techniques
- inspection
- palpation
- percussion
- auscultation

Assessing related body structures

Because signs and symptoms of immune and blood disorders typically are nonspecific, begin the assessment by observing the client's general physical appearance. Look for signs of acute illness, such as grimacing or profuse perspiration, and of chronic illness, such as emaciation and listlessness.

Your assessment must also include vital signs and physical effects in such areas as the skin, hair, nails, head and neck, eyes and ears, respiratory system, cardiovascular system, GI system, urinary system, nervous system, and musculoskeletal system.

Vital signs. Elevated temperature suggests infection; tachycardia could be related to anemia or bleeding; tachypnea could be related to a disorder that compromises the blood's oxygen-carrying capacity; orthostatic hypotension could be related to hypovolemia or infection.

Skin. Pallor may be related to anemia or another blood disorder that disrupts oxygen delivery. Pallor and jaundice may accompany hemolytic anemia. Petechiae or ecchymoses may indicate a bleeding disorder, such as thrombocytopenia. A butterfly-shaped rash over the nose and cheeks may indicate SLE; palpable, nonpainful, purplish lesions on the lower extremities may be Kaposi's sarcoma, which occurs with AIDS.

Hair. Alopecia on the arms, legs, or head or broken hairs above the forehead occur in SLE.

Nails. Pale nail beds may reflect compromised oxygen-carrying capacity (in anemia). Longitudinal striations also indicate anemia. Koilonychia (spoon-shaped nails) may occur in a client with iron-deficiency anemia. Onycholysis (nail separation from the nail bed) may result from Hashimoto's disease. In fact, the nail angle may change from 160 degrees to 180 degrees or more. This abnormality, known as finger clubbing, indicates chronic hypoxia, which sometimes occurs with an immune or blood disorder.

Head and neck. Nasal mucosa ulceration may indicate SLE. Pale, boggy turbinates suggest chronic allergy. Red mucous membranes suggest polycythemia; petechiae and ecchymoses suggest bleeding disorders. Fluffy white patches scattered throughout the mouth may be candidiasis, a fungal infection. Lacy white plaques on the buccal mucosa may be caused by hairy leukoplakia, associated with AIDS. Such lesions occur in a client who who has immunosuppressive disorders or who receives chemotherapy. Gingival swelling, redness, oozing, bleeding, or ulcerations can signal bleeding disorders. The tongue may appear smooth and beefy red in folic-acid deficiency states or enlarged in Hashimoto's disease and multiple myeloma. It may lack papillae in pernicious anemia.

Eyes. The client with myasthenia gravis may exhibit transient eye muscle weakness, especially when fatigued. Conjunctival pallor may accompany anemia or a bleeding disorder. Scleral icterus may occur with blood disorders that cause jaundice—for example, hemolytic anemia—or with liver dysfunction, and may be noted before skin color changes. Drooping eyelids occur in myasthenia gravis, and swelling, redness, or lesions are signs of infection or inflammation. Ophthalmoscopic inspection revealing vessel tortuosity may indicate sickle cell anemia; hemorrhage or infiltration may point to hemorrhagic leukemia, vasculitis, or thrombocytopenia.

Ears. Hearing acuity is reduced in Hashimoto's disease. Otoscopic examination of the tympanic membrane revealing erythema, bulging, indistinct landmarks, and a displaced light reflex may indicate otitis media, an infection that may affect a client with an immune disorder.

Assessment checklist

The nurse should ask herself or himself these questions before beginning the assessment:
- ☐ Have I gathered all the necessary equipment?
- ☐ Have I washed my hands?
- ☐ Have I asked health history questions pertaining to many different systems to cover the immune system and blood?
- ☐ Have I reviewed all relevant laboratory data?

Respiratory system. During an asthma attack, the client may sit up to use every accessory muscle of respiration. Chest expansion may be limited in a client with scleroderma. Exertional dyspnea, tachypnea, and orthopnea (difficulty breathing except in an upright position) commonly accompany the cardiac effort needed to supply oxygen to hypoxic tissues. On chest percussion, a dull sound indicates consolidation, which may occur with pneumonia; hyperresonance may result from trapped air, which occurs with bronchial asthma. Wheezing suggests asthma or an allergic response. Crackles may denote a respiratory infection, such as pneumonia, which may affect a client with an immunodeficiency.

Cardiovascular system. The point of maximal impulse (PMI), normally located in the fifth intercostal space at the midclavicular line, may be broadened, displaced, or less distinct because of ventricular enlargement, the body's compensatory mechanism for severe anemia. Any auscultated apical systolic murmurs may signify severe anemia; mitral, aortic, and pulmonic murmurs, sickle cell anemia; pericardial friction rub, endocarditis or pericardial effusion—which occurs in about 50% of clients with SLE. Raynaud's phenomenon (intermittent arteriolar vasospasm of the fingers or toes and sometimes of the ears and nose), which may be caused by SLE or scleroderma, produces blanching in the affected area followed by cyanosis, pallor, and then, reddening. Weak, irregular peripheral pulses may indicate anemia.

GI system. In autoimmune disorders that cause diarrhea, such as ulcerative colitis, bowel sounds increase. In scleroderma and in autoimmune disorders that cause constipation, bowel sounds decrease. Hepatomegaly (liver enlargement) may accompany many immune disorders, such as hemolytic anemia. An enlarged liver that feels smooth and tender suggests hepatitis; one that feels hard and nodular suggests a neoplasm. Hepatomegaly may occur in immune disorders that cause congestion by blood cell overproduction or by excessive demand for cell destruction. Abdominal tenderness may result from infections, commonly seen in clients with immunodeficiency disorders.

Urinary system. Normal urine appears clear and amber or straw colored. Slightly aromatic, it may look pink or grossly bloody from bladder capillary hemorrhages in a client with a coagulation disorder. Cloudy, malodorous urine may result from a urinary tract infection. In a client with a WBC deficiency or immunodeficiency, the external genitalia may be focal points for inflammation. Discharge or bleeding related to infection may be noted, too.

Nervous system. Impaired neurologic function may occur secondary to hypoxia, fever, or, more drastically, from intracranial hemorrhage related to a coagulation defect. Thus, an anemic client may not be able to concentrate or may become confused; this likelihood increases for an elderly client. Hemorrhage also compromises oxygen supply to nerve tissues, resulting in similar symptoms. If bleeding occurs within the cranial vault, disorientation, progressive loss of consciousness, changes in motor and sensory capabilities, changes in pupillary responses, and seizures may result. (These responses depend on the hemorrhage site.) Other neurologic effects may occur in a client with an immune disorder. For example, a client with SLE may experience altered mentation, depression, or psychosis; a client with rheumatoid arthritis may have peripheral neuropathies, such as numbness or tingling of fingers.

Musculoskeletal system. Autoimmune disorders, such as SLE, rheumatoid arthritis, and hemarthrosis, can limit range of motion and cause joint enlargement. If palpation reveals bone tenderness in the sternum, the cause may be bone marrow hyperactivity, a compensatory mechanism for oxygen-carrying deficits prevalent in anemias. Bone tenderness may also result from a leukemic or immunoproliferative disorder, such as plasma cell myeloma, that causes cell packing in the marrow. Skeletal pain also may be from direct disease invasion of the marrow in some leukemias or immunoproliferative disorders—for example, plasma cell myeloma.

Inspecting the lymph nodes

● The first step in regional lymph node assessment is to inspect areas where the client reports "swollen glands" or "lumps" for color abnormalities and visible lymph node enlargement. Then inspect all other nodal regions. Proceed from head to toe to avoid missing any region. Normally, lymph nodes cannot be seen.

Palpating the lymph nodes

● When assessing a client for signs of an immune or blood disorder, the nurse should palpate the superficial lymph nodes of the head and neck, axillary, epitrochlear, inguinal, and popliteal areas, using the pads of the index and middle fingers. Always palpate gently; begin with light pressure and gradually increase the pressure.

Head and neck node palpation

● Head and neck nodes are best palpated with the client in a sitting position.

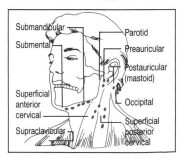

Submandibular
Submental
Superficial anterior cervical
Supraclavicular
Parotid
Preauricular
Postauricular (mastoid)
Occipital
Superficial posterior cervical

• To palpate the preauricular, parotid, and mastoid nodes, position your fingers as shown.

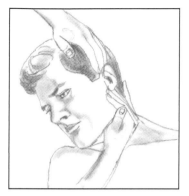

• To palpate the submandibular, submental, anterior cervical, and occipital nodes, position your fingers as shown. Palpate over the mandibular surface and continue moving up and down the entire neck. Flex the head forward or to the side being examined. This relaxes the tissues and makes enlarged nodes more palpable. Reverse your hand position to palpate the opposite side.

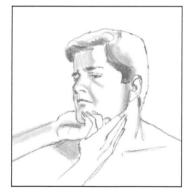

• To palpate the supraclavicular nodes, encourage the client to relax so the clavicles drop. To relax the soft tissues of the anterior neck, flex the client's head slightly forward with your free hand. Then hook your left index finger over the clavicle lateral to the sternocleidomastoid muscle. Rotate your fingers deeply into this area to feel these nodes.

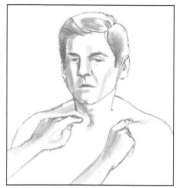

• To palpate the posterior cervical nodes and spinal nerve chain, place your fingertip pads along the anterior surface of the trapezius muscle. Then move your fingertips toward the posterior surface of the sternocleidomastoid muscle.

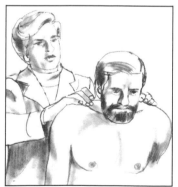

Axillary and epitrochlear node palpation

• Axillary and epitrochlear nodes are best palpated with the client in a sitting position. Axillary nodes may also be palpated with the client lying supine.

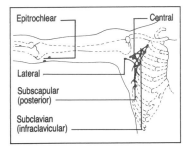

- To palpate the axillary nodes, use your nondominant hand to support the client's relaxed right arm, and put your other hand as high in the client's right axilla as possible.

Then palpate the axillary nodes, gently pressing the soft tissues against the chest wall and the muscles surrounding the axilla. Repeat this procedure for the left axilla.

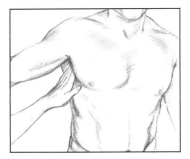

- To palpate the epitrochlear lymph nodes, place your fingertips in the depression above and posterior to the medial area of the elbow and palpate gently.

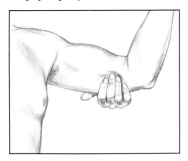

Inguinal and popliteal node palpation

- Inguinal and popliteal nodes are best palpated with the client lying supine. Popliteal nodes may also be assessed with the client sitting or standing.

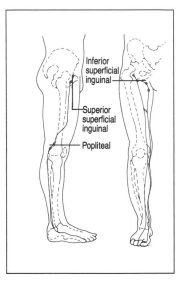

- To palpate the inferior superficial inguinal (femoral) lymph nodes, gently press below the junction of the saphenous and femoral veins.

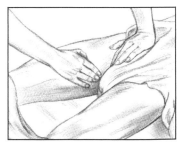

- To palpate the superior superficial inguinal lymph nodes, press along the course of the saphenous veins from the inguinal area to the abdomen.

(Text continues on page 232.)

Common laboratory studies

For a client with signs and symptoms of an immune or blood disorder, various laboratory studies can provide the nurse with valuable clues to the possible cause. This chart lists common laboratory studies along with normal values or findings. Remember that values differ among laboratories, and check the normal value range for the specific laboratory.

TEST	NORMAL VALUES OR FINDINGS
Bone marrow test	
Bone marrow aspiration	*Normoblasts, total* Adult: 25.6% Child: 23.1% Infant: 8%
	Neutrophils, total Adult: 56.5% Child: 57.1% Infant: 32.4%
	Eosinophils Adult: 3.1% Child: 3.6% Infant: 2.6%
	Basophils Adult: 0.01% Child: 0.06% Infant: 0.07%
	Lymphocytes Adult: 16.2% Child: 16% Infant: 49%
	Plasma cells Adult: 1.3% Child: 0.4% Infant: 0.02%
	Megakaryocytes Adult: 0.1% Child: 0.1% Infant: 0.05%
	Myeloiderythroid ratio Adult: 2:3 Child: 2:9 Infant: 4:4

continued

Common laboratory studies continued

TEST	NORMAL VALUES OR FINDINGS
Blood tests	
Peripheral blood smear	Anucleated biconcave RBC disks 6 to 8 microns in diameter and uniform in size, shape, and staining characteristics
Complete blood count (CBC)	*Erythrocyte (RBC) count* Man: 4.5 to 6.2 million/mm³ Woman: 4.2 to 5.4 million/mm³ Child: 4.6 to 4.8 million/mm³ Full-term neonate: 4.4 to 5.8 million/mm³
	Hematocrit *(HCT or packed RBC volume)* Man: 42% to 54% Woman: 38% to 46% Child: 36% to 40% Neonate: 55% to 68%
	Hemoglobin (Hb) Man: 14 to 18 g/dl; 12.4 to 14.9 g/dl (after middle age) Woman: 12 to 16 g/dl; 11.7 to 13.8 g/dl (after middle age) Child: 11 to 13 g/dl Neonate: 17 to 22 g/dl
Red blood cell (RBC) indices	*Mean corpuscular volume (MCV)* 84 to 99 mcm³/RBC
	Mean corpuscular Hb (MCH) 26 to 32 pg/RBC
	Mean corpuscular Hb concentration (MCHC) 30% to 36%
Leukocyte (WBC) count	4,100 to 10,900/ mm³
Differential WBC count	*Neutrophils* 47.6% to 76.8%
	Eosinophils 0.3% to 7%
	Basophils 0.3% to 2%

Common laboratory studies continued

TEST	NORMAL VALUES OR FINDINGS
Differential WBC count continued	*Monocytes* 0.6% to 9.6%
	Lymphocytes 16.2% to 43%
Erythrocyte (osmotic) fragility	Normal curve as plotted against known normals
Erythrocyte sedimentation rate (ESR)	0 to 20 mm/hour Rates gradually increase with age.
Platelet (thrombocyte) count	130,000 to 370,000/mm³
Activated partial thromboplastin time (APTT)	25 to 36 seconds
Prothrombin time (PT)	Male: 9.6 to 11.8 seconds Female: 9.5 to 11.3 seconds
Plasma thrombin time (thrombin clotting time)	10 to 15 seconds
Plasma fibrinogen (Factor I)	195 to 365 mg/dl
Fibrin split products (fibrinogen degradation products, FDP)	*Screening assay* <10 mcg/ml
	Quantitative assay <3 mcg/ml
Direct antiglobulin test (DAGT, direct Coombs' test)	Negative (neither antibodies nor complement appear on RBCs)
Immunoelectrophoresis	*IgG* 6.4 to 14.3 mg/ml
	IgA 0.3 to 3 mg/ml
	IgM 0.2 to 1.4 mg/ml
Enzyme-linked immunosorbent assay (ELISA)	Negative for antibodies

• To palpate the popliteal nodes, press gently along the posterior muscles at the back of the knee.

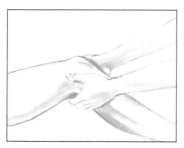

Advanced assessment skills: Spleen percussion and palpation

• To assess the spleen—an advanced assessment skill—the nurse can use percussion to estimate its size and palpation to detect tenderness and enlargement.

• Percuss the lowest intercostal space in the left anterior axillary line; percussion notes should be tympanic.

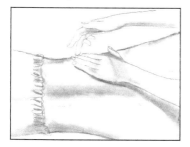

• Ask the client to take a deep breath, then percuss this area again. If the spleen is normal in size, the area will remain tympanic. If the tympanic percussion note changes on inspiration to dullness, the spleen is probably enlarged.

• To estimate spleen size, outline the spleen's edges by percussing in several directions from areas of tympany to areas of dullness.

• Stand on the right side of the supine client. Then reach across the client to support the posterior lower left rib cage with your left hand. Place your right hand below the left costal margin and press inward.

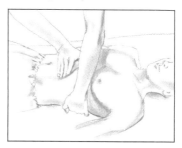

• Instruct the client to take a deep breath. The spleen normally should not descend on deep inspiration below the ninth or tenth intercostal space in the posterior midaxillary line. If the spleen is enlarged, you will feel its rigid border. Do not overpalpate the spleen; an enlarged spleen can rupture easily.

DOCUMENTATION

The SOAPIE method of documentation includes the following components: subjective (history) data, objective (physical) data, assessment, planning, implementation, and evaluation. The following example shows how to document nursing care for a client with chronic fatigue.

Case history

Ms. Delaney, age 38, who was admitted to the hospital this morning, is an unmarried, white woman who enjoyed good health until 3 weeks ago when she began to suffer chronic fatigue. She lives alone and works as a real estate broker.

S	O	A	P	I	E

Client states, "I'm tired all the time. I have to make an effort to go to work each morning." Client reports recent prolonged menses lasting 9 days; intermittent, localized, dull sternal pain; and poor appetite; 15-lb weight loss over past 3 weeks. Client denies recent acute illness, headache, and dyspnea.

Selected nursing diagnosis categories

The nurse can use these diagnosis categories to formulate nursing diagnoses for a client with an immune system or blood problem.
- Activity intolerance
- Decreased cardiac output
- High risk for altered body temperature
- High risk for infection
- High risk for injury
- Impaired adjustment
- Impaired skin integrity
- Impaired tissue integrity
- Ineffective individual coping

SUGGESTED READINGS

Corbett, J. (1993). Interpreting the immunoglobulins. *American Journal of Nursing*, 93(3), 16F-16H.

Gawlikowski, J. (1992). White cells at war. *American Journal of Nursing*, 92(3), 44-51.

Holzemer, W. (1992). Nursing effectiveness research and patient outcomes: A challenge for the second HIV/AIDS decade. *Critical Care Nursing Clinics of North America*, 4(3), 429-435.

Ungvarski, P., and Schmidt, J. (1992). AIDS patients under attack ... opportunistic infections. *RN*, 55(11), 36-45.

S   **O**   A   P   I   E

Temperature 100° F., pulse 100 and regular, respirations 22 and regular, blood pressure 126/84. CBC: HCT 29%, Hb 10 g/dl. Pale skin with scattered, bilateral ecchymoses on legs and petechiae on upper arm, around waist, and under breasts bilaterally. Markedly red and inflamed gingivae. Petechiae on buccal mucosa.

S   O   **A**   P   I   E

High risk for infection related to alteration in protective mechanisms. Client appears pale and lethargic. CBC results show low hemoglobin and hematocrit.

S   O   A   **P**   I   E

Teach client how to prevent infection. Also teach family and friends to avoid infecting the client. Teach client to use soft toothbrush. Monitor laboratory results.

S   O   A   P   **I**   E

Instructed client about personal hygiene techniques that reduce infection risk. Monitor blood transfusion ordered by physician.

S   O   A   P   I   **E**

Client demonstrates regular use of soft toothbrush.

18

Endocrine System

The endocrine system, together with the nervous system, regulates important body functions, including growth and development of body tissue, reproduction, energy production, metabolism, and the ability to adapt to stress. For this reason, endocrine dysfunction can affect virtually every body system and profoundly influence a person's health and sense of well-being.

HEALTH HISTORY

When collecting health history information about a client's endocrine function, the nurse should keep in mind that endocrine system components function interdependently with each other and with other body organs. Therefore, assessment requires a holistic approach. Complaints related to endocrine dysfunction may result from, or be the cause of, problems in other body systems. Often, the systemic effects of endocrine dysfunction are readily apparent, related to the effects of hormone deficiency or excess regardless of the cause or location of the original defect. Sometimes, however, endocrine dysfunction manifests itself in nonspecific ways—particularly in early phases. The nurse also should remember that endocrine problems can alter a client's life-style dramatically. For example, a client with diabetes mellitus must make lifelong adjustments to maintain blood glucose levels

within normal limits; a young woman with Cushing's syndrome may have difficulty coping with her altered appearance.

Three groups of sample questions follow. Those on *health and illness patterns* help the nurse identify actual or potential endocrine-related health problems; those on *health promotion and protection patterns* help the nurse determine how the client's life-style and behavior may affect endocrine system function; and those on *role and relationship patterns* help the nurse determine how the problem affects the client's self-image and relationships with others.

Health and illness patterns

Do you feel tired, lethargic, or weak?
(RATIONALE: Decreased energy level may result from hypopituitarism, hypothyroidism, or altered blood glucose levels from excessive or insufficient insulin.)

If you feel weak, is the weakness generalized or confined to a specific area or areas?
(RATIONALE: Generalized weakness occurs in various endocrine disorders, including diabetes mellitus, hyperparathyroidism, and Addison's disease. Weakness in a specific area seldom results from an endocrine disorder.)

Have you noticed any muscle twitching?
(RATIONALE: Muscle twitching may result from increased secretion of antidiuretic hormone or decreased secretion of parathormone or aldosterone.)

Do you feel any numbness or tingling in your arms or legs?
(RATIONALE: These sensations may indicate sensory peripheral neuropathy, an abnormal condition characterized by biochemical abnormalities and degeneration of the peripheral nerves that often occurs in diabetes mellitus.)

Have you recently gained or lost weight unintentionally? If so, how much and over what time period?
(RATIONALE: Weight gain may result from hypothyroidism, syndrome of inappropriate antidiuretic hormone [SIADH] secretion, or Cushing's syndrome. Weight loss may be seen in panhypopituitarism, hyperthyroidism, Addison's disease, and hyperglycemia.)

Have you recently experienced any changes in your normal behavior, such as nervousness or mood swings?
(RATIONALE: Endocrine disorders that alter thyroid hormone, insulin, or corticosteroid levels can alter behavior and cause emotional lability.)

How would you rate your memory and attention span?
(RATIONALE: Memory loss can result from hypothyroidism or hypoparathyroidism; shortened attention span, from hyperthyroidism or hyperparathyroidism.)

Have you noticed an increase in the amount of urine you pass, or have you been feeling unusually thirsty lately?
(RATIONALE: Increased urination [polyuria] and increased thirst [polydipsia] are classic signs of diabetes mellitus and diabetes insipidis.)

Do you often feel hot or cold when other people in the same room are comfortable?
(RATIONALE: Heat intolerance often is associated with hyperthyroidism; cold intolerance, with hypothyroidism.)

Have you ever had radiation treatments? If so, what for?
(RATIONALE: Radiation exposure can cause endocrine glands to atrophy, resulting in dysfunction.)

Have you ever had a brain infection, such as meningitis or encephalitis?
(RATIONALE: These infections can cause hypothalamic disturbances, which can disrupt the hypothalamic-pituitary-target gland axis.)

What was your growth pattern? Were you considered tall or short for your age? Did you have any growth spurts? If so, when and to what degree?
(RATIONALE: A slow growth rate could indicate hypopituitarism or hypothyroidism; a rapid growth rate, hyperpituitarism, hyperthyroidism, or gonadal hormone excess.)

Have you ever been diagnosed as having an endocrine, or glandular, problem? If so, what was the problem, when was it diagnosed, and how has it been treated?
(RATIONALE: Most endocrine disorders are chronic, requiring lifelong treatment.)

Does anyone in your family have diabetes mellitus, thyroid disease, hypertension (high blood pressure) or elevated blood fats?
(RATIONALE: Diabetes mellitus [particularly Type II] and thyroid disease show familial tendencies. Pheochromocytoma, a rare tumor of the adrenal medulla that secretes excessive amounts of catecholamines and elevates blood pressure, may result from an autosomal dominant trait. Lipid abnormalities are often inherited.)

Have you noticed any changes in your skin, such as acne, increased or decreased oiliness or dryness, or changes in color?
(RATIONALE: Many endocrine problems produce cutaneous manifestations. For example, in adults, acne may result from Cushing's syndrome. Increased oiliness may be related to acromegaly or androgen excess. Dry, thick skin may result from hypothyroidism; scaly skin, from hypoparathyroidism.)

Do you bruise more easily than you used to?
(RATIONALE: Abnormal susceptibility to bruising may be associated with hypothyroidism or Cushing's syndrome.)
(Text continues on page 238.)

Anatomy review

The illustrations below show the endocrine system glands in a male and in a female.

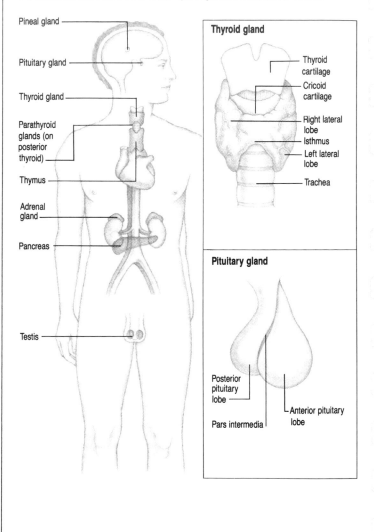

Pineal gland

Pituitary gland

Thyroid gland

Parathyroid glands (on posterior thyroid)

Thymus

Adrenal gland

Pancreas

Testis

Thyroid gland

Thyroid cartilage

Cricoid cartilage

Right lateral lobe

Isthmus

Left lateral lobe

Trachea

Pituitary gland

Posterior pituitary lobe

Pars intermedia

Anterior pituitary lobe

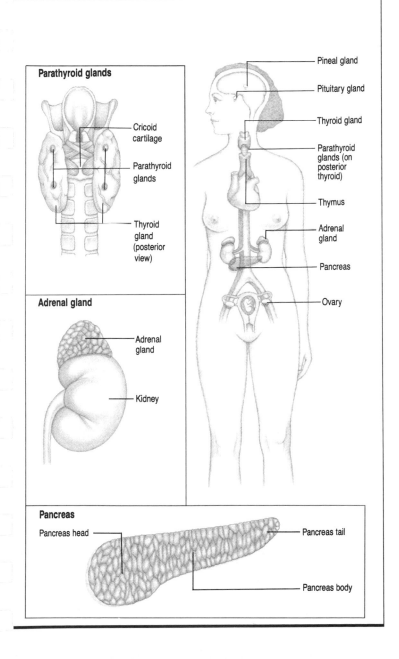

Parathyroid glands

Cricoid cartilage

Parathyroid glands

Thyroid gland (posterior view)

Adrenal gland

Adrenal gland

Kidney

Pineal gland

Pituitary gland

Thyroid gland

Parathyroid glands (on posterior thyroid)

Thymus

Adrenal gland

Pancreas

Ovary

Pancreas

Pancreas head

Pancreas tail

Pancreas body

Have you noticed any increase in the size of your hands or feet?
(RATIONALE: In adults, widening of the hand and foot bones may result from acromegaly.)

Do your fingernails and toenails seem brittle? Have they thickened or separated from your fingers and toes?
(RATIONALE: Nail brittleness may result from hypoparathyroidism or hypothyroidism. Separation of the distal end of the nail from the nail bed [onycholysis] may occur in hyperthyroidism.)

Have you noticed any change in the amount and distribution of your body hair?
(RATIONALE: An overall decrease in hair growth can be related to hyperthyroidism. In males, decreased axillary and pubic hair growth often points to androgen deficiency. In females, excessive androgen levels can cause increased axillary and facial hair growth and a masculine pubic hair pattern [hirsutism].)

Has your voice deepened or otherwise changed recently?
(RATIONALE: Vocal hoarseness can result from hypothyroidism. Deepening of the voice in females may indicate excess testosterone or, in both sexes, excess growth hormone.)

Are you experiencing any visual problems, especially double vision (diplopia) or blurred vision?
(RATIONALE: Diplopia may point to a pituitary adenoma putting pressure on the optic nerve or to Graves' ophthalmopathy, a disorder commonly associated with hyperthyroidism. Blurred vision can be an early sign of hyperglycemia.)

Do your eyes burn or feel "gritty" when you close them?
(RATIONALE: Such sensations often occur with exophthalmos [protruding eyeballs], a common manifestation of Graves' disease.)

Have you ever felt as though your heart was racing, even when you hadn't been exerting yourself?
(RATIONALE: Tachycardia [a heart rate in excess of 100 beats per minute] may be associated with hyperthyroidism, diabetes insipidus, or Addison's disease.)

Have you ever been told that you have high blood pressure?
(RATIONALE: Excessive catecholamine levels resulting from pheochromocytoma often cause episodic hypertension.)

Has your appetite increased or decreased recently?
(RATIONALE: Increased appetite [polyphagia] may indicate hyperthyroidism or diabetes mellitus. Decreased appetite [anorexia] often occurs in hypothyroidism and Addison's disease.)

Do you often experience constipation or diarrhea?
(RATIONALE: Constipation can result from hypopituitarism, hypothyroidism, decreased antidiuretic hormone [ADH], hyperparathyroidism, or pheochromocytoma. Frequent defecation often occurs in hyperthyroidism. Constipation may alternate with diarrhea in diabetic autonomic neuropathy.)

Do you have less interest in people, things, and activities that once interested you? Do you ever feel depressed for no particular reason?
(RATIONALE: Apathy and depression may be related to hypopituitarism, hypothyroidism, hyperthyroidism, or increased or decreased levels of ADH, glucocorticoids, insulin, or parathyroid hormone [PTH].)

Pediatric client

Pose these questions to the child's parent or guardian.

Have you ever been told that the child's growth and development are above or below normal rates?
(RATIONALE: Altered growth and development may indicate a disturbance in growth, thyroid, or gonadal hormone levels.)

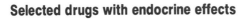

Selected drugs with endocrine effects

The commonly used drugs listed below may adversely affect the endocrine system.

ANTICONVULSANTS
- carbamazepine
- phenytoin

ANTIFUNGALS
- ketoconazole

ANTIHYPERTENSIVES
- clonidine hydrochloride
- methyldopa
- minoxidil

ANTINEOPLASTICS
- busulfan
- cyclophosphamide
- tamoxifen citrate
- vinblastine sulfate

ANTIPSYCHOTICS
- chlorpromazine hydrochloride
- haloperidol

BETA BLOCKERS
- atenolol
- labetalol hydrochloride
- metoprolol tartrate
- nadolol
- pindolol
- propranolol hydrochloride
- timolol maleate

CORTICOSTEROIDS
- methylprednisolone
- prednisone

DIURETICS
- bumetanide
- furosemide
- thiazides

ORAL CONTRACEPTIVES
- conjugated estrogens
- estrogen-progestin combinations

MISCELLANEOUS AGENTS
- chlorpropamide
- clofibrate
- lithium carbonate
- metoclopramide hydrochloride

Has the child had a recent history of weight loss and excessive thirst, hunger, and urination?
(RATIONALE: These classic signs of Type I diabetes mellitus commonly occur in children.)

Pregnant client

Have you ever been told you had diabetes during this or any previous pregnancy?
(RATIONALE: Women who have had gestational diabetes mellitus [diabetes associated only with pregnancy] have an increased risk of developing Type II diabetes mellitus later in life.)

Have you ever given birth to an infant weighing more than 10 lb (4.5 kg)?
(RATIONALE: A high-birth-weight infant may indicate a maternal predisposition to diabetes.)

Health promotion and protection patterns

What prescription drugs do you currently take?
(RATIONALE: Many drugs can increase or decrease hormone levels and cause endocrine system dysfunctions; some can mask signs

and symptoms of endocrine dysfunctions. For a list, see *Selected drugs with endocrine effects.*)

Have you been sleeping more or less than usual?
(RATIONALE: Sleep disturbances often occur in endocrine disorders. Disorders such as hyperthyroidism, Cushing's syndrome, pheochromocytoma, diabetes mellitus, and diabetes insipidus may lead to restlessness and insomnia or the inability to sleep related to nocturia.)

Have you been feeling under more stress lately? Can you talk about what may be causing this stress? Does your current problem seem to be related to this stress?
(RATIONALE: Many endocrine disorders, such as diabetes mellitus, can be exacerbated by stress. Also, treatment of certain endocrine disorders—for instance, diabetes mellitus, Addison's disease, and hypothyroidism—may require lifelong hormone replacement therapy and changes in life-style, which may increase stress.)

Role and relationship patterns

What is your image of yourself? Do you think that the problem you are experiencing will get better or worse? What bothers you most about this problem?

(RATIONALE: A client with an endocrine disorder often has a poor self-image related to such effects as altered metabolism, increased susceptibility to and inability to cope with stress, and disfigurement or disability.)

Do you have family members or close friends that you can ask for help when you need it?

(RATIONALE: A client receiving treatment for an endocrine disorder may need another person's help in administering prescribed medications, complying with life-style changes, or performing normal activities of daily living.)

Have you noticed any changes in your sexual interest or sexual functioning?

(RATIONALE: Changes in libido [psychic energy or instinctual drive associated with sexual drive or pleasure] may occur in hypothyroidism or acromegaly. Diabetes mellitus may cause impotence in males and dyspareunia in females.)

PHYSICAL ASSESSMENT

The nurse uses the following equipment and techniques when assessing the endocrine system.

Equipment
- tape measure
- scale
- stethoscope
- glass of water with a straw

Techniques
- inspection
- palpation
- auscultation

Assessing related body structures

Because of the interrelationship of the endocrine system with all other body systems, physical assessment of a client with a known or suspected endocrine problem must include a total body evaluation, focusing on the areas described in the following sections. It also must include a complete neurologic assessment because of the role of the hypothalamus in regulating endocrine function through the pituitary gland. (For detailed information on neurologic assessment steps, see Chapter 15, Nervous System.)

Vital signs, height, and weight. Vital sign changes may provide important clues to the presence and nature of an endocrine disorder. For example, hypertension develops in many endocrine disorders, particularly pheochromocytoma, Cushing's syndrome, and hyperthyroidism. Hypotension commonly occurs in hypothyroidism. Fever may be related to excessive glucocorticoid levels or insufficient insulin levels; hypothermia may develop in hypoglycemia. Bradycardia (a heart rate of less than 60 beats/minute) occurs in myxedema and hypopituitarism. Tachycardia occurs in thyroid tumors and hyperthyroidism.

Weight gain unexplained by overeating or lack of exercise may point to Cushing's syndrome or hypothyroidism. In Cushing's syndrome, excessive glucocorticoid secretion may trigger hyperinsulinemia, causing excessive fat deposition on the face, neck, and trunk. In hypothyroidism, a decreased thyroxin level slows metabolic rate and decreases nutrient use, leading to weight gain.

In children, height that is consistently above or below normal for a sustained time could point to an increase or decrease in growth hormone production by the anterior pituitary. When assessing a child, keep in mind that the normal growth rate averages roughly 3″ per year between ages 1 through 7, and 2″ per year between ages 8 through 15. Hypopituitary dwarfism related to growth hormone deficiency usually becomes apparent at about age 2.

In hyperthyroidism, an increased metabolic rate can accelerate the body's use of nutrients and lead to weight loss. Weight loss can also accompany uncontrolled diabetes mellitus as a result of osmotic diuresis and the inability to use ingested nutrients. A weight gain or loss of 2 to 3 pounds within 48 hours may result from altered ADH levels. Weight gain occurs from oversecretion of ADH; weight loss, from insufficient secretion with resultant alterations in fluid balance.

General appearance. Initial observation may identify the effects of a major endocrine disorder, such as hyperthyroidism or hypothyroidism, dwarfism, or acromegaly. Evaluation of the client's overall affect, clarity and quality of speech, and activity level may provide more insight. For example, a client with hyperthyroidism may speak rapidly, perhaps incoherently at times; a client with hypothyroidism may speak slowly and deliberately; and a client with myxedema may slur words and sound hoarse. In an adult male client, a high-pitched voice may point to hypogonadism; in an adult female, an abnormally deep voice may point to excessive androgen secretion related to Cushing's syndrome, acromegaly, congenital adrenal hyperplasia or tumors, polycystic ovaries, or ovarian tumors.

A client's body development also may provide important clues to the presence and nature of an endocrine problem. For example, an outward-curved spine (kyphosis) may indicate compression fractures related to osteoporosis, which often occurs with hyperparathyroidism. Osteoporosis also may manifest itself as a sharp angular deformity caused by collapsed vertebrae. In a client with Cushing's syndrome, fat deposits typically concentrate on the face (moon facies), neck, interscapular area (buffalo hump), trunk, and pelvic girdle. Thyroid hormone deficiency in infants (cretinism) is characterized by a stocky build.

Even the client's dress may provide clues to an endocrine problem. For instance, inappropriately heavy clothing in warm weather may indicate cold sensitivity from hypothyroidism, and a lack of outer garments in cold weather may indicate heat intolerance from hyperthyroidism.

Skin, hair, and nails. Hyperpigmentation of joints, genitalia, buccal mucosa, palmar creases, recent scars, and sun-exposed body areas occurs in most clients with Addison's

---

Assessment checklist

The nurse should ask herself or himself these questions before beginning the assessment:
☐ Have I gathered all the necessary equipment?
☐ Have I washed my hands?
☐ Have I reviewed all relevant laboratory data?

---

disease. In a client who has undergone adrenalectomy, this hyperpigmentation usually indicates an adrenocorticotropic hormone (ACTH)-producing pituitary tumor or may indicate growth hormone excess. Gray-brown pigmentation of the neck and axillae (acanthosis nigricans) may occur in a client with polycystic ovaries, growth hormone excess, or Cushing's syndrome. Yellow pigmentation in the palmar creases can indicate hyperlipidemia; a yellowish cast to the skin may point to hypothyroidism. An overall decrease in skin pigmentation typically occurs in panhypopituitarism.

Dry, coarse, rough, and scaly skin can indicate hypothyroidism or hypoparathyroidism. Coarse, leathery, moist skin and enlarged sweat glands usually occur in acromegaly. Warm, moist, tissue-thin skin may point to hyperthyroidism. In an adult client, acne frequently develops in Cushing's syndrome or from androgen excess. Yellowish nodules on extensor surfaces of the elbows and knees and on the buttocks typically occur in severe hypertriglyceridemia. Purple striae, typically on the abdomen, and bruises (ecchymoses) are common signs of Cushing's syndrome. Edema often occurs in hypothyroidism and Cushing's syndrome. Dry mucous membranes and poor skin turgor may occur in diabetes mellitus.

Coarse, dry, brittle hair usually is associated with hypothyroidism; fine, silky, thinly distributed hair, with hyperthyroidism. In an adult female client, excessive facial, chest, abdominal, or pubic hair (hirsutism) may point to growth hormone or androgen excess. Hair loss or thinning in the axillae, pubic area, and the outer third of the eyebrows may indicate hypopituitarism, hypothyroidism, or hypogonadism.

Thick, brittle nails may suggest hypothyroidism; thin, brittle nails may result from hyperthyroidism. Increased nail pigmentation occurs in Addison's disease.

Head and neck. Eyelid tremors may indicate hyperthyroidism. Eyeball protrusion (exophthalmos) and incomplete eyelid closure, usually bilateral, are associated with Graves' disease, a common cause of severe hyperthyroidism, or thyrotoxicosis. A visible increase in tongue size may indicate hypothyroidism or acromegaly; in acromegaly, an enlarged tongue may have a furrowed appearance. A fine, rhythmic tremor of the tongue may occur in hyperthyroidism; fine, fascicular (twitching) tremors, in hyperparathyroidism. A mass at the base of the anterior neck or a visible thyroid gland may indicate thyroid hyperplasia.

Chest. In an adult male client, gynecomastia may be related to hypogonadism, hypothyroidism, thyrotoxicosis, estrogen excess from an adrenal tumor, or Cushing's syndrome. (Keep in mind, however, that transient gynecomastia may develop during puberty.) In a nonlactating female, nipple discharge could indicate prolactin or estrogen excess, hypothyroidism, diabetes mellitus, or Cushing's syndrome. Breast (areolar) hyperpigmentation may accompany excess ACTH production, as in Cushing's disease or an ACTH-secreting pituitary tumor.

Genitalia. In an adult male, abnormally small testes suggest hypogonadism. In an adult female, an enlarged clitoris may indicate masculinization. Vaginitis may occur in uncontrolled diabetes mellitus.

Extremities. Muscle atrophy in the arms and legs usually occurs in Cushing's syndrome, hypothyroidism, and hyperthyroidism. A fine, rhythmic tremor of the

extremities also may occur in hyperthyroidism. Muscle atrophy between the thumb and index finger (thenar wasting) and contracture of the palmar fascia (Dupuytren's contracture) may develop in long-term diabetes mellitus. Abnormally large fingers and hands may indicate acromegaly; finger clubbing may be associated with thyroid abnormalities. In the lower legs, dependent redness or bluish coloration and absence of hair may indicate vascular insufficiency related to diabetes mellitus.

Palpating the thyroid

● Usually, you will not be able to palpate the client's thyroid, but you may feel the isthmus (center portion connecting the two lobes of the thyroid). You may, however, see or feel a normal thyroid in a client with an extremely thin neck.

● To palpate the thyroid from the front, face the client and locate the cricoid cartilage with the pads of your index and middle fingers. Ask the client to swallow as you palpate the thyroid isthmus just below the cricoid cartilage, using the same two fingers. (Swallowing raises the larynx, the trachea, and the thyroid gland, but not the lymph nodes or other structures.)

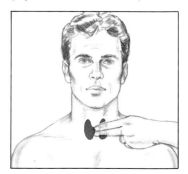

● To palpate the right lobe using the anterior approach, displace the client's trachea to the right with your right hand while you palpate with the fingers of your left hand. (See illustration on page 244.)

Common laboratory studies

For a client with signs and symptoms of an endocrine disorder, various laboratory studies can provide the nurse with valuable clues to the possible cause. This chart lists common laboratory studies along with their normal values or findings. Remember that values differ among laboratories, and check the normal range for the specific laboratory.

TEST	NORMAL VALUES OR FINDINGS
Blood tests	
Cortisol	*8 a.m.:* 7 to 28 mcg/dl *4 p.m.:* 2 to 18 mcg/dl (The 4 p.m. level is usually half the 8 a.m. level.)
Catecholamines 　Epinephrine, basal supine 　Epinephrine, standing 　Norepinephrine, basal supine 　Norephinephrine, standing	 30 to 95 pg/ml 0 to 140 pg/ml 70 to 750 pg/ml 15 to 475 pg/ml
Parathyroid hormone (PTH)	10 to 65 pg/ml
Total calcium	8.9 to 10.1 mg/dl
Phosphorus	2.5 to 4.5 mg/dl
Oral glucose tolerance test	160 to 180 mg/dl 30 to 60 min after oral glucose dose; fasting levels or lower in 2 to 3 hr
Glycosylated hemoglobin (GHB, glycohemoglobin)	5.5% to 9% of total hemoglobin
HGH radioimmunoassay (RIA)	*Males:* < 5 ng/ml *Females:* < 10 ng/ml
Insulin-induced hypoglycemia	Rise in growth hormone 2- to 3-fold over baseline
Thyroid stimulating hormone (TSH)	0.6 to 4.6 IU/ml
Gonadotropins (FSH, LH)	*Females* FSH: follicular phase, 5 to 20 mIU/ml; mid-cycle peak, 15 to 30 mIU/ml; luteal phase, 5 to 15 mIU/ml; postmenopausal, 50 to 100 mIU/ml LH: follicular phase, 5 to 25 mIU/ml; mid-cycle peak, 30 to 60 mIU/ml; luteal phase, 5 to 15 mIU/ml; postmenopausal > 50 mIU/ml *Males* FSH: 5 to 20 mIU/ml LH: 5 to 20 mIU/ml

continued

Common laboratory studies continued

TEST	NORMAL VALUES OR FINDINGS
T₄ RIA	4 to 11 mcg/dl
T₃ RIA	75 to 220 ng/dl
Urine studies	
Free cortisol	0 to 110 mcg/24 hr

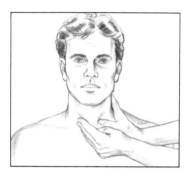

• Grasp the sternocleidomastoid muscle with your left hand (place the tips of your index and middle fingers behind the muscle, your thumb in front), and palpate for the posterior of the right lobe of the thyroid between your left fingers. To palpate the left lobe, use your left hand to move the thyroid cartilage and your right hand to palpate.

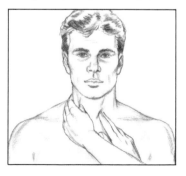

• To palpate the thyroid from behind the client, gently place the fingers of both hands on either side of the trachea, just below the cricoid cartilage. Ask the client to swallow as you palpate the thyroid isthmus.

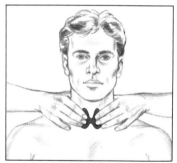

• Palpating one lobe at a time, ask the client to lower the chin and flex the neck slightly to the side you are assessing. To palpate the right lobe, place your left hand on the neck and move the thyroid cartilage to the right.

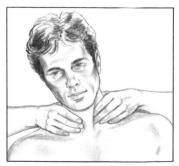

• Grasp the sternocleidomastoid muscle with your right hand, while placing your middle fingers deep into and in front of the muscle; palpate for the right border of the right lobe. For the left lobe, use your right hand to move the cartilage to the left and your left hand to palpate.

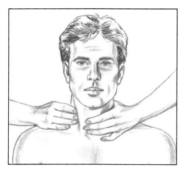

Auscultating the thyroid

• If you palpate an enlarged thyroid gland, auscultate it. In a client with an enlarged thyroid, auscultation may detect systolic bruits. Such bruits, caused by vibrations produced by accelerated blood flow through the thyroid arteries, may indicate hyperthyroidism.

• To auscultate for bruits, place the bell of the stethoscope over one of the lateral lobes of the thyroid, then listen carefully for a low, soft, rushing sound. To ensure that tracheal sounds do not obscure any bruits, have the client hold his or her breath while you auscultate.

DOCUMENTATION

The SOAPIE method of documentation includes the following components: subjective (history) data, objective (physical) data, assessment, planning, implementation, and evaluation. The following example shows how to document nursing care for a client with diabetes.

Case history

Jacob Smith, age 52, has Type II diabetes mellitus. Until recently, when Mr. Smith experienced stress related to his wife's death,

---

Selected nursing diagnosis categories

The nurse can use these diagnosis categories to formulate nursing diagnoses for a client with an endocrine problem.
• Activity intolerance
• Altered growth and development
• Altered sexuality patterns
• Body image disturbance
• Hyperthermia
• Hypothermia
• Impaired adjustment
• Impaired home maintenance management
• Ineffective family coping: Compromised
• Ineffective individual coping
• Ineffective thermoregulation

---

his diabetes was well controlled by diet and glyburide (DiaBeta), 10 mg twice daily. Mr. Smith has come for a follow-up evaluation of his blood glucose level, which was 260 mg/dl at his last visit.

S   O   A   P   I   E

Client states, "I'm urinating a lot, drinking a lot, and I'm always hungry." Client also states, "I hope my blood sugar is down. I can't give myself insulin....my hands shake every time I pick up the needle. The thought of sticking the needle in my leg makes me want to vomit."

S   **O**   A   P   I   E

Weight loss of 6 lb in past 2 weeks. Fasting blood glucose level 310 mg/dl. Urine glucose and ketones negative. Skin flushed and dry. Poor skin turgor noted, as evidenced by tenting. Urine is dilute in appearance.

S   O   **A**   P   I   E

Anxiety related to self-injection of insulin. Client has lost weight and is dehydrated.

S   O   A   **P**   I   E

Allow time for client to verbalize fear about self-injection of insulin. Teach client about drawing up insulin into a syringe, injecting insulin, rotating injection sites within a selected anatomic region (such as the abdomen), storing and caring for insulin and syringes, identifying signs and symptoms of low blood glucose levels, and identifying treatment measures.

S   O   A   P   **I**   E

Spent time with client, allowing him to express his fears and anxiety about self-injection of insulin. Gave client printed information about insulin injection and hypoglycemia to take home. Client viewed film on insulin injection before leaving. Taught client self-injection of insulin.

S   O   A   P   I   **E**

Client self-injected 10 units of saline S.Q. in right lower abdominal quadrant after drawing it up correctly. Although nervous, client stated, "That didn't really hurt. I can't believe I did it!" Client stated that film was good reinforcement.

Yalow, R. (1992). Radioimmunoassay of hormones. In J. Wilson and D. Foster (Eds.), *William's textbook on endocrinology* (8th ed.). (pp. 1635-1646). Philadelphia: W.B. Saunders.

SUGGESTED READINGS

Brown, S. (1990). Studies of educational interventions and outcomes in diabetic adults: A meta-analysis revisited. *Patient Education and Counseling*, 16(3), 189-215.

Greenspan, S., and Resnick, N. (1990). Geriatric endocrinology. In F. Greenspan (Ed.), *Basic and clinical endocrinology* (3rd ed.). (pp. 741-756). Norwalk, CT: Appleton and Lange.

Griffin, J. (1992). Dynamic tests of endocrine function. In J. Wilson and D. Foster (Eds.), *William's textbook on endocrinology* (8th ed.). (pp. 1663-1670). Philadelphia: W.B. Saunders.

Haas, L. (1991). Drug therapy for diabetes. *Nurse Practitioner Forum*, 2(3), 166-174.

Katzung, B. (1992). Endocrine drugs. In B. Katzung (Ed.), *Basic and clinical pharmacology* (5th ed.). (pp. 513-616). Norwalk, CT: Appleton and Lange.

Steil, C., and Deakins, D. (1990). Today's insulins: What you and your patient need to know. *Nursing90*, 20(8), 34-40.

UNIT FOUR

Performing Special Assessments

19

Complete and Partial Assessments

The main elements of the nursing assessment—health history, physical assessment, and review of laboratory and other diagnostic studies—provide the information needed to formulate nursing diagnoses, which in turn serve as the basis for planning, implementing, and evaluating client care. This chapter describes how the nurse can carry out these tasks efficiently by performing a complete assessment effectively and by performing a properly focused partial assessment.

COMPLETE ASSESSMENT

The nurse's complete assessment includes three essential components: the health history, physical assessment, and review of laboratory and other diagnostic studies.

Health history

The client's health history is the most important part of the complete assessment. It provides information about the client's physical and environmental background and investigates the client's cultural, social, emotional, intellectual, philosophical, and spiritual views. Also, it indicates whether a complete or partial physical assessment is necessary.

The complete history consists of five basic components: biographic data, health and illness patterns, health promotion and protection patterns, role and relationship patterns, and a summary of health data. Each component seeks information about a different aspect of the client's life and health. To obtain a complete health history, explore each component with the client during the interview.

Physical assessment

A complete physical assessment may be needed during a client's first visit to an outpatient setting (if the client does not need emergency or urgent care) or as a periodic checkup. To perform a complete physical assessment for routine screening, follow the guidelines below. Keep in mind that this physical assessment format is just one of many possible formats. Modify it, as needed, to meet the client's needs and abilities.

Preparing for the complete physical assessment

For the complete physical assessment, plan to use all four assessment techniques: inspection, palpation, percussion, and auscultation. Also employ the gentle art of listening to the client. Throughout the examination, be sensitive to the client's needs. Provide proper instruction and information to help the client feel comfortable with the examination, and drape the client appropriately, exposing only the body area to be examined.

Before beginning the complete assessment, check the room to make sure it has an examination table with stirrups, stool, gooseneck lamp, desk with two chairs, counter or stand to hold supplies, scale, and sink. (If the assessment takes place in the client's home, adapt available furnishings, as needed.) Then gather the following supplies and equipment:

• thermometer
• watch with a second hand
• stethoscope with diaphragm and bell heads
• sphygmomanometer
• visual acuity chart, page of newsprint, and color perception pages or plates
• ophthalmoscope
• otoscope or an ophthalmoscope with an otoscopic tip
• nasoscope, an ophthalmoscope with a nasal tip, or a nasal speculum and a penlight
• penlight
• transilluminator
• ruler and measuring tape
• marking pencil
• gloves
• tongue depressors
• cotton balls
• cotton-tipped applicators
• 4" x 4" gauze pads
• tuning fork
• reflex hammer
• vaginal speculum and Papanicolaou (Pap) smear materials
• lubricant
• fecal testing materials
• goniometer
• test tubes of hot and cold water (optional)
• test tubes of odorous materials, such as coffee, chocolate, or other familiar substances (optional)

• substances for taste assessment, such as sugar, salt, vinegar, and quinine (optional)
• coin
• paper clip
• pin and cotton to test sharp and dull sensations
• gown and drapes.

After gathering the necessary equipment, warm the room and the instruments. Instruct the client to empty the bladder (and provide a urine specimen, if needed), remove all clothing, and put on the gown. Ensure privacy by closing the examination room door or pulling the bed curtains closed, and draping the client appropriately. To prevent contamination of the client, yourself, or another client, wear gloves during examination of the mucous membranes, genitals, rectum, and any area with lesions or signs of infection or infestation.

General survey

Make a general survey to obtain fundamental information about the client's overall health and mental status. Observe the client and listen closely to develop an overall picture that will guide subsequent assessment.

To obtain general survey information, begin by noting the client's sex, race, and approximate age. Then check for obvious signs of physical or emotional distress and adjust your assessment accordingly.

If the client is not in severe distress, continue the general survey by observing the client's face for expression, contour, and symmetry; noting the client's body type, posture, and movement; assessing the client's speech for tone, clarity, strength, vocabulary, sentence structure, and pace; and noting the client's dress, grooming, and personal hygiene. Finally, assess the client's mental state, especially noting level of consciousness and behavior.

Height, weight, and vital signs

First, measure the client's height and weight, which should fall within the norms for adults and children. Keep in mind that body weight not only provides information about nutrition, but also is a valuable indicator of fluid balance and hydration. For an infant, also measure the head and chest circumference

(Text continues on page 278.)

Performing physical assessments

The chart on the following pages provides guidelines for the complete assessment. It presents an approach that moves systematically from head to toe and concludes with the reproductive system—the most potentially embarrassing or sensitive part of the assessment. It groups assessment techniques by body region and nurse-client positioning to make the assessment as efficient as possible and to avoid tiring the client. In this chart, the first column describes the assessment technique to be used, the second column lists the normal findings for adults, and the third column reviews special considerations, including the purpose of the technique as well as nursing and developmental considerations. Where a change in nurse-client positioning is essential, it appears as the first item under special considerations. Before beginning, take and record the client's vital signs, height, and weight.

TECHNIQUE	NORMAL FINDINGS	SPECIAL CONSIDERATIONS
Head and neck		
Inspect the hair and scalp color and condition.	Normal hair color (black, brown, red, blond, gray) and texture with full distribution over scalp; pink, smooth, mobile scalp without lesions	• This assessment can provide information about the client's body systems, such as the endocrine system. • An elderly client may have thin hair. • An infant commonly has fine, thin hair or no hair.
Inspect the head. Then palpate from the forehead to the posterior triangle of the neck for the posterior cervical lymph nodes.	Symmetrical, rounded normocephalic head positioned at midline and erect with no lumps or ridges	• This technique can detect asymmetry, size changes, enlarged lymph nodes, and tenderness. • Inspect and gently palpate the fontanelles and sutures in an infant. Fontanelles should feel soft, yet firm, and be flush with the scalp; sutures should be smooth and not override one another or feel separated. • A neonate's head may be asymmetrical from molding during vaginal delivery. • Measure head circumference of an infant.
Palpate in front of and behind the ears, under the chin, and in the anterior triangle for the anterior cervical lymph nodes.	Nonpalpable lymph nodes or small, round, soft, mobile, nontender lymph nodes	• This technique can detect enlarged lymph nodes. • If nodes are enlarged, note their size, location, consistency, tenderness, temperature, and mobility. • A client under age 12 may normally have palpable lymph nodes that may range from $\frac{1}{8}''$ to $\frac{3}{8}''$ (3 mm to 1 cm) across. • Palpate only one side of the anterior neck at a time to avoid pressing both carotid arteries and reducing blood supply to the brain.

Performing physical assessments continued

TECHNIQUE	NORMAL FINDINGS	SPECIAL CONSIDERATIONS
Palpate the left and then the right carotid artery.	Bilateral equality in pulse amplitude and rhythm	• Palpate gently using the index and middle fingers. Check only one side of the neck at a time.
Auscultate the carotid arteries.	No bruit on auscultation	• Auscultation in this area can detect a bruit, a sign of turbulent blood flow.
Palpate the trachea.	Straight, midline trachea	• This technique evaluates the position of an important respiratory system structure. • Palpate by placing a thumb or forefinger on either side of the trachea at the sternocleidomastoid inner border above the suprasternal notch.
Palpate the suprasternal notch.	Palpable pulsations with an even rhythm	• Palpation in this area allows evaluation of aortic arch pulsations. • Palpate using only one index finger.
Palpate the supraclavicular area.	Nonpalpable lymph nodes	• This technique can detect enlarged lymph nodes.
Palpate the thyroid gland.	Thin, mobile thyroid isthmus; nonpalpable thyroid lobes	• Palpation can detect thyroid gland enlargement, tenderness, or nodules. • Palpate with the pads of your index and middle fingers, assessing the left lobe with your right hand and the right lobe with your left hand. Palpate inside of the sternocleidomastoid muscle and below the cricoid and thyroid cartilages. • If the client's thyroid is difficult to palpate, try palpating from behind the client or asking the client to drink some water while you feel for thyroid movement. The thyroid normally rises with swallowing. • If the thyroid is enlarged, auscultate for bruits.
Have the client touch the chin to the chest and to each shoulder, each ear to one shoulder, then tip the head back as far as possible.	Symmetrical strength and movement of neck muscles	• These maneuvers evaluate range of motion (ROM) in the neck. • Increased cervical flexion may make head tilting difficult for an elderly client. Have such a client move only to the point of discomfort. Record the degree of motion.

continued

Performing physical assessments continued

TECHNIQUE	NORMAL FINDINGS	SPECIAL CONSIDERATIONS
Place your hands on the client's shoulders while the client shrugs the shoulders against this resistance.	Symmetrical strength and movement of neck muscles	• This procedure checks cranial nerve XI (accessory nerve) functioning and trapezius muscle strength.
Place your hand on the client's left cheek while the client pushes against this resistance. Repeat this procedure on the client's right side.	Symmetrical strength of neck muscles	• This procedure checks cranial nerve XI (accessory nerve) functioning and sternocleidomastoid muscle strength.
Inspect the facial structures.	Symmetrical structures without edema, deformities, or lesions	• Face the client. • This technique evaluates the overall condition of the face.
Have the client smile, frown, wrinkle the forehead, and puff out the cheeks.	Symmetrical smile, frown, and forehead wrinkles; equal puffing out of the cheeks	• This maneuver evaluates the motor portion of cranial nerve VII (facial nerve).
Inspect the external appearance of the nose.	Symmetrical nose without edema, deformity, drainage, discoloration, or nostril flaring	• This technique evaluates the overall condition of the nose. • The external appearance of the nose can vary among individuals. • An infant's nose usually is slightly flattened.
Occlude one nostril externally with your finger, while the client breathes through the other. Repeat this procedure on the client's other nostril.	Patent nostrils	• This technique checks patency of the nasal passages.
Inspect the internal nostrils, using a nasal illuminator or nasal speculum.	Moist, pink-to-red nasal mucosa without lesions or polyps	• This technique can detect excessive drainage, edema, inflammation, and other abnormalities. • Steady the client's head with your opposite hand. • The nasal mucosa normally appears slightly enlarged in a pregnant client. • Use only a flashlight to inspect an infant's or toddler's nostrils; a nasal speculum is too sharp.

Performing physical assessments continued

TECHNIQUE	NORMAL FINDINGS	SPECIAL CONSIDERATIONS
Palpate the nose.	Nose without bumps, lesions, edema, or tenderness	• This technique assesses for structural abnormalities in the nose. • Palpate gently with the pads of your index and middle fingers. • Nose deviation to one side may be caused by asymmetrical bones or cartilages, which can be palpated. Such deviation may be normal if the nostrils are patent.
Palpate and percuss the frontal and maxillary sinuses.	No tenderness on palpation or percussion	• These techniques are used to elicit tenderness, which may indicate sinus congestion or infection. • When percussing the sinuses, use immediate percussion. • In a client under age 8, the frontal sinuses commonly are too small to assess. • If palpation and percussion elicit tenderness, assess further by transilluminating the sinuses.
Palpate the temporomandibular joints as the client opens and closes the jaws.	Smooth joint movement without pain; good approximation (bones line up where they meet)	• This action assesses the temporomandibular joints and the motor portion of cranial nerve V (trigeminal nerve). • Use the middle three fingers of each hand to palpate properly.
Inspect the oral mucosa, gingivae, teeth, and salivary gland openings, using a tongue depressor and a penlight.	Pink, moist, smooth oral mucosa without lesions; pink, moist slightly irregular gingivae without sponginess or edema; 32 bright white to ivory-colored teeth with smooth edges and correct occlusion; small, white-rimmed salivary gland openings without tenderness or inflammation	• Have the client open the mouth and remove any dentures. • Wear examination gloves. • This technique evaluates the condition of several oral structures. • Move the tongue depressor from the molar area to the front of the mouth, being careful not to bump the frenula. • The oral mucosa normally appears bluish or patchily pigmented in a dark-skinned client. • A child may have up to 20 temporary (baby) teeth. • Slight gingival swelling may be normal during pregnancy.

continued

Performing physical assessments continued

TECHNIQUE	NORMAL FINDINGS	SPECIAL CONSIDERATIONS
Observe the tongue and hard and soft palates.	Pink, slightly rough tongue with a midline depression and comfortable fit in floor of mouth; pink to light red palates with symmetrical lines	• Observation provides information about the client's hydration and the condition of these oral structures. • If necessary, flatten the top of the tongue with the tongue depressor. • Mucous membrane inspection is especially important to assessing hydration in a child.
Ask the client to stick out the tongue.	Midline tongue without tremors	• This procedure tests cranial nerve XII (hypoglossal nerve), which controls the motor function of the tongue.
Ask the client to say "Ahh" while sticking out the tongue. Inspect the visible oral structures.	Symmetrical rise in soft palate and uvula during phonation; pink, midline, cone-shaped uvula; +1 tonsils (both tonsils behind the pillars)	• Phonation ("Ahh") checks portions of cranial nerves IX and X (glossopharyngeal and vagus nerves). It also lowers the tongue, providing a good view of the anterior and posterior uvula, pillars, and tonsils.
Test the gag reflex using a tongue depressor.	Gagging	• Gagging during this procedure indicates that cranial nerves IX and X are intact. • Use this procedure cautiously in a client with nausea; it may cause vomiting. • Use a light touch on the back of the tongue to elicit this reflex.
Place the tongue depressor at the side of the tongue while the client pushes it to the left and right with the tongue.	Symmetrical ability to push tongue depressor to left and right	• This action tests cranial nerve XII (hypoglossal nerve). • If the client reports impaired taste, test cranial nerves VII and IX using moist cotton swabs flavored with sugar, salt, vinegar, and quinine.
Test the sense of smell using a test tube of coffee, chocolate, or another familiar substance.	Correct identification of all smells in both nostrils	• This action tests cranial nerve I (olfactory nerve). • Make sure the client keeps both eyes closed as you test one nostril at a time.

Performing physical assessments continued

TECHNIQUE	NORMAL FINDINGS	SPECIAL CONSIDERATIONS
Eyes and ears		
Perform a visual acuity test using the standard Snellen eye chart.	20/20 vision	• Stand 20′ away from the seated client. • This test assesses the client's distance vision and evaluates cranial nerve II. • Note whether the client's visual acuity was tested with or without corrective lenses. • Visual acuity varies with age. For example, 20/30 is normal for a toddler. • In an elderly client, decreased lens elasticity commonly causes presbyopia, which reduces near vision. • Refer client with decreased or increased acuity to an ophthalmologist or optometrist for evaluation.
Hold a page of newsprint 12″ to 14″ (30.5 to 35.5 cm) from the client while the client reads it aloud.	Correct reading of newsprint without difficulty	• Sit directly in front of the seated client. • This test assesses the client's near vision. • Make sure that a client who normally wears corrective lenses for reading does so for this test. • For an illiterate client, use the Snellen E chart.
Ask the client to identify the pattern in a specially prepared page of color dots or plates.	Correct identification of pattern	• This test assesses the client's color perception. • Early detection of color blindness is important for a child. It allows the child to compensate for the difficulty and alerts teachers to the child's needs.
Perform the six cardinal positions of gaze test.	Bilaterally equal eye movement without nystagmus	• This test evaluates the function of each of the six extraocular muscles and tests cranial nerves III, IV, and VI (oculomotor, trochlear, and abducens nerves). • A child who fails this test requires immediate referral to an ophthalmologist. • An adult client who fails this test and one of the other extraocular muscle tests requires immediate referral to an ophthalmologist. continued

Performing physical assessments continued

TECHNIQUE	NORMAL FINDINGS	SPECIAL CONSIDERATIONS
Perform the cover-uncover test.	Steady eyes without movement, wandering, or jerking	• This extraocular muscle function test assesses the fusion reflex, which makes binocular vision possible. • A child who fails this test requires immediate referral to an ophthalmologist to correct strabismus (crossed eyes). • An adult client who fails this test and one of the other extraocular muscle tests requires immediate referral to an ophthalmologist.
Perform the corneal light reflex test.	Light reflection by cornea in exactly the same place in both eyes	• This test checks the ability of extraocular muscles to hold the eyes steady, or parallel, when fixed on an object. • A child who fails this test requires immediate referral to an ophthalmologist to correct strabismus (crossed eyes). • An adult client who fails this test and one of the other extraocular muscle tests requires immediate referral to an ophthalmologist.
Test the peripheral vision by comparing it with your own.	A field of vision that is 50 degrees from the top, 60 medially, 70 downward, and 110 laterally	• This test assesses the peripheral vision portion of cranial nerve II (optic nerve) and measures the ability of the retina to receive stimuli from the periphery of the client's vision. • The nurse must have normal vision; otherwise, the test will be inaccurate. • This test discovers only large peripheral vision defects, such as blindness in one quarter of the visual field. • Peripheral vision normally decreases in an elderly client.
Inspect the external structures of the eyeball (eyelids, eyelashes, and lacrimal apparatus).	Bright, clear, symmetrical eyes without nystagmus; ability to close eyelids completely over the sclera; eyelids that match the client's	• This portion of the assessment allows the nurse to detect common problems, such as ptosis (lid lag), ectropion (outward-turning eyelids), entropion (inward-turning eyelids), and styes (purulent infection of sebaceous gland of the eyelid).

Performing physical assessments continued

TECHNIQUE	NORMAL FINDINGS	SPECIAL CONSIDERATIONS
External structures of the eyeball continued	complexion and are free from edema, scaling, and lesions; equally distributed eyelashes that curve outward; smooth lacrimal apparatus without signs of inflammation	• An Asian client may have epicanthal folds in the eyelids. • An elderly client may have thin eyelashes and lackluster eyes.
Palpate the lacrimal apparatus.	No tenderness or masses on palpation	• This technique evaluates the condition of the tear ducts. • Palpate gently by pressing your index finger against the lower orbital rim near the nose. • If palpation causes excessive tearing or expresses purulent material, suspect a blockage or infection.
Inspect the conjunctiva and sclera.	Pink palpebral conjunctiva and clear bulbar conjunctiva without swelling, drainage, or hyperemic blood vessels; white, clear sclera	• This technique detects conjunctivitis and the scleral color changes that may occur with systemic disorders. • A dark-skinned client may have small, dark spots on the sclera. • An elderly client may have a thickened bulbar conjuctiva on the nasal side (pinguecula).
Inspect the cornea, iris, and anterior chamber by shining a penlight tangentially across the eye.	Clear, transparent cornea and anterior chamber; illumination of total iris	• This technique assesses anterior chamber depth and the condition of the cornea and iris. • A black or elderly client may exhibit a thin, grayish ring in the cornea (corneal arcus).
Examine the pupils for equality of size, shape, reaction to light, and accommodation.	Pupils equal, round, reactive to light, and accommodation (PERRLA), directly and consensually	• Testing the pupillary response to light and accommodation assesses cranial nerves III, IV, and VI. • A client over age 85 may show almost no pupil reaction to accommodation.
Observe the red reflex using an ophthalmoscope.	Sharp, distinct orange-red glow	• Presence of the red reflex indicates that the cornea, anterior chamber, and lens are free from opacity and clouding. • For information about the complete ophthalmoscopic examination, see Chapter 7.

continued

Performing physical assessments continued

TECHNIQUE	NORMAL FINDINGS	SPECIAL CONSIDERATIONS
Inspect the ear.	Nearly vertical–positioned ears that line up with the eye, match the facial color, are similarly shaped, and are in proportion to the face; no drainage, nodules, or lesions	• Sit or stand at the client's side facing the ear. • This technique determines the general condition and positioning of the ears. • Ear size and shape vary greatly. Obtain information about other family members' ears for comparison. • In an elderly client, the external ear structure may have lost adipose tissue and the cartilage may be harder. • A dark-skinned client may have darker orange or brown cerumen (earwax); a fair-skinned client will have yellow cerumen.
Palpate the ear and mastoid process.	No pain, swelling, nodules, or lesions	• These techniques can detect any areas of tenderness or edema, which may indicate an inflammation or infection. They may also uncover other abnormalities, such as nodules or lesions. • If the client has pain or swelling on palpation, use extreme care when performing an otoscopic examination. If otitis externa is present, this examination may not be possible.
Perform the whispered voice test or the watch-tick test on one ear at a time.	Whispered voice heard at a distance of 1' to 2' (30.5 to 61 cm); watch-tick heard at a distance of 5" (12.7 cm)	• Stand 1' to 2' (30.5 to 61 cm) behind the client. • Record the number of feet or inches you stand away from the client during the test. • Perform a complete otoscopic examination. (See Chapter 7.)
Perform Weber's test using a 512 or 1024 cycles/second (CPS) tuning fork.	Tuning fork vibrations heard equally in both ears or in the middle of the head	• This test helps differentiate any conductive or sensorineural hearing loss. • The sound is heard best in the ear with a conductive loss.
Perform the Rinne test using a 512 or 1024 CPS tuning fork.	Tuning fork vibrations heard in front of the ear for at least as long as they are heard on the mastoid process	• This test helps differentiate any conductive or sensorineural hearing loss.

Performing physical assessments continued

TECHNIQUE	NORMAL FINDINGS	SPECIAL CONSIDERATIONS
Posterior thorax		
Observe the skin, bones, and muscles of the spine, shoulder blades, and back as well as symmetry of expansion and accessory muscle use.	Even skin tone; symmetrical placement of all structures; bilaterally equal shoulder height; symmetrical expansion with inhalation; no accessory muscle use	• Stand behind the seated client, slightly to the client's right if you are right-handed or to the client's left if you are left-handed. • Expose the posterior thorax. • Ensure that your hands and the stethoscope are warm. • Observation provides information about lung expansion and accessory muscle use during respiration. It may also detect a deformity that can alter ventilation, such as scoliosis.
Assess the anteroposterior and lateral diameters of the thorax.	Lateral diameter up to twice the anteroposterior diameter (2:1)	• This assessment may detect abnormalities, such as an increased anteroposterior diameter (barrel chest as low as 1:1) associated with chronic obstructive pulmonary disease (COPD). • An infant's anteroposterior diameter may equal or exceed the lateral diameter; a toddler's should be smaller than the lateral diameter. • An elderly client's anteroposterior diameter may increase in relation to the lateral diameter, creating a rounded chest. • Measure an infant's chest circumference at the nipple line.
Palpate down the spine.	Properly aligned spinous processes without lesions or tenderness; firm, symmetrical, evenly spaced muscles	• This technique detects pain in the spine and paraspinous muscles. It also evaluates their consistency. • Use the pads of your middle three fingers to palpate the spine.
Palpate over the posterior thorax.	Smooth surface; no lesions, lumps, or pain	• This technique helps detect musculoskeletal inflammation and other abnormalities. • Use the palmar surfaces of your fingertips and hands to palpate the posterior thorax.
Percuss the costovertebral area.	Thudding sensation without pain or tenderness	• This action evaluates the condition of the kidneys. • Perform blunt percussion in this area using the ulnar surface of your fist.

continued

Performing physical assessments continued

TECHNIQUE	NORMAL FINDINGS	SPECIAL CONSIDERATIONS
Assess respiratory excursion.	Symmetrical expansion and contraction of the thorax	• This technique checks for equal expansion of the lungs. • Assess for respiratory excursion in two locations posteriorly: at T10 and at the level of the axilla just below the scapula.
Palpate for tactile fremitus as the client repeats *ninety-nine*.	Equally intense vibrations of both sides of the chest	• Palpation provides information about the content of the lungs; vibrations increase over consolidated or fluid-filled areas and decrease over gas-filled areas. • Use the ulnar or palmar surface of your hands to detect fremitus. • Palpate at the apices, inside the scapulae, down the back, and under the axillae, using a systematic palpation sequence and comparing each side to the other. • Vibration intensity varies with chest thickness and underlying thoracic structures.
Percuss over the posterior and lateral lung fields.	Resonant percussion note over the lungs that changes to a dull note at the diaphragm	• This technique helps identify the density and location of the lungs, diaphragm, and other anatomic structures. • Use mediate percussion in all areas of the posterior and lateral thorax. • Follow a systematic percussion sequence and compare each side with the other. • Percussion is unreliable in an infant because of the relative size of the infant's chest and the adult's fingers. • Percussion may produce hyperresonant sounds in a client with COPD or an elderly client because of hyperinflation of lung tissue.
Percuss for diaphragmatic excursion on each side of the posterior thorax.	Excursion from 1¼″ to 2¼″ (3 to 6 cm)	• This technique evaluates diaphragm movement during respiration. • Keep in mind that the diaphragm normally is slightly higher on the right side than on the left.

Performing physical assessments continued

TECHNIQUE	NORMAL FINDINGS	SPECIAL CONSIDERATIONS
Auscultate the lungs through the posterior thorax as the client breathes slowly and deeply through the mouth. Also auscultate lateral areas.	Bronchovesicular sounds (soft, breezy sounds) between the scapulae; vesicular sounds (soft, swishy sounds about two notes lower than bronchovesicular sounds) in the lung periphery	• Lung auscultation helps detect abnormal fluid or mucus accumulation as well as obstructed passages. It also helps determine the condition of the alveoli and surrounding pleura. • Use the diaphragm of the stethoscope for an adult. For a pediatric client, use the bell of an adult stethoscope (if you do not have a pediatric one), pressing it firmly to create a small diaphragm. • Follow the same systematic sequence as for percussion. • For a client with significant hair growth over the area to be auscultated, wet the hair to decrease sound blurring. • Auscultate a child's lungs before performing other assessment techniques that may cause crying, which increases the respiratory rate and interferes with clear auscultation. • Auscultate at fewer sites for a pediatric client. • Because a child's chest is thinner and more resonant than an adult's, breath sounds are normally harsher or more bronchial.
Anterior thorax		
Observe the skin, bones, and muscles of the anterior thoracic structures as well as symmetry of expansion and accessory muscle use.	Even skin tone; symmetrical placement of all structures; symmetrical costal angle of less than 90 degrees; symmetrical expansion with inhalation; no accessory muscle use	• Stand in front of the seated client and expose the anterior thorax. • Observation provides information about lung expansion and accessory muscle use during respiration. It may also detect a deformity that can prevent full lung expansion, such as pigeon chest. • Women tend to use their upper chest muscles to breathe; men and children tend to breathe diaphragmatically.
Inspect the anterior thorax for lift, heaves, or thrusts and for the point of maximum impulse (PMI).	PMI not usually visible; no lifts, heaves, or thrusts	• PMI may be visible in a thin or young client.

continued

Performing physical assessments continued

TECHNIQUE	NORMAL FINDINGS	SPECIAL CONSIDERATIONS
Palpate over the anterior thorax.	Smooth surface; no lesions, lumps, or pain	• This technique helps detect musculoskeletal inflammation and other abnormalities. • Use the palmar surfaces of your fingertips and hands to palpate the anterior thorax. • Compare the left side with the right side during palpation.
Assess respiratory excursion.	Symmetrical expansion and contraction of the thorax	• This technique checks for equal expansion of the lungs. • Assess for respiratory excursion in three locations anteriorly: at the 2nd, 5th, and 10th intercostal spaces. • For a client with pendulous breasts, do not assess respiratory excursion at the 6th intercostal space anteriorly. Instead check posterior excursion at this level.
Palpate for tactile fremitus as the client repeats *ninety-nine*.	Equally intense vibrations of both sides of the chest, with more vibrations in the upper chest than in the lower chest	• Palpation provides information about the content of the lungs; vibrations increase over consolidated or fluid-filled areas and decrease over gas-filled areas. • Use the ulnar or palmar surface of your hands to detect fremitus. • Use a systematic palpation sequence and compare one side with the other. • Vibration intensity varies with chest thickness and underlying thoracic structures.
Percuss over the anterior thorax.	Resonant percussion note over lung fields that changes to a dull note over ribs and other bones	• This technique helps identify the density and location of the lungs, diaphragm, and other anatomic structures. • Use mediate percussion in all areas of the anterior thorax. • Follow a systematic percussion sequence and compare one side with the other. • Percussion is unreliable in an infant because of the relative size of the infant's chest and the adult's fingers. • Percussion may produce hyperresonant sounds in an elderly client because of hyperinflation of lung tissue.

Performing physical assessments continued

TECHNIQUE	NORMAL FINDINGS	SPECIAL CONSIDERATIONS
Auscultate the lungs through the anterior thorax as the client breathes slowly and deeply through the mouth. Also auscultate lateral areas.	Bronchovesicular sounds (soft, breezy sounds) on either side of the sternum at the 2nd to 4th intercostal spaces; vesicular sounds (soft, swishy sounds about two notes lower than bronchovesicular sounds) in the lung periphery	• Lung auscultation helps detect abnormal fluid or mucus accumulation as well as obstructed passages. It also helps determine the condition of the alveoli and pleura. • Use the diaphragm of the stethoscope for an adult. For a pediatric client, use the bell of an adult stethoscope (if you do not have a pediatric one), pressing it firmly to create a small diaphragm. • Follow the same systematic sequence as for percussion. • For a client with significant hair growth over the area to be auscultated, wet the hair to decrease sound blurring. • Auscultate a child's lungs before performing other assessment techniques that may cause crying. • Auscultate at fewer sites for a pediatric client. • Because a child's chest is thinner and more resonant than an adult's, breath sounds are normally harsher or more bronchial.
Inspect the breasts and axillae with the client's hands resting at his or her side, placed on the hips, and raised above the head.	Symmetrical, convex, similar-looking breasts with soft, smooth skin and bilaterally similar venous patterns; symmetrical axillae with varying amounts of hair, but no lesions; nipples at same level on chest, and same color	• This technique evaluates the general condition of the breasts and axillae and detects abnormalities. • If the client's breasts are large or pendulous, observe them with the client leaning forward. • Some women have a congenital anomaly in which extra breast tissue, nipples, or breasts appear along the milk lines. • Assess the breasts of a female adolescent according to the stage of breast development. • Reassure a young male adolescent that gynecomastia normally disappears within a year. • Expect to see enlarged breasts with darkened nipples and areola and purplish linear streaks in a pregnant client. • On the breasts of a lactating client, check for abnormalities, such as cracks, fissures, redness, tenderness, blisters, and petechiae.

continued

Performing physical assessments continued

TECHNIQUE	NORMAL FINDINGS	SPECIAL CONSIDERATIONS
Palpate the axillae with the client's arms resting against the side of the body.	Nonpalpable nodes	• This technique detects nodular enlargements and other abnormalities. • Assess the central axilla as well as the anterior and posterior axillary folds and the lateral nodes. • Palpate deep in the axilla, using the fingerpads.
Palpate the breasts and nipples.	Smooth, relatively elastic tissue without masses, cracks, fissures, areas of induration (hardness), or discharge	• Help the client lie down and place her hands above her head. Stand at the right side if you are right-handed; at the left, if you are left-handed. • Place a small pad or pillow under the client's shoulder on the side to be assessed to spread the breast tissue evenly. • This technique evaluates the consistency and elasticity of the breasts and nipples and may detect nipple discharge. • Employ circular or wedge palpation, using your fingerpads and overlapping the finger movements. • Make a cytologic smear of any nipple discharge not caused by pregnancy or lactation. • Some neonates exhibit palpable breast enlargement and nipple discharge ("witch's milk"). • A mature breast may feel more granular or stringy than a youthful breast. • Premenstrually, the client may exhibit breast tenderness, nodularity, and fullness. • A pregnant client may discharge colostrum from the nipple and may exhibit nodular breasts with prominent venous patterns. • A lactating client may have breast engorgement, with hard, warm, reddened breasts.
Inspect the neck for jugular vein distention.	No visible pulsations	• Help the client into a supine position at a 45-degree angle. • This technique roughly assesses right-sided heart pressure. • Note the angle at which the client is reclining when you inspect. (A 45-degree angle is most common.)

Performing physical assessments continued

TECHNIQUE	NORMAL FINDINGS	SPECIAL CONSIDERATIONS
Palpate the precordium for the PMI.	PMI in the apical area (fifth intercostal space at the midclavicular line)	• This technique helps evaluate the size and location of the left ventricle.
Auscultate the aortic, pulmonic, tricuspid, and mitral areas for heart sounds.	S_1 and S_2 heart sounds with a regular rhythm and an age-appropriate rate	• Auscultation over the precordium with the bell and diaphragm evaluates the heart rate and rhythm and can detect extra sounds, murmurs, and other abnormal heart sounds. • Note any extra heart sounds (S_3 or S_4), murmurs, clicks, snaps, or rubs. • If you detect a murmur, recheck it with the client sitting leaning forward or lying on one side. If a murmur is still present, document its timing (in systole, diastole, or both), location, intensity, pitch, radiation, and quality. • A child may have functional (innocent) heart murmurs.

Abdomen

Observe the abdominal contour.	Symmetrical flat or rounded contour	• Stand on the client's right if you are right-handed; on the left, if you are left-handed. • Expose the abdomen from the breast to the groin. Keep a female client's breasts covered, and place a drape at the pubic hair line. • Normal abdominal contour may vary with body type. • An infant or toddler will have a rounded abdomen. • An emaciated client will have a scaphoid abdomen.
Inspect the abdomen for skin characteristics, symmetry, contour, peristalsis, and pulsations.	Symmetrical contour with no lesions, striae, rash, or visible peristaltic waves	• A slender client may have a flat or concave abdomen. • To detect an incisional or umbilical hernia, observe for a protrusion while the supine client lifts his or her head. • Expect to see a potbelly in a child under age 4.

continued

Performing physical assessments continued

TECHNIQUE	NORMAL FINDINGS	SPECIAL CONSIDERATIONS
Auscultate all four abdominal quadrants.	Normal bowel sounds in all four quadrants	• Abdominal auscultation can detect abnormal bowel sounds and other abnormal sounds. • Always auscultate the abdomen before palpating and percussing it to avoid creating unusual sounds or rupturing an aneurysm. • Apply the diaphragm of the stethoscope lightly to the abdomen. You may need to listen for up to 5 minutes to detect bowel sounds. • Note any bruits, especially over the aorta, iliac arteries, and femoral arteries. • Promote cooperation in an infant or young child by auscultating with the child on the parent's lap.
Percuss from below the right breast to the inguinal area down the right midclavicular line.	Dull percussion note over the liver; tympanic note over the rest of the abdomen	• Percussion in this area helps evaluate the size of the liver. • Gas in the colon or consolidation in the right lower lung lobe can mask liver border dullness.
Percuss from below the left breast to the inguinal area down the left midclavicular line.	Tympanic percussion note	• Percussion in this area that elicits a dull note can detect an enlarged spleen. • If percussion elicits a dull note, turn the client on the right side and percuss along the left midaxillary line between the 6th and 11th ribs to assess the degree of splenic dullness. • Percussion sounds may be difficult to assess in an obese client.
Palpate all four abdominal quadrants, moving from the upper quadrants to the inguinal areas down the midclavicular lines.	Nontender organs without masses	• Ask the client to bend his or her knees while remaining supine. This helps relax the abdominal muscles for palpation and percussion. • Palpation provides information about the location, size, and condition of the underlying structures. • Palpate in a systematic sequence, using light palpation first and repeating the process with deep palpation, which may be done with one or two hands. • Plan to palpate and percuss any painful area last to prevent guarding.

Performing physical assessments continued

TECHNIQUE	NORMAL FINDINGS	SPECIAL CONSIDERATIONS
Abdominal palpation continued		• Have a ticklish client place his or her hand over yours during palpation as a distraction. • If palpation reveals bladder distention above the symphysis pubis, percuss and palpate the bladder.
Palpate for the kidneys on each side of the abdomen.	Nonpalpable kidneys or solid, firm, smooth kidneys (if palpable)	• This technique evaluates the general condition of the kidneys. • Keep in mind that the right kidney lies lower than the left, and that it may be palpable in a thin client or a client with reduced abdominal muscle mass. • If you cannot feel the kidneys, try capturing the kidney, an advanced palpation technique.
Palpate the liver at the right costal border.	Nonpalpable liver or smooth, firm, nontender liver with a rounded, regular edge (if palpable)	• This technique evaluates the general condition of the liver. • Perform deep palpation with one or both hands while the client takes a deep breath. • The liver may be palpable in a thin client. • An alternative technique requires "hooking" your fingerpads under the costal margin to palpate the liver. This technique may give the client pain. • In a child, the liver is proportionally larger and easier to palpate.
Palpate for the spleen at the left costal border.	Nonpalpable spleen	• This procedure detects any splenomegaly (spleen enlargement). • Perform deep palpation with one or both hands while the client takes a deep breath. • An alternative technique requires "hooking" your fingerpads under the edge of the costal margin to palpate the spleen. This technique may give the client pain.
Palpate the femoral pulses in the groin area.	Strong, regular pulse	• This technique assesses vascular patency. • This is an important pulse point in a child.

continued

Performing physical assessments continued

TECHNIQUE	NORMAL FINDINGS	SPECIAL CONSIDERATIONS
Upper extremities		
Observe the skin and muscle mass of the upper extremities.	Uniform color and texture with no lesions; elastic turgor; muscle mass equal bilaterally	• Stand in front of the seated client. • Beginning the assessment with the hands puts the client at ease. • The skin provides information about hydration, circulation, and the status of body systems, such as the urinary system. • Continue to observe the client's skin throughout the assessment. • If lesions are present, note their size, shape, color, location, and elevation. • An elderly client may have dry, thin skin with reduced turgor. • An infant can become dehydrated quickly, so assessing turgor is important.
Ask the client to extend the arms forward and then rapidly turn the palms up and down.	Steady hands with no tremors or pronator drift	• This maneuver tests proprioception and cerebellar function.
Place your hands on the client's upturned forearms while the client pushes up against resistance. Then place your hands under the forearms while the client pushes down.	Symmetrical strength and ability to push up and down against resistance	• This procedure checks the muscle strength of the arms.
Inspect and palpate the fingers, wrists, and elbow joints.	Smooth, freely movable joints with no swelling	• This procedure provides information about the status of the joints. • An elderly client may exhibit osteoarthritic changes that cause enlarged, stiff, and painful joints.
Palpate the client's hands to assess skin temperature.	Warm, moist skin with bilaterally even temperature	• Skin temperature assessment provides data about circulation to the area. • Particularly note cool, clammy skin or warm, dry skin.
Palpate the radial and brachial pulses.	Bilaterally equal rate and rhythm	• Palpation of pulses helps evaluate peripheral vascular status.

Performing physical assessments continued

TECHNIQUE	NORMAL FINDINGS	SPECIAL CONSIDERATIONS
Inspect the color, shape, and condition of the fingernails, and test for capillary refill.	Pink nail beds with smooth, rounded nails; 160-degree angle where nail meets the cuticle; brisk capillary refill	• Nail assessment provides data about the integumentary, cardiovascular, and respiratory systems.
Place two fingers in each of the client's palms while the client squeezes your fingers.	Bilaterally equal hand strength	• This maneuver tests muscle strength in the hands.
Lower extremities		
Inspect the legs and feet for color, lesions, varicosities, hair growth, nail growth, edema, and muscle mass.	Skin color that matches rest of complexion; symmetrical hair and nail growth; no lesions, varicosities, or edema; muscle mass equal bilaterally	• Stand near the supine client. • Inspection assesses adequate circulatory function.
Test for pitting edema in the pretibial area midway between the knee and ankle and in the pedal area.	No pitting edema	• This test checks for and evaluates pitting edema, which results from excess sodium and water in interstitial spaces. • If edema is present, grade it according to the scale approved by your health care facility.
Palpate for pulses and skin temperature in the posterior tibial area behind the ankle and the dorsalis pedis area on the foot.	Bilaterally even pulse rate, rhythm, and skin temperature	• Palpation of pulses and temperature in these areas helps evaluate peripheral vascular status. • If the posterior tibial and the dorsalis pedis pulses are normal, you do not need to check the popliteal pulse. If they are abnormal, ask the client to bend the knees slightly. Then palpate the popliteal pulse.
Perform the straight leg test on one leg at a time.	Painless leg lifting	• Stand to one side of the client. • This test checks for vertebral disk problems. • Remind the client to keep the knee straight and the foot comfortably dorsiflexed. • If the client has difficulty with this test, you may help by steadying the leg being raised.

continued

Performing physical assessments continued

TECHNIQUE	NORMAL FINDINGS	SPECIAL CONSIDERATIONS
Palpate for crepitus as the client abducts and adducts the hip. Repeat this procedure on the opposite leg.	No crepitus	• Place one hand on the client's hip and the other on the knee. • This test assesses ROM of the hip. • To assess hip movement, have the client bring the knee over the abdomen as far as possible. • Help the client cross the knee over the abdomen and away from you. • Perform Ortolani's maneuver on an infant to assess hip abduction and adduction.
Ask the client to raise his or her thigh against the resistance of your hands. Repeat this procedure on the opposite thigh.	Each thigh lifts easily against resistance	• Help the client sit up. Place both hands on the client's thigh. • This maneuver tests the motor strength of the upper legs. • Have a preschooler or school-age child hop on each foot to test motor strength in the legs.
Ask the client to push outward against the resistance of your hands.	Each leg pushes easily against resistance	• Place one hand on each leg in the tibial area below the knee. • This maneuver tests the motor strength of the lower legs. • Have a preschooler or school-age child hop on each foot to test motor strength in the legs.
Ask the client to pull backward against the resistance of your hands.	Each leg pulls easily against resistance	• Place one hand on each calf. • This maneuver tests the motor strength of the lower legs. • Have a preschooler or school-age child hop on each foot to test motor strength in the legs.
Nervous system		
Lightly touch the ophthalmic, maxillary, and mandibular areas on each side of the client's face with a cotton swab and a pin. Ask what the client feels with each touch.	Correct identification of sensation and location	• Have the client remain seated with eyes closed. • This test evaluates the function of cranial nerve V (trigeminal nerve). • Test the three different areas randomly so that the client does not notice a pattern, but be sure to check all three areas with both the pin and the swab. • Temperature sensitivity does not need to be tested if the client exhibits pain sensitivity. (Pain and

Performing physical assessments continued

TECHNIQUE	NORMAL FINDINGS	SPECIAL CONSIDERATIONS
		temperature travel on the same tracts in the nervous system.) If pain sensitivity is not elicited, test temperature sensitivity using test tubes of warm and cold water.
Touch several areas on the dorsal and palmar surfaces of the arms, hands, and fingers with the cotton swab and pin. Ask what the client feels with each touch.	Correct identification of sensation and location	• This test evaluates the function of the ulnar, radial, and medial nerves (the dermatomes). • Do not break the skin with the pin. • The wooden end of a broken cotton swab will serve instead of a pin, if desired. • Do not perform this test on a young child, who may be frightened by the pinpricks.
Touch several nerve distribution areas on the legs, feet, and toes with the cotton swab and pin. Ask what the client feels with each touch.	Correct identification of sensation and location	• This test evaluates the function of the dermatome areas randomly. • If the client does not perceive a sensation in a particular area, evaluate that area in greater detail. • Do not perform this test on a young child, who may be frightened by the pinpricks. • This test may take more time for an elderly client.
Tap the styloid process of the radius, about 1" to 2" (2.5 to 5 cm) above the wrist, using a reflex hammer. Repeat this procedure on the opposite arm.	Elbow flexion, forearm supination, and finger and hand flexion	• Have the client place both hands thumbs up in his or her lap. Place two fingers of one of your hands over the client's radius about 1⅛" to 2" (3 to 5 cm) above the wrist. As an alternate position, hold the client's thumb up and away from the body, and have the client "let go" of the weight in the arm during the procedure. • This procedure elicits the brachioradialis deep tendon reflex (DTR). • Manipulate the client's hand and tap in several areas over the wrist, if necessary, to elicit the reflex. continued

Performing physical assessments continued

TECHNIQUE	NORMAL FINDINGS	SPECIAL CONSIDERATIONS
Place your thumb or finger over the biceps tendon. Then tap lightly over your thumb or finger, using a reflex hammer. Repeat this procedure on the opposite arm.	Brisk elbow flexion	• Have the client place both hands in his or her lap and relax both arms. Place two fingers of one of your hands in the client's antecubital fossa. • This procedure elicits the biceps DTR. • Manipulate the joint and tap in several areas, if necessary, to elicit the reflex. • If you have difficulty eliciting this DTR, ask the client to squeeze both thighs together during the procedure. This should distract the client's attention from the area being assessed.
Tap the triceps tendon area (about 1″ to 2″ [2.5 to 5 cm] above the elbow on the olecranon process of the ulnar bone) using a reflex hammer. Repeat this procedure on the opposite arm.	Brisk elbow extension and triceps muscle contraction	• Have the client place both hands on his or her hips. Place two fingers of one of your hands over the client's triceps tendon area. As an alternate position, hold the client's upper arm in a flexed position and have the client "let go" of the weight in the arm during the procedure. • This procedure elicits the triceps DTR. • Manipulate the joint and tap in several areas, if necessary, to elicit the reflex. • If you have difficulty eliciting this DTR, ask the client to squeeze both thighs together during the procedure. This should distract the client's attention from the area being assessed.
Tap just below the patella, using a reflex hammer. Repeat this procedure on the opposite patella.	Knee extension and quadriceps muscle contraction	• Have the client sit at the edge of the table, knees flexed. • This procedure elicits the patellar DTR. • Manipulate the joint and tap in several areas, if necessary, to elicit the reflex. • If you have difficulty eliciting this DTR, ask the client to link both hands together tightly and try to pull them apart against resistance. This should distract the client's attention from the area being assessed.

Performing physical assessments continued

TECHNIQUE	NORMAL FINDINGS	SPECIAL CONSIDERATIONS
Tap over the Achilles tendon area, using a reflex hammer. Repeat this procedure on the opposite ankle.	Plantar flexion followed by muscle relaxation	• Crouch in front of the seated client. Hold the client's dorsiflexed foot in your hand. As an alternate position, have the client kneel on a stable chair, with both feet dangling over the edge. • This procedure elicits the Achilles DTR. • Manipulate the joint and tap in several areas, if necessary, to elicit the reflex. • If you have difficulty eliciting this DTR, ask the client to link both hands together tightly and try to pull them apart against resistance.
Stroke the sole of the foot using the end of the reflex hammer handle. Stroke on the little toe side from the heel to the toe; then stroke across the ball of the foot.	Toe flexion	• This procedure elicits a superficial reflex, known as the plantar reflex, which is plantar flexion of all toes. Babinski's sign occurs as dorsiflexion of the great toe with or without fanning of the other toes. Expect Babinski's sign in children under age 2; later, it is abnormal.
Ask the client to dorsiflex both feet against the resistance of your hands.	Both feet lift easily against resistance	• Place your hands on the dorsal surfaces of the client's feet. • This procedure tests foot strength and ROM.
Ask the client to plantarflex both feet against the resistance of your hands.	Both feet push down easily against resistance	• Place your hands, palms up, on the plantar surfaces of the client's feet. • This procedure tests foot strength and ROM. • Wash your hands or remove your gloves when you complete assessing the client's feet.
Inspect the feet and toes for lesions. Palpate for dorsalis pedis pulses.	No lesions or lumps; equal bilateral pulses	• Pulses and hair distribution help evaluate peripheral vascular status.
Trace a one-digit number in the palm of the client's hand using your finger. Ask the client to identify the number.	Correct identification of number	• Stand in front of the seated client. Have the client close both eyes. • This procedure evaluates the client's tactile discrimination through graphesthesia. continued

Performing physical assessments continued

TECHNIQUE	NORMAL FINDINGS	SPECIAL CONSIDERATIONS
Place a familiar object, such as a key or a coin, in the client's hand. Ask the client to identify it.	Correct identification of object	• This procedure evaluates the client's tactile discrimination through stereognosis.
Observe the client walk across the room in four ways: with a regular gait, on the toes, on the heels, and heel-to-toe.	Steady gait, good balance, and no signs of muscle weakness or pain in any style of walking	• Ask the client to stand up. Stand several feet away from the client. • This technique evaluates the cerebellum and motor system, and checks for vertebral disk problems.
Inspect the scapulae, spine, back, and hips as the client bends forward as far as possible; bends backward; and bends from side to side.	Full ROM, easy flexibility, and no signs of scoliosis or varicosities	• Stand in back of the client. • Open the client's gown in the back. • Inspection evaluates the client's ROM and detects musculoskeletal abnormalities, such as scoliosis.
Perform the Romberg test. Ask the client to stand straight with both eyes closed and both feet together.	Steady stance with minimal weaving	• Stand facing the client. • This test checks cerebellar functioning and evaluates balance and coordination. • Do not touch the client unless the client is about to lose balance. • If the client begins to lose balance, stop the test.

Male reproductive system

Inspect the penis.	Loose, wrinkled skin over the shaft and taut, smooth skin over the glans penis with no lesions, ulcers, or breaks; appropriate size of penis for developmental age	• Stand facing the standing male client. • Put on surgical gloves. • Minimize client embarrassment by explaining each assessment step before doing it and projecting a professional demeanor. • This technique assesses the general condition of the penis and detects abnormalities such as lesions and ulcers. • Lift the penis to inspect its dorsal and ventral surfaces, or alternatively, ask the client to lift his penis. • If lesions are present, document their location, size, color, and presence of any exudate. Obtain an exudate sample to culture, if necessary. • If the client is uncircumcised,

Performing physical assessments continued

TECHNIQUE	NORMAL FINDINGS	SPECIAL CONSIDERATIONS
		have him retract the foreskin to allow inspection of the glans penis. • An infant's penis usually appears pink and smooth. An uncircumcised infant's foreskin usually is tight for 2 to 3 months after birth and does not retract easily. • During childhood, the penis remains completely hairless. During puberty, the genitals enlarge and secondary sex characteristics appear.
Palpate the penis.	Palpable dorsal vein and ridges of internal structures; no lumps, induration, or tender areas	• This technique allows detection of structural abnormalities or lumpy, indurated, or tender areas. • To palpate the penis properly, gently grasp the shaft between the thumb and first two fingers and palpate its length.
Inspect the urethral meatus.	Opening at tip of the glans penis free of redness or discharge	• Inspection evaluates the overall condition of the urethral meatus and detects signs of infection. • If a discharge is present, obtain a sample to culture. If necessary, have the client "milk" his penis to obtain a sample. To maintain asepsis, avoid touching the culture plate with your gloved (contaminated) hand.
Inspect the scrotum.	Symmetrical distribution of pubic hair over the symphysis pubis and scrotum; scrotal skin free of lesions, ulcers, or redness; appropriate size of scrotum for the client's developmental age, with the left testicle slightly lower than the right	• Inspection of these structures checks for male sex characteristics and hair distribution patterns. • A child's scrotum should be hairless. • An elderly client may have gray or white pubic hair. His scrotal skin may be less taut, giving the scrotum a pendulous appearance.
Palpate the scrotum.	Rough, rugated skin; symmetrical, smooth, freely movable, oval-shaped testes; palpable ridge of tissue lying vertically on the testicular surface (epi-	• This technique allows detection of lumps or tender areas. • To palpate a testicle properly, place your thumb in front and your first two fingers behind the scrotal sac. • Absence of one or both testes

continued

Performing physical assessments continued

TECHNIQUE	NORMAL FINDINGS	SPECIAL CONSIDERATIONS
Scrotum palpation continued	didymis); smooth, freely movable vas deferens	(undescended testes) in an infant over a few months old should be referred to a physician. When the cremasteric muscle relaxes, the testes resume their normal position. • Transilluminate any lumps, nodular areas, or areas of swelling.
Inspect and palpate the inguinal area.	Smooth skin without visible bulges or palpable lymph nodes	• These techniques can detect femoral hernias and enlarged inguinal lymph nodes. • To make a suspected hernia more visible, ask the client to bear down as if passing a stool. • Keep in mind that the hand used for palpation is contaminated.
Palpate the groin as the client coughs or bears down.	No palpable lumps	• This procedure can detect a hernia, which will feel like a bump, mass, or bulge when the client coughs or bears down. • To palpate for an inguinal hernia in an adult, gently insert the middle or index finger into the inguinal canal and up to Hesselbach's triangle. • To palpate for an inguinal hernia in a child, use your little finger. • To palpate for a femoral hernia, palpate near the femoral artery. • If you have had special preparation, perform a prostate examination. (See Chapter 14.)
Female reproductive system		
Inspect the vulva and other visible structures.	Female hair distribution pattern; skin without lesions	• Help the client into the lithotomy position. Sit on a stool at the base of the examination table. • Drape the client appropriately. • Focus the light before you put on gloves. • If necessary, call in an assistant before proceeding with this part of the assessment. • Inspection evaluates the development of female sex characteristics. • Compare a pediatric client's development with her developmental stage. • An elderly client may have little pubic hair.

Performing physical assessments continued

TECHNIQUE	NORMAL FINDINGS	SPECIAL CONSIDERATIONS
Palpate the vulva and labia.	Smooth surfaces free of lumps and lesions	• This technique checks the vulva and labia for abnormalities, such as lumps and lesions. • To palpate properly, use your dominant thumb and index finger. • Do not palpate a child's vulva and labia unless abuse is suspected. • An elderly client may have decreased fat in the labia and mons pubis.
Palpate the Bartholin's glands.	No swelling	• Palpation can detect signs of infection, such as swelling or discharge. • To palpate properly, use your thumb (at the posterior-lateral area of the vaginal opening) and index finger (in the vagina). • If a discharge is present, obtain a sample for culture. • Do not palpate a child's Bartholin's glands unless abuse is suspected.
Inspect the structures inside the labia minora.	Pink urethral meatus without redness or swelling; intact clitoris; vaginal orifice free of swelling, redness, or discharge	• To perform this inspection, turn your palm up with your index finger still in the vagina. Part the labia with your middle finger and thumb. • For a pediatric client, inspect the orifice for lesions.
Withdraw the index finger from the vagina while gently "stripping down" the urethra about ¾″ (2 cm).	No discharge	• This procedure checks for discharge from the Skene's glands and urethra. • If a discharge is present, obtain a sample for culture.
Press your fingers down just inside the vaginal introitus as the client bears down.	Pressure on finger, but no protrusion of bladder	• This maneuver checks for cystocele. • To palpate properly, use your index and middle fingers.
Withdraw the fingers as the client bears down. Help the client to a comfortable position. Then leave the examination room to allow the client to dress in private.	Gentle tightening of the vaginal walls; no bulges or masses	• This maneuver checks for uterine prolapse and rectocele. • Ask the client to bear down more than once, if necessary. • Glove both hands if the client is heavy. • If you have had special preparation, perform a complete pelvic examination. (See Chapter 13.)

and compare the findings to a chart of standard measurements.

Next, assess the client's vital signs, which include temperature, pulse, respirations, and blood pressure.

Body structures and systems

To begin the "hands on" part of the assessment, make sure the client is seated comfortably. Then assess each body structure and system in an integrated fashion, using a body region approach rather than a body system approach. For example, assess the posterior thorax—which includes portions of the respiratory, urinary, and musculoskeletal systems—and then assess the anterior thorax—which includes portions of the respiratory, cardiovascular, musculoskeletal, and gastrointestinal systems as well as the breasts. After the physical assessment, however, plan to organize and document your findings by body system.

Many health care professionals use a head-to-toe approach when performing a complete assessment. However, most health care professionals develop their own variations. Whether you perform a head-to-toe assessment or some other type, take a systematic approach that will provide consistency and aid documentation. It should minimize the number of changes in nurse-client positioning, avoid tiring the client unnecessarily, allow you to work most efficiently, and ensure that no assessment area is overlooked.

Documentation

To understand the significance of assessment findings and form a clear picture of the client's health status, carefully review the physical assessment information as well as the health history findings and the results of any laboratory studies and diagnostic tests that may have been ordered. Laboratory studies will depend on the client's condition, but usually include blood and urine tests. Based on these data, formulate appropriate nursing diagnoses, which determine how to plan, implement, and evaluate nursing care.

The ability to organize data is essential for proper documentation. To document a complete physical examination, organize and record assessment findings by body system. This provides easier access to more concise assessment data for the entire health care team. Remember to document all data completely, including normal and abnormal findings, and to be specific. Be sure to document negative findings, rather than not mentioning them.

The following documentation sample illustrates the proper way to document normal and abnormal physical assessment findings for an adult.

Height. 5'3"

Weight. 120 lb

Vital signs. Temperature 98.6° F. (oral), pulse 82 (radial) and regular, respirations 16 and regular, blood pressure 120/80 L sitting.

General survey. Caucasian female, age 34, well-dressed, well-nourished, in no apparent distress. Relaxed facial expression, clear, strong, non-pressured speech. Moves well. Dress and grooming appropriate. Alert and oriented to person, place, time, situation. Emotional status slightly anxious, but appears in good mood; no suicidal ideation.

Skin, hair, and nails. Skin warm and dry with good turgor. Few freckles over bridge of nose; small (5 mm) round, brown maculopapular mole above right breast; 2-cm scar beneath right knee (from a fall as a child). Hair auburn, clean, fine-textured. Scalp free of lesions. Nails pink, firm, well-trimmed, without lesions or clubbing. Right fourth toe has 1-cm corn.

Head and neck. Skull and face symmetrical; facial sensation intact to pin and cotton. Smiles, grimaces, wrinkles forehead, and closes eyelids tightly. No maxillary or frontal sinus tenderness on palpation or percussion. Clenches jaw without pain. Bilateral tonsillar nodes, 1 cm, nontender, mobile, discrete. Nonpalpable occipital, postauricular, preauricular, submaxillary, submental, posterior cervical, anterior cervical, and supraclavicular lymph nodes. Trachea midline. Carotid pulses bilaterally full and equal; no bruits. No jugular vein distention. Thyroid without masses, enlargement, tenderness; rises with swallowing. Full ROM of neck with equal, bilateral strength to resistance.

Nose. Straight septum without lesions; patent nostrils. Nasal mucosa free of lesions with scant clear discharge; bright pink, nonswollen turbinates.

Mouth and throat. 32 teeth, clean and in good repair; gums intact. Tongue and uvula midline. Palate rises with phonation. Gag reflex present. Tonsils absent. Tongue, palate, mucosa, and throat without lesions or exudate. Tongue pushes easily against resistance of tongue depressor.

Eyes. Symmetrical and free of lesions, discharge, pain, exophthalmos. Visual acuity with Snellen— left eye 20/25, right eye 20/20, both eyes 20/20 with corrective lenses. Lids and lashes intact. Sclera white; bulbar conjunctiva and corneas clear; palpebral conjunctiva deep pink; irises equally round and brown; pupils equal, round, reactive to light and accommodation. Extraocular movement intact without nystagmus. Visual fields grossly intact by confrontation. Ophthalmoscopic examination: red reflex present; background pink without lesions; optic disks creamy white with sharp margins; cup less than half of disk; vessels show no narrowing or A-V nicking; A-V ratio 2:3; bright foveal reflection in macula.

Ears. Pinna symmetrical without lesions or tenderness. Gross hearing intact. Weber heard equally in both ears; Rinne air conduction > bone conduction. Small amount of reddish cerumen in ear canals. Tympanic membranes pearly gray; light reflexes and landmarks appropriately placed bilaterally.

Respiratory system. Respirations unlabored. No bony abnormalities or tenderness. Anteroposterior: lateral diameter 1:2. Re-

spiratory expansion equal; diaphragmatic excursion 5 cm bilaterally. No increased fremitus. Lung fields resonant. Breath sounds vesicular through most of lung fields.

Breasts. Left breast slightly larger than right (has been this way since puberty). No skin changes, tenderness, masses, nipple discharge, or axillary or supraclavicular adenopathy. Does breast self-examination about once a month.

Cardiovascular system. No lifts or heaves. Point of maximum impulse visible and palpable at left midclavicular line at the 5th intercostal space. S_1 and S_2 regular rate and rhythm. No murmurs, extra sounds, or rubs on auscultation. No pretibial edema or varicosities. Radial, posterior tibial, and dorsalis pedis pulses normal amplitude and equal. Normal hair distribution on feet and toes.

Abdomen. Contour flat without lesions or pulsations. Bowel sounds auscultated in all four quadrants. No bruits. No masses, tenderness, hepatomegaly, or splenomegaly. Tympany throughout abdomen on percussion. Liver span of 8 cm percussed at right midclavicular line from costal angle to 6th ICS. No costovertebral angle tenderness. Femoral pulses equal bilaterally. One 1-cm, mobile, nontender node in right inguinal area.

Musculoskeletal system. Spine without abnormalities; full ROM. Fingers, wrists, elbows, shoulders, hips, knees, and ankles full ROM. No joint abnormalities or pain palpated. Muscle size and strength equal bilaterally.

Nervous system. Reasoning intact and judgment appropriate. (Answers questions appropriately and can list alternatives for a stressful situation, choosing appropriate action.) Immediate, recent, and remote memory intact. Intellect appears superior to educational level; can do serial sevens. Cranial nerves II through XII intact. Deep tendon reflexes—brachioradialis, biceps, triceps, patellar, Achilles, 2 + and equal. Plantar reflex intact. Sensory function intact to pin and cotton over face, hands, forearms, lower legs, and feet. Motor function adequate with equal hand, arm, leg, and foot strength. Gait intact. Cerebellar function intact—Romberg negative, heel-to-toe intact, no pronator drift.

Reproductive system. Vulva and Bartholin's glands, urethral meatus, and Skene's glands without lesions, discharge, or atrophy. Normal female hair distribution. Vaginal wall with rugae and small amount of whitish, thin, nonodorous discharge. No cystocele or rectocele. Cervix nontender and without lesions. Squamocolumnar junction on exocervix. Slightly friable with Pap. Uterus firm, midline, anteflexed, mobile, nontender, and nonpregnant in size. Adnexae have no masses or tenderness. Ovaries nonpalpable. No rectal lesions or masses; confirms bimanual examination; brown stool; guaiac negative.

PARTIAL ASSESSMENT

Like the complete assessment, the nurse's partial assessment includes a health history, a physical examination, and a review of the results of laboratory and diagnostic studies. However, the partial assessment focuses on a specific client concern or problem. More commonly performed than a complete assessment, it may be done in many different health care settings.

Health history

For an outpatient, an inpatient, or a distressed client, expect to take a partial history, or episodic write-up. For this type of health history, obtain full biographic data and detailed information only about the reason for seeking health care. (Use the PQRST method.)

Combine other health history components, such as past health status, family health status, status of physiologic systems, and health promotion and protection patterns, as needed. For example, combine past history and family history by asking the client, "Have you or anyone in your family had any of the following disorders?" Then list specific disorders. Be sure to determine the presence or absence of five prevalent diseases (alcoholism, cancer, diabetes, heart disease, and hypertension) and others appropriate to the client or culture.

Physical assessment

Although you might perform a complete physical assessment on the client's first visit or during a periodic checkup, most of the time you will perform episodic (partial) physical assessments to evaluate the specific symptoms reported in the health history.

Use the health history information as a guide when assessing a client with a specific problem or when tracking the progress of a regular client. For example, partial assessment techniques for a child with an allergic reaction to a medication might include temperature assessment; skin inspection; evaluation of breathing and respirations; auscultation of the lungs and heart; and evaluation of the ears, nose, and throat. Partial assessment techniques for a client recovering from abdominal surgery might include vital sign measurements, weight measurement, inspection of the incision, auscultation of bowel sounds, and abdominal palpation.

No matter what the client's condition, however, a partial assessment should include a general survey, vital sign measurements, and evaluation of certain body structures and systems.

General survey and vital signs

Make a general survey by assessing the client's mental status during the health history interview and by observing the client walk into the room and sit down (or move around in bed). Assess any additional mental status elements by talking with the client during the physical examination.

Next, evaluate the client's vital signs, combining assessments when possible. For example, take the client's blood pressure while an oral thermometer registers the client's temperature.

Partial assessment checklist

When a client needs a partial assessment, use the following checklist to evaluate basic structures and systems. Then list any additional areas that need to be assessed based on the client's reason for seeking health care.

☐ Make a general survey.
☐ Assess mental status.
☐ Take temperature.
☐ Assess pulse rate and rhythm.
☐ Assess the respiratory rate and rhythm.
☐ Measure blood pressure.
☐ Observe skin color, texture, and turgor.
☐ Test gross motor coordination.
☐ Examine the pupils (PERRLA).
☐ Assess gross vision and hearing.
☐ Examine oral structures as client says "Ahh."
☐ Auscultate breath sounds in the posterior thorax.
☐ Auscultate breath sounds in the anterior thorax.
☐ Auscultate the heart for apical rate, rhythm, and irregularities.
☐ Auscultate the abdomen.
☐ Percuss the abdomen.
☐ Palpate the abdomen.
☐ Palpate for pretibial edema.
☐ Palpate the dorsalis pedis pulse.
☐ Additional areas for assessment based on reason for seeking health care: ____

---

turn are the foundation for planning, implementing, and evaluating the client's care.

Finally, document all partial assessment findings, using the same concise, accurate documentation style as for a complete assessment.

SUGGESTED READINGS

Cobble, J. (1992). Trauma assessment. *Emergency, 24*(6), 24-28.

Milner, E., and Collins, M. (1992). A tool to improve systematic client assessment in undergraduate nursing education. *Journal of Nursing Education, 31*(4), 186-187.

Morton, P. (1993). *Health assessment in nursing* (2nd ed.). Springhouse, PA: Springhouse Corp.

Nettina, S., and Gregonis, S. (1990). Triage: Assigning priorities. *Nursing90, 20*(11), 86.

Stark, J. (1991). Streamline your discharge planning. *Nursing91, 21*(6), 32I, 32L.

Body structures and systems

During this part of the physical assessment, evaluate certain basic structures and systems. (For additional information, see *Partial assessment checklist*.) Then, based on the client's needs and health history data, assess additional pertinent areas.

Documentation

If laboratory or diagnostic studies have been ordered for a client, consider the results along with the health history and partial physical assessment findings. As with the complete assessment, use this information as the basis for nursing diagnoses, which in

20

Perinatal and Neonatal Assessments

Because pregnancy affects a woman's entire body, the prenatal assessment must be comprehensive. It should evaluate common complaints and include a complete assessment of each body system. It should also assess the client's emotional status, including her acceptance of the pregnancy, her preparation for motherhood, and the pregnancy's impact on the family.

For postpartum assessment, collect data on the client's response to delivery and to the neonate as well as her adjustment to the puerperium (the 6 weeks after childbirth). Also, teach the client about the changes occurring in her body.

Neonatal assessment begins immediately after birth and continues for the duration of the neonate's nursery stay. The nurse is usually the first health care professional to examine the neonate in the delivery room. To conduct such an examination, you will need to know how to calculate an Apgar score and how to make general—but crucial—observations about the neonate's appearance and behavior. This information, coupled with pertinent maternal and fetal history data, provides an initial data base for nursery personnel and pediatricians to use during subsequent examinations.

PRENATAL ASSESSMENT

Prenatal assessment begins when the client first seeks medical care because she suspects she may be pregnant, and continues until labor and delivery.

Health history

Help put the client at ease by conducting the health history interview in a quiet, comfortable, and private environment. Proceed at an unhurried pace to allow the client time to answer all questions thoroughly and accurately. Begin by obtaining all relevant biographic data. Then ask questions about the pregnancy and the client's health status.

Three groups of sample questions follow. Those on *health and illness patterns* help the nurse identify actual or potential pregnancy-related health problems; those on *health promotion and protection patterns* help the nurse determine how the cient's life-style and behavior may affect her health and the health of her developing fetus; and those on *role and relationship patterns* help the nurse determine how the pregnancy is affecting the client's body image, life-style, and relationships with others.

Health and illness patterns

When was the first day of your last menstrual period?
(RATIONALE: Knowing the date of the last menstrual period helps diagnose pregnancy and determine the approximate delivery date.)

Was this menstrual period like the previous ones?
(RATIONALE: A pregnant client may seem to have a period, but with different characteristics. The client could interpret as a period changes that include spotting [scant bloody discharge from the vagina], which could indicate an ectopic pregnancy, a cervical infection, or a problem with hormonal support of the endometrium.)

How is your overall health? Have you experienced any problems during this pregnancy?
(RATIONALE: These questions allow the client to discuss her general health status and any specific complaints related to pregnancy or other conditions.)

Have you had uterine or pelvic surgery or injury?
(RATIONALE: Previous uterine or pelvic surgery or injury may necessitate cesarean delivery.)

Have you ever had a sexually transmitted disease? If so, which one and when? What treatment did you receive?
(RATIONALE: An untreated sexually transmitted disease places the fetus at risk for infection during passage through the birth canal.)

Have you been pregnant before? If so, how would you describe the pregnancy and its outcome?
(RATIONALE: Knowing the history of the client's previous pregnancies can help identify any potential problems with the current pregnancy.)

Have you ever had an abortion?
(RATIONALE: Abortion may result in cervical incompetency or adhesions that could cause problems during pregnancy and delivery.)

If you have given birth before, have you breast-fed or bottle-fed your infant(s)?
(RATIONALE: This question allows the client to discuss her plans for feeding her infant and any problems she might have experienced with feeding previous infants.)

Is your blood Rh negative? If so, did you receive Rh_o immunoglobulin (RhoGAM) after your first delivery?
(RATIONALE: An Rh-negative woman who has delivered an Rh-positive infant becomes sensitized to the Rh factor and needs RhoGAM to prevent complications with subsequent deliveries.)

Family health status

Has anyone in your family experienced any complications during pregnancy, labor, or delivery? If so, what were the complications and how were they resolved?
(RATIONALE: A family history of pregnancy or childbirth complications—such as spontaneous abortion, multiple births, or difficult labor—suggests a predisposition to such problems.)

Has anyone in your family had hypertension, diabetes mellitus, gestational diabetes (diabetes during pregnancy only), obesity, or heart disease?
(RATIONALE: Such familial conditions can adversely affect the health of a pregnant client or her fetus.)

Health promotion and protection patterns

Are you currently using any street drugs or alcohol? If so, which ones, in what amounts, and for how long?
(RATIONALE: During pregnancy, a client's use of illicit drugs—such as cocaine and heroin—can cause severe drug withdrawal symptoms and possible long-term neurologic effects in the neonate. Alcohol abuse during pregnancy can cause fetal birth defects.)

Did you use a contraceptive before this pregnancy? If so, which type? When did you stop using it?
(RATIONALE: The answer to this question provides information about the effectiveness of contraception and pregnancy planning.)

Do you smoke cigarettes? If so, how many do you smoke per day and how long have you been smoking?
(RATIONALE: Smoking during pregnancy is associated with fetal growth retardation and increased fetal and neonatal morbidity and mortality.)

When did you last have a Papanicolaou (Pap) test? What were the results?
(RATIONALE: The answer provides information about the client's health promotion and protection patterns. It also indicates whether the Pap test was normal.)

What is your typical daily diet? Which types and what amounts of food do you eat at each meal and between meals?
(RATIONALE: This question helps assess the client's nutritional status. It also gives the client an opportunity to discuss any concerns about food and gives you an opportunity to clear up any misconceptions she may have, such as "eating for two.")

Do you exercise regularly? If so, which type of exercise and how often?
(RATIONALE: Unless contraindicated, regular moderate exercise can improve or maintain muscle tone, which can help ease delivery and speed the body's return to its prepregnant state.)

How much sleep do you usually get per day? Do you feel well rested?
(RATIONALE: A pregnant client may require more sleep, particularly during the first and third trimesters. Inadequate sleep can cause increased stress and stress-related problems.)

Have you thought about what type of delivery you would like? Have you attended any prenatal classes?

(RATIONALE: These questions help assess the client's preparation for labor and delivery as well as her attitudes toward the pregnancy. They also provide an opportunity to explain available learning resources.)

Do you have any questions about any aspect of pregnancy or childbirth?
(RATIONALE: This open-ended question gives the client an opportunity to discuss any concerns and explore any areas not yet covered in the interview.)

Role and relationship patterns
How do you feel about being pregnant? How do you feel about having and caring for your baby? Is the pregnancy (or the anticipated baby) causing any problems in such areas as family relationships, finances, career, or living accommodations? Do you feel that you are receiving sufficient support from your family and friends during your pregnancy?
(RATIONALE: These questions provide an opening for the client to express her concerns.)

Have you been engaging in sexual intercourse during this pregnancy? How do you feel about sexual activity during pregnancy?
(RATIONALE: Normally, sexual activity need not be restricted during pregnancy. The client may experience increased sexual desire after the first trimester as a result of pelvic vasocongestion.)

Physical assessment
Pregnancy affects almost all body systems and major organs. The nurse who assesses a pregnant client needs to know these effects, along with normal findings.

Skin
First, inspect the client's skin, particularly noting any color changes. Examples include a brownish hyperpigmentation of the facial skin (chloasma, also called melasma, or the mask of pregnancy) and a brownish black pigmented line on the abdominal midline (the linea nigra). The areolae, nipples, and vulva also may darken from hyperpigmentation. Most of these color changes fade gradually after delivery.

Assessing the fundus

To estimate the size of the uterus—and fetal growth—palpate and measure the fundus. Before the 12th gestational week, when the gravid uterus moves into the abdominal cavity, estimate uterine size by bimanual assessment. After the 12th week, use fundal palpation to determine fundal height.

To palpate fundal height, stand at the supine client's right side and place the palm of your left hand about 1⅛″ to 1⅝″ (3 to 4 cm) above where the fundus should be. Palpating toward the symphysis pubis, find the point where the soft abdomen ends and the firm round fundal edge begins.

Next, using a measuring tape, determine the distance along the anterior abdominal wall from the top of the fundus to the notch at the inferior edge of the symphysis pubis. At 12 to 13 weeks, the fundus can be felt just above the symphysis pubis; at 16 weeks, the fundus is about midway between the symphysis pubis and the umbilicus; at 20 weeks, it can be felt at the umbilical level.

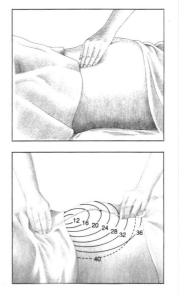

Thyroid gland
When assessing the head and neck, be sure to palpate the thyroid. In about 50% of all pregnant women, the thyroid gland enlarges because of increased vascularity and hyperplasia of this glandular tissue.

Respiratory system
As you observe the client's chest, note the breathing pattern and respiratory rate. During pregnancy, the thoracic cage shortens, widening at the base. The pregnant client may change from abdominal breathing to thoracic breathing as pregnancy progresses.

Cardiovascular system
Auscultate the client's cardiovascular system, keeping in mind that a 30% to 50%

increase in blood volume occurs during pregnancy, commonly accentuating heart sounds. In fact, systolic murmurs occur in about 90% of pregnant women. The heart is displaced upward and laterally, secondary to the pressure exerted by the gravid (pregnant) uterus on the diaphragm, sometimes causing the point of maximum impulse (PMI) to be displaced laterally.

Observe the condition of the client's veins. Pelvic congestion predisposes the client to venous varicosities in the legs and vulva. Edema in the arms and legs is also common.

Breasts
Inspect and palpate the breasts. In about the 8th week, they enlarge. The nipples become

larger and more erect. Montgomery's tubercles (sebaceous glands on the areolae) become more prominent. Colostrum, the precursor of milk, can be expressed as early as the 24th gestational week. Initially clear to yellowish, colostrum becomes cloudy later in the pregnancy. Striae (streaks or stretch marks caused by rapidly increasing skin tension) on the breast may become more visible as vascularity and venous engorgement increase.

Abdomen

Inspect and auscultate the abdomen. Striae gravidarum, varying from one pregnant woman to another, appear as the skin stretches to accommodate the growing uterus. The umbilicus may flatten or protrude. Peristalsis (rhythmic motion of smooth-muscle bowel) slows during pregnancy, so bowel sounds may decrease. The gravid uterus displaces the colon laterally upward and posteriorly.

Auscultate the fetal heart, which can be heard with a Doppler system as early as the 10th gestational week. In early pregnancy, the fetal heart beats loudest (area of maximum intensity) just above the mother's symphysis pubis at midline. Later in pregnancy, the fetal heart is best heard through the fetal back; optimum auscultation location depends on fetal position.

Musculoskeletal system

Observe the client's posture and gait during the assessment. Posture and gait changes result from the gravid uterus thrusting forward and changing the woman's center of gravity. To compensate for these changes, the woman throws her shoulders backward and hyperextends the vertebral column. The abnormal lordosis (curve of the spine) will return to normal after delivery. During the third trimester, the pelvic joints and ligaments relax in preparation for delivery. The pelvis becomes slightly broader.

Documentation

To complete the prenatal assessment, document your history and physical assessment findings as well as the results of any laboratory studies that may have been ordered.

The following example shows how to document some normal assessment findings.

Height. 5'6"

Weight. 136 lb

The client, a 23-year-old primigravida, states that she has not had a period in 2 months. She reports nausea and vomiting upon awakening and complains of tenderness and fullness in her breasts. Physical assessment reveals brownish discoloration around the areolae of both breasts. The client reports tenderness when the breasts are palpated. The breasts feel firm and full. Abdominal palpation finds the uterus at the level of the symphysis pubis. Gynecologic assessment shows dark-blue discoloration of the vaginal mucosa.

POSTPARTUM ASSESSMENT

The postpartum period represents a time of great change in the mother, the neonate, and the family. The nurse's postpartum assessment of the client evaluates the physiologic and psychological changes that occur as her body returns to its prepregnant state. It also assesses the client's and family's adjustment to these changes.

Health history

The postpartum health history collects data on the client's responses to delivery and to the neonate as well as on her adjustment to the puerperium. Take this opportunity to teach the client about the changes in her body.

Three groups of sample questions follow. Those on *health and illness patterns* help the nurse identify actual or potential postpartum problems; those on *health promotion and protection patterns* help the nurse evaluate personal habits and activities that may affect the client's recovery from childbirth and adjustment to the neonate; and those on *role and relationship patterns* help the nurse determine how the client and her family are adjusting to the neonate.

Health and illness patterns

How do you feel? Are you experiencing any specific problems you would like to discuss?
(RATIONALE: The client's physical health and comfort can directly affect her mental and emotional adjustment. These questions also give the client a chance to discuss any issues that she may be reluctant to bring up.)

How is your energy level?
(RATIONALE: Postpartum fatigue normally results from disrupted sleep patterns and the emotional stress of adjusting to the neonate and to motherhood.)

Do you have any pain or discomfort in your abdominal or genital areas?
(RATIONALE: For 2 or 3 days after delivery, periodic uterine contractions commonly produce afterpains. Vaginal bruising and edema caused by vaginal delivery also may produce discomfort for several days. Pain or discomfort also is likely if the client had an episiotomy.)

Do you have any discomfort in your breasts or nipples?
(RATIONALE: Breast milk production, which begins around the third day after delivery, commonly causes painful breast engorgement. In a breast-feeding woman, the nipples may be tender for the first few days of nursing.)

Do you have difficulty urinating or feel any pain or discomfort in your bladder or urinary tract?
(RATIONALE: Bladder trauma during birth can cause overdistention and incomplete bladder emptying during voiding. These effects may persist for several days.)

Have you had a bowel movement yet?
(RATIONALE: After delivery, decreased bowel motility, fluid loss, and perineal discomfort commonly delay resumption of normal bowel function for up to a week.)

Do you have any weakness or decreased sensations in your legs and feet?

(RATIONALE: A transient decrease in leg muscle strength may result from the muscle strain and exertion associated with labor and delivery. Use of regional anesthesia during labor and delivery may lead to diminished sensations in the legs and feet for up to 24 hours.)

Health promotion and protection patterns

What is your typical daily diet? Which types and what amounts of food do you eat at each meal and between meals?
(RATIONALE: When caring for the neonate, the client may ignore her own health. Encourage the client to eat properly, especially if she is breast-feeding.)

How much sleep are you getting? Do you feel well rested or tired?
(RATIONALE: A woman often has difficulty sleeping after delivery; excitement, discomfort, and problems of adjusting to the neonate's demands may seriously disrupt sleep patterns.)

Have you been walking? If not, why not?
(RATIONALE: Early ambulation in the postpartum period can help promote healing and decrease the risk of thrombophlebitis.)

Do you feel that the baby is increasing your stress?
(RATIONALE: A neonate may seriously disrupt the tranquility of a household. Assess the client's ability to cope with this disruption and teach stress-management techniques, if appropriate.)

Do you know the signs and symptoms of postpartum problems that require immediate medical attention?
(RATIONALE: Make sure that the client and her family can recognize the warning signs and symptoms of serious postpartum complications, such as hemorrhage, infection, thromboembolism, and hypertension.)

Are you aware of community agencies and other resources that could help you care for the baby at home?

(RATIONALE: Social service and other agencies may provide assistance in caring for the neonate at home.)

Have you scheduled a follow-up examination?
(RATIONALE: A maternal follow-up examination should be performed 4 to 6 weeks after delivery.)

Do you have a car seat to take the baby home from the hospital?
(RATIONALE: Most hospitals require that the parents have an approved car seat for transporting the neonate home.)

Role and relationship patterns
How do you feel about the new baby and your role as mother?
(RATIONALE: The client may experience "postpartum blues" during the first 10 days or so after delivery. Symptoms include crying, irritability, loss of appetite, and difficulty sleeping. Usually, this condition is transient; persistence for more than 2 weeks may indicate postpartum depression.)

Is your partner supportive and is he taking an active role in caring for the baby?
(RATIONALE: A new father may feel ignored and may withdraw as the client focuses her attention on the neonate.)

Do you feel that you are receiving enough help and support from family and friends?
(RATIONALE: The client's psychological well-being depends heavily on how her family and friends respond to the neonate.)

Physical assessment
Postpartum physical assessment begins with the client supine. Throughout the assessment, the nurse collects data on the client's responses to delivery and to the neonate, as well as on her adjustment to the puerperium. The nurse also teaches the client about her physical changes. Usually, postpartum physical assessment proceeds from head to toe.

Breasts
Inspect the nipples for signs of infection, bleeding, or crusting. On palpation, the breasts should be soft and nontender. However, many women experience engorgement secondary to the increased breast vascularity that occurs in preparation for lactation. Engorged breasts become enlarged, firm, and usually tender. Look for any reddened or warm areas, which could indicate mastitis.

Abdomen
After delivery, the abdomen is soft, lacking appreciable muscle tone, but muscle tone usually returns to the prepregnant level by 6 weeks postpartum.

Instruct the client to urinate before you begin the fundal height assessment. Immediately after delivery, the fundus should be firm and positioned at the umbilicus. As normal involution (decrease in uterine size) progresses, the fundus gradually moves from below the umbilicus to just above the symphysis pubis. The fundus can be palpated after childbirth for 10 to 14 days, when the uterus again becomes a nonpalpable pelvic organ.

Throughout the postpartum period, the uterus should remain rounded and firm.

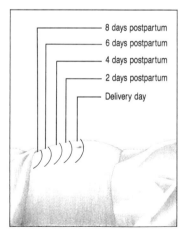

- 8 days postpartum
- 6 days postpartum
- 4 days postpartum
- 2 days postpartum
- Delivery day

Perineum and rectum
Inspect the perineum and episiotomy (incision made in the perineum to enlarge the vaginal opening for delivery) site for signs of erythema, edema, ecchymoses (bruising), or hematoma (blood clot).

Assess the lochia for consistency, amount, color, and odor. Lochia rubra, the dark-red vaginal drainage occurring the first 3 days after delivery, contains red blood cells, placental and decidual debris, and plasma. As the placental site heals, fewer red blood cells are shed and the lochia becomes serosanguineous. Called lochia serosa (pale pink or brown), the serosanguineous matter continues sloughing for 4 to 10 days after delivery. After about 10 days, the lochia is called lochia alba (yellow or white) and consists mostly of plasma and leukocytes.

After assessing the perineum, assess the rectum for hemorrhoids, which may result from engorged pelvic tissue during pregnancy and pressure on the rectum during vaginal delivery.

Extremities

Assess the arms and legs for signs of edema, varicosities, or thrombophlebitis. Edema in the legs requires a complete assessment of leg pulses and skin temperature.

Documentation

To complete the postpartum assessment, document your health history and physical assessment findings as well as any laboratory studies that may have been ordered.

NEONATAL ASSESSMENT

Neonatal assessment begins immediately after delivery and continues throughout the nursery stay. The nurse's complete neonatal assessment includes a perinatal history (covering such factors as maternal health history, duration of labor, use of analgesia or anesthesia during labor, and any complications of labor and delivery), determination of gestational age, behavioral assessment, and physical assessment.

Behavioral assessment

Begin the assessment by observing the neonate's interactions with the environment. To do this, observe the state of alertness: Is the neonate sleeping deeply or lightly? Is the ne-

onate drowsy or alert? Are the eyes open? Is the neonate crying? The time that the neonate spends in each state and the ease of transition from one state of alertness to another varies between individuals. Recording the state of alertness is an important part of the collected neonatal assessment data.

Physical assessment

Knowing the perinatal history and observing astutely are essential skills for the nurse's complete neonatal assessment. Systematic inspection of the neonate usually proceeds from head to toe, beginning with observing the pulse and respiratory rates while the neonate sleeps. Use a radiant warmer or take other precautions, such as exposing only those areas of the neonate that are being assessed, to ensure thermoregulation.

Respirations and pulse rate

Immediately after the neonate's birth, assess respirations. The normal irregular and shallow respiratory rate ranges from 30 to 60 breaths/minute. Brief (15-second) apnea (absence of respiration), also called periodic breathing, occurs characteristically. The chest and abdomen should rise simultaneously with respiration. Auscultated breath sounds are bronchial and loud.

Then evaluate the pulse rate and heart sounds. The pulse rate changes and usually follows a pattern similar to the respiratory rate. Auscultated apically with a stethoscope for a full minute, the normal pulse rate is 120 to 160 beats/minute, increasing to 180 beats/minute during crying and motor activity. During deep sleep, the pulse rate may drop to 100 beats/minute. A slower heartbeat should be reported to the physician. Neonatal heart sounds have a higher pitch, shorter duration, and greater intensity than adult heart sounds.

General appearance

Assess overall skin color. Is the neonate jaundiced (yellow), pale, cyanotic (blue), or ruddy? To determine muscle tone and level of consciousness, observe position and motor ac-

Assessment findings during the periods of neonatal reactivity

During the first hours after birth, the neonate experiences gradual, predictable changes in physiologic characteristics and behavioral responses, reflecting the periods of neonatal reactivity (which are separated by a sleep stage). This chart shows the normal assessment findings associated with each reactivity period.

PARAMETER	FIRST PERIOD	SECOND PERIOD
Skin color	Fluctuates from pale pink to cyanotic (blue)	Fluctuates from pale pink to cyanotic, with periods of mottling
Alertness level	Awake and alert, progressing to sleep	Hyperactive, with exaggerated responses
Cry	Rigorous, diminishing with sleep	Periodic
Respiratory rate	Up to 80 breaths/minute	40 to 60 breaths/minute, with periods of more rapid respirations
Respiratory effort	Irregular and labored	Usually unlabored
Heart rate	Up to 180 beats/minute	120 to 160 beats/minute, with periods of more rapid beating
Heart rhythm	Irregular, progressing to regular	Irregular as sleep begins, progressing to regular
Bowel sounds	Absent	Present
Stool	May not be passed	Meconium passed
Voiding	Rare	Usually begins
Mucus production	Minimal, diminishing gradually	Present, may be excessive
Sucking reflex	Strong, diminishing as sleep begins	Strong

tivity. Is the neonate crying? What type of cry? Is it high-pitched, weak, or lusty? Is the neonate moving all extremities? Are movements symmetrical? Continue these observations throughout the assessment.

Weight ranges from 5 lb, 8 oz to 8 lb, 13 oz (2,500 to 4,000 g). To weigh the neonate, calibrate the scale at zero, drape a protective covering on the weighing platform, and place the unclothed neonate on it. Weigh at the same time each day. A neonate may lose

up to 10% of birth weight within the first 3 or 4 days of life. Height assessment usually accompanies weight assessment. Measure the neonate from crown to heel. The normal range is 18″ to 22″ (45 to 55 cm).

Skin and hair

Observe the skin for color and condition. Large amounts of vernix caseosa (a graywhite, cheeselike, protective skin covering) is normally seen immediately after birth, dimin-

Neonatal reflex assessment

The nurse assesses several reflexes to help determine whether the neonate's neuromuscular system is intact. Keep in mind that gestational age and neonatal muscle tone can alter the reflex responses and that some reflexes are not as age-specific as others.

REFLEX	ELICITING THE REFLEX	NORMAL RESPONSE
Sucking or rooting	Touch neonate's lip, cheek, or corner of mouth.	Neonate will turn head toward stimulation and open mouth; sucking activity noted.
Extrusion	Touch or depress tongue.	Neonate will force tongue outward.
Tonic neck or "fencing"	Turn head of supine neonate from midline to one side.	Extremities will extend on side toward which neonate is turned; opposite extremities will flex.
Palmar grasp	Apply pressure to palm of hand.	Neonate's fingers will curl around examiner's finger.
Plantar (Babinski)	Stroke the side of the foot from heel to toe and across the ball of the foot.	Neonate will hyperextend the toes, dorsiflex the great toe, and fan the toes outward.
Moro or "startle"	Apply a sudden stimulus, such as a hand clap, when neonate is lying quietly.	Neonate will draw up legs and bring arms up in an embracing motion; extremity movements should be symmetrical.
Stepping or "walking"	Hold neonate vertically; allow soles of feet to touch table surface.	Neonate will step, simulating walking.

ishing after several days. Vernix residues cling to the neck and groin creases and to the genital region. Skin tones range from pink in Caucasian neonates to creamy tan in darker-skinned, Black, Hispanic, or Asian neonates. Acrocyanosis (blue and red discoloration), resulting from sluggish peripheral circulation or from chilling, commonly appears during the first 24 hours. Also, when the neonate is cold, mottling (a patchy, purplish skin discoloration) may appear. Milia, white papules caused by accumulated sebum in the sebaceous glands, frequently occur across the nose, cheeks, and chin. These disappear within 2 to 3 weeks.

Note the type and amount of hair. The full-term neonate should have some head hair, but the amount varies. Lanugo (downy fetal hair) normally covers the face, shoulders, and back.

Head

Within a couple of hours of the neonate's birth, measure the head circumference at its greatest diameter, usually the occipitofrontal circumference. The normal size range is about 12¾" to 14½" (32 to 36 cm).

Next, palpate, inspect, and measure the fontanels. The diamond-shaped anterior fontanel normally measures 1⅛" to 1⅝" (3 to 4 cm) long and ¾" to 1⅛" (2 to 3 cm) wide and may enlarge as molding resolves. The triangle-shaped posterior fontanel may be closed at birth (from molding) but can remain palpable for about 3 months. The anterior fontanel is flat and should remain open for about 18 months.

Inspect the face for overall appearance and symmetry. Features should be appropriately placed and proportionate. Structures, muscle tone, and expression should be symmetrical.

Eyes, symmetrically sized and shaped, should be framed by eyebrows and eyelashes. Eyeballs should be round and firm. Watch for the neonate to focus momentarily, follow an object to the midline, and face toward a speaking voice. Nystagmus (involuntary oscillating eye movements) and strabismus (crossed eyes) are common in the first 2 to 3 months. Because of immature lacrimal glands, tears or discharge may appear. Occasionally, an exudate or swelling results from prophylactic drugs used to prevent ophthalmia neonatorum (neonatal conjunctivitis).

Check the ears for proper placement. The pinnas should intercept an imaginary line from the outer canthus of the eyes. Palpate for cartilage in the pinnas, and confirm hearing by eliciting the neonatal startle response to a sudden loud noise.

The nose should be midline, usually flat and broad. Some mucus may appear but no drainage. Because a neonate is an obligatory nose breather, check nostril patency by occluding one nostril at a time and observe for respiratory distress signs, such as sternal retraction.

Chest

Measure the chest at the nipple line. The average chest circumference is 12" to 13" (30 to 33 cm) or ¾" to 1½" less than the head circumference.

Palpate the normally rounded chest for signs of fracture, such as asymmetrical movement and crepitus. Symmetrical, the nipples normally measure less than ½" (5 to 10 mm) in a full-term neonate. Related to maternal estrogen in utero, breast engorgement may occur in either sex.

Ortolani's maneuver

With the neonate supine, flex the hips and knees at right angles; abduct them until the lateral aspects of the knees touch the examination table.

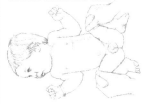

Next, bring the knees together, keeping the hips and knees flexed, and attempt to rotate the hips clockwise and counterclockwise to evaluate symmetry of movement.

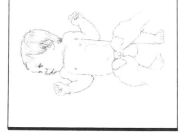

Abdomen

Inspect, auscultate, and palpate the abdomen, which should be rounded and dome-shaped, and soft with no masses. Bowel sounds should exist 1 to 2 hours after birth. Meconium (the thick, sticky, green or black first stool) should pass within the first 24 to 48 hours, indicating an intact and functioning gastrointestinal tract.

The umbilical stump falls midline at the lower abdomen. The umbilical cord – at birth moist, soft, and creamy white – should be securely clamped, nonbleeding, and free of signs of infection. It should remain dry and odorless. Then it progressively shrinks, turns black, and detaches in approximately 2 weeks.

Back

To inspect the back, turn the neonate to a prone position with the head to the side to prevent occluding the nostrils. Look first for a straight spine and planar alignment of shoulders, scapulae, and iliac crests; then palpate the spine. It should be intact, without indentations or dimpling.

Extremities

Note positions and movements of the arms and legs. The neonate usually assumes a position reflecting its normal position in utero. Motor activity should include a full range of motion with all four extremities moving spontaneously and equally. Often the fist is clenched with the thumb under the fingers. Fingernails and toenails should extend slightly beyond the tips of the fingers and toes. The legs should be equally long with comparable gluteal folds. Because the lateral muscles are more developed than the medial muscles, the legs should appear bowed.

Test hip joint stability by using Ortolani's maneuver. You may hear and feel a click or popping sound if the joint is unstable.

Anus and genitalia

Take the temperature rectally to assess anal patency in either sex.

In the male neonate, palpate the two pendulous and wrinkled scrotal sacs for evidence of a testis in each. Then observe that the prepuce (the foreskin, which does not retract easily) covers the glans penis and that the urinary meatus appears as a slit at the penile tip.

In the female neonate, the external genitalia usually look edematous and hyperpigmented. The labia majora dominate and cover the labia minora. The clitoris, also edematous, is noticeable. A grayish white mucus discharge (smegma), which is normal, or a blood-tinged discharge (pseudomenstruation), caused by maternal hormones in utero, may be present. The urinary meatus, positioned beneath the clitoris, is difficult to see.

Assess the frequency and amount of urination in neonates of both sexes. Because the fetal kidneys function, the neonate commonly voids within 24 hours of birth. Urine voided in the first few days may be scant and infrequent (two to six times daily); however, as dietary intake increases, the frequency of daily voidings also increases (15 to 20 times daily).

Documentation

To complete the neonatal assessment, document your findings, including the results of any laboratory studies that may have been ordered.

SUGGESTED READINGS

Cohen, S., et al. (1991). *Maternal, neonatal, and women's health nursing*, Springhouse, PA: Springhouse Corp.

Kenner, C. (1990). Measuring neonatal assessment. *Neonatal Network,* 9(4), 17-22.

Shrago, L. (1992). The breastfeeding dyad: Early assessment, documentation, and intervention. *NAACOG's Clinical Issues in Perinatal and Women's Health Nursing,* 3(4), 583-597.

Whaley, L., and Wong, D. (1991). *Nursing care of infants and children* (4th ed.). St. Louis: Mosby.

Appendices, Master Glossary, and Index

Appendix 1

NANDA taxonomy of nursing diagnoses

The currently accepted classification system for nursing diagnoses is that of the North American Nursing Diagnosis Association (NANDA), as shown in *NANDA Nursing Diagnoses: Definitions and Classification 1992-1993*. It is organized around nine human response patterns: exchanging, communicating, relating, valuing, choosing, moving, perceiving, knowing, and feeling.

The complete taxonomic structure is listed here. The series of numbers before each diagnosis is its classification number, used to determine the placement of the diagnosis within the taxonomy. The number of digits delineates the level of abstraction of the nursing diagnosis (more specific diagnoses are assigned longer numbers).

Pattern 1. Exchanging (Mutual giving and receiving)

1.1.2.1	Altered nutrition: More than body requirements
1.1.2.2	Altered nutrition: Less than body requirements
1.1.2.3	Altered nutrition: Potential for more than body requirements
1.2.1.1	High risk for infection
1.2.2.1	High risk for altered body temperature
1.2.2.2	Hypothermia
1.2.2.3	Hyperthermia
1.2.2.4	Ineffective thermoregulation
1.2.3.1	Dysreflexia
1.3.1.1	Constipation
1.3.1.1.1	Perceived constipation
1.3.1.1.2	Colonic constipation
1.3.1.2	Diarrhea
1.3.1.3	Bowel incontinence
1.3.2	Altered urinary elimination
1.3.2.1.1	Stress incontinence
1.3.2.1.2	Reflex incontinence
1.3.2.1.3	Urge incontinence
1.3.2.1.4	Functional incontinence
1.3.2.1.5	Total incontinence
1.3.2.2	Urinary retention
1.4.1.1	Altered (specify type) tissue perfusion (renal, cerebral, cardiopulmonary, gastrointestinal, peripheral)

1.4.1.2.1	Fluid volume excess
1.4.1.2.2.1	Fluid volume deficit
1.4.1.2.2.2	High risk for fluid volume deficit
1.4.2.1	Decreased cardiac output
1.5.1.1	Impaired gas exchange
1.5.1.2	Ineffective airway clearance
1.5.1.3	Ineffective breathing pattern
1.5.1.3.1	Inability to sustain spontaneous ventilation
1.5.1.3.2	Dysfunctional ventilatory weaning response
1.6.1	High risk for injury
1.6.1.1	High risk for suffocation
1.6.1.2	High risk for poisoning
1.6.1.3	High risk for trauma
1.6.1.4	High risk for aspiration
1.6.1.5	High risk for disuse syndrome
1.6.2	Altered protection
1.6.2.1	Impaired tissue integrity
1.6.2.1.1	Altered oral mucous membrane
1.6.2.1.2.1	Impaired skin integrity
1.6.2.1.2.2	High risk for impaired skin integrity

Pattern 2. Communicating (Sending messages)

2.1.1.1	Impaired verbal communication

continued

NANDA taxonomy of nursing diagnoses   continued

Pattern 3. Relating (Establishing bonds)

3.1.1	Impaired social interaction
3.1.2	Social isolation
3.2.1	Altered role performance
3.2.1.1.1	Altered parenting
3.2.1.1.2	High risk for altered parenting
3.2.1.2.1	Sexual dysfunction
3.2.2	Altered family processes
3.2.2.1	Caregiver role strain
3.2.2.2	High risk for caregiver role strain
3.2.3.1	Parental role conflict
3.3	Altered sexuality patterns

Pattern 4. Valuing (Assigning relative worth)

4.1.1	Spiritual distress (distress of the human spirit)

Pattern 5. Choosing (Selecting alternatives)

5.1.1.1	Ineffective individual coping
5.1.1.1.1	Impaired adjustment
5.1.1.1.2	Defensive coping
5.1.1.1.3	Ineffective denial
5.1.2.1.1	Ineffective family coping: Disabling
5.1.2.1.2	Ineffective family coping: Compromised
5.1.2.2	Family coping: Potential for growth
5.2.1	Ineffective management of therapeutic regimen (individual)
5.2.1.1	Noncompliance (specify)
5.3.1.1	Decisional conflict (specify)
5.4	Health-seeking behaviors (specify)

Pattern 6. Moving (Involving activity)

6.1.1.1	Impaired physical mobility
6.1.1.1.1	High risk for peripheral neurovascular dysfunction
6.1.1.2	Activity intolerance
6.1.1.2.1	Fatigue
6.1.1.3	High risk for activity intolerance
6.2.1	Sleep pattern disturbance
6.3.1.1	Diversional activity deficit
6.4.1.1	Impaired home maintenance management
6.4.2	Altered health maintenance
6.5.1	Feeding self-care deficit
6.5.1.1	Impaired swallowing
6.5.1.2	Ineffective breast-feeding
6.5.1.2.1	Interrupted breast-feeding
6.5.1.3	Effective breast-feeding
6.5.1.4	Ineffective infant feeding pattern
6.5.2	Bathing or hygiene self-care deficit
6.5.3	Dressing or grooming self-care deficit
6.5.4	Toileting self-care deficit
6.6	Altered growth and development
6.7	Relocation stress syndrome

Pattern 7. Perceiving (Receiving information)

7.1.1	Body image disturbance
7.1.2	Self-esteem disturbance
7.1.2.1	Chronic low self-esteem
7.1.2.2	Situational low self-esteem
7.1.3	Personal identity disturbance

NANDA taxonomy of nursing diagnoses continued

Pattern 7. Perceiving (Receiving information) continued

7.2	Sensory or perceptual alterations (specify visual, auditory, kinesthetic, gustatory, tactile, olfactory)
7.2.1.1	Unilateral neglect
7.3.1	Hopelessness
7.3.2	Powerlessness

Pattern 8. Knowing (Associating meaning with information)

8.1.1	Knowledge deficit (specify)
8.3	Altered thought processes

Pattern 9. Feeling (Being subjectively aware of information)

9.1.1	Pain
9.1.1.1	Chronic pain
9.2.1.1	Dysfunctional grieving
9.2 1.2	Anticipatory grieving
9.2.2	High risk for violence: Self-directed or directed at others
9.2.2.1	High risk for self-mutilation
9.2.3	Post-trauma response
9.2.3.1	Rape-trauma syndrome
9.2.3.1.1	Rape-trauma syndrome: Compound reaction
9.2.3.1.2	Rape-trauma syndrome: Silent reaction
9.3.1	Anxiety
9.3.2	Fear

Appendix 2

Common Laboratory Studies

TEST AND SIGNIFICANCE	NORMAL VALUES OR FINDINGS	ABNORMAL FINDINGS AND POSSIBLE CAUSES
Blood tests		
Acid phosphatase, serum By measuring the phosphatase enzymes produced by prostatic tumors, this test helps detect prostatic cancer.	0 to 1.1 Bodansky units/ml; 1 to 4 King Arm-strong units/ml; 0.13 to 0.63 Bessey-Lowery-Brock units/ml	• Above-normal level: Prostatic cancer, some drugs • Below-normal level: Some drugs
Activated partial thromboplastin time (APTT) This test evaluates intrinsic pathway clotting factors, except for Factors VII and XIII, by measuring the time required for fibrin clot formation after adding calcium and phospholipid emulsion to a plasma sample.	25 to 36 seconds	• Prolonged time: Deficiency of plasma clotting factors other than VII and XIII; presence of heparin; presence of fibrin split products, fibrinolysins, or circulating antibodies that are specific to the clotting factors • Shortened time: Extensive cancer (except liver cancer), hemorrhage, early stage of disseminated intravascular coagulation (DIC)
Albumin, serum This test measures serum levels of albumin, which maintains oncotic pressure and transports substances, such as fatty acids, that are insoluble in water.	3.3 to 4.5 g/dl	• Above-normal level: Underhydration; in all cases, results may mask nutritional implications • Below normal level: Possible visceral protein depletion, overhydration, pregnancy, decreased muscle mass, nephrotic syndrome
Alkaline phosphatase Measuring this enzyme helps detect focal hepatic lesions and skeletal diseases, primarily those characterized by marked osteoblastic activity.	1.5 to 4 Bodansky units/dl *Males:* 90 to 239 units/liter *Females under age 45:* 76 to 196 units/liter *Females over age 45:* 87 to 250 units/liter	• Above-normal level: Liver disease, obstructive biliary disease, osteomalacia, metastatic bone tumors, Paget's disease of bone, bone fracture healing • Below-normal level: Hypophosphatasia, malnutrition, hypothyroidism, pernicious anemia, placental insufficiency, dwarfism
Alpha-fetoprotein Detecting this glycoprotein may indicate hepatocellular carcinoma, testicular cancer, or fetal neural tube defects (in a pregnant client).	< 30 ng/ml (levels vary throughout pregnancy)	• Above-normal level: Primary liver cancer, testicular cancer, ineffective treatment, neural tube defect in fetus • Below-normal level: No clinical significance
Amylase and lipase Measuring these pancreatic enzymes is the most valuable indicator of pancreatic function.	*Amylase:* 60 to 80 Somogyi units/dl *Lipase:* 32 to 80 units/liter	• Above-normal level of both enzymes: Pancreatic inflammation or obstruction, gastrointestinal (GI) ulceration

Common Laboratory Studies continued

TEST AND SIGNIFICANCE	NORMAL VALUES OR FINDINGS	ABNORMAL FINDINGS AND POSSIBLE CAUSES
Blood tests continued		
Amylase and lipase continued		• Below-normal level of amylase: Chronic pancreatitis, hepatitis, cirrhosis, toxemia of pregnancy, severe burn, some drugs • Below-normal level of lipase: Some drugs, advanced age
Arterial blood gas (ABG) analysis This test evaluates gas exchange in the lungs by measuring the partial pressures of oxygen (Pao_2) and carbon dioxide ($Paco_2$) and the pH of arterial blood. Pao_2 indicates how much oxygen the lungs deliver to the blood, and $Paco_2$ indicates how efficiently the lungs eliminate carbon dioxide. The pH indicates the acid-base level of the blood by measuring the hydrogen ion concentration. ABG measurements also show the amount of bicarbonate ions (HCO_3^-) and the oxygen (O_2) saturation of the blood.	*Pao_2:* 75 to 100 mm Hg *$Paco_2$:* 35 to 45 mm Hg *pH:* 7.35 to 7.42 *HCO_3^-:* 22 to 26 mEq/liter *O_2 saturation:* 94% to 100%	• pH less than 7.35, $Paco_2$ greater than 45 mm Hg (respiratory acidosis): Central nervous system (CNS) depression from drugs, injury, or disease; asphyxia; hypoventilation • pH greater than 7.42, $Paco_2$ less than 35 mm Hg (respiratory alkalosis): Hyperventilation respiratory stimulation by drugs, disease, hypoxia, fever, or high room temperature • pH less than 7.35, HCO_3^- less than 22 mEq/liter (metabolic acidosis): HCO_3^- depletion caused by renal disease, diarrhea, excess production of organic acids related to hepatic disease, endocrine disorders, hypoxia, or shock • pH greater than 7.42, HCO_3^- greater than 26 mEq/liter (metabolic alkalosis): Loss of hydrochloric acid from prolonged gastric suctioning, loss of potassium from increased renal excretion, excessive alkali ingestion
Bilirubin Measuring direct (prehepatic) and indirect (posthepatic) bilirubin helps evaluate hepatobiliary and erythropoietic functions.	*Direct:* 0.5 mg/dl or less *Indirect:* 1.1 mg/dl or less *Total:* 1 to 12 mg/dl (in neonates) or 0.2 to 1.0 mg/dl (in others)	• Above-normal level: Hepatitis, biliary tract obstruction (direct and indirect); fasting (total and direct); hemolytic disease (indirect) • Below-normal level: No clinical significance
Blood urea nitrogen (BUN) This test reflects protein intake and renal excretory capacity and helps identify uremia.	8 to 20 mg/dl	• Above-normal level: Renal disease, reduced renal blood flow, urinary tract obstruction • Below-normal level: Liver failure, malnutrition, celiac disease, overhydration, pregnancy

continued

Common Laboratory Studies continued

TEST AND SIGNIFICANCE	NORMAL VALUES OR FINDINGS	ABNORMAL FINDINGS AND POSSIBLE CAUSES
Blood tests continued		
Carcinoembryonic antigen (CEA) Normally, production of this glycoprotein halts shortly after birth; it may begin again later if a neoplasm develops.	5 ng/dl	• Above-normal level: Colorectal cancer • Below-normal level: No clinical significance
Catecholamines This test assesses adrenal medulla function.	*Epinephrine, basal supine:* 0 to 110 pg/ml *Epinephrine, standing:* 0 to 140 pg/ml *Norepinephrine, basal supine:* 70 to 750 pg/ml *Norepinephrine, standing:* 200 to 1,700 pg/ml	• Above-normal level: Pheochromocytoma, neuroblastoma, electroshock therapy, shock caused by hemorrhage, endotoxins, anaphylaxis • Below-normal level: No clinical significance
Cholesterol, total This test measures the circulating levels of free cholesterol and cholesterol esters and reflects the body's fat metabolism.	120 to 220 mg/dl	• Above-normal level: Increased risk of coronary artery disease, obstructive biliary disease, fatty liver degeneration • Below-normal level: Chronic liver disease
Complete blood count (CBC) This test determines the actual number of blood elements in relation to volume and quantifies abnormalities.	*Erythrocyte (red blood cell [RBC]) count* *Males:* 4.5 to 6.2 million/mm^3 *Females:* 4.2 to 5.4 million/mm^3 *Children:* 4.6 to 4.8 million/mm^3 *Full-term neonates:* 4.4 to 5.8 million/mm^3	• Above-normal level: Primary or secondary polycythemia, dehydration • Below-normal level: Anemia, fluid overload, recent hemorrhage
	Hematocrit (Hct or packed RBC volume) *Males:* 42% to 54% *Females:* 38% to 46% *Children:* 36% to 40% *Neonates:* 55% to 68%	• Above-normal level: Polycythemia, hemoconcentration related to blood loss, dehydration • Below-normal level: Anemia, hemodilution

Common Laboratory Studies continued

TEST AND SIGNIFICANCE	NORMAL VALUES OR FINDINGS	ABNORMAL FINDINGS AND POSSIBLE CAUSES
Blood tests continued		
Complete blood count (CBC) continued	*Hemoglobin (Hgb)* *Males:* 14 to 18 g/dl; 12.4 to 14.9 g/dl (after middle age) *Females:* 12 to 16 g/dl; 11.7 to 13.8 g/dl (after middle age) *Children:* 11 to 13 g/dl *Neonates:* 17 to 22 g/dl	• Above-normal level: Hemoconcentration from polycythemia or dehydration • Below-normal level: Anemia, recent hemorrhage or fluid retention causing hemodilution
Creatine kinase (CK) This enzyme reflects tissue catabolism. Its isoenzyme CK-MB is used to evaluate cardiac tissue. Its isoenzyme CK-MM is used to measure skeletal muscle damage.	*Total CK* *Males:* 25 to 130 units/liter *Females:* 10 to 150 units/liter	• Above-normal level: Postconvulsions; alcoholic cardiomyopathy; pulmonary, cerebral, or myocardial infarction; severe hypokalemia; carbon monoxide poisoning; malignant hyperthermia • Below-normal level: No clinical significance
	CK-MB: Undetectable to 7 units/liter	• Above-normal level: Myocardial infarction (MI), severe skeletal muscle injury • Below-normal level: No clinical significance
	CK-MM: 5 to 70 units/liter	• Above-normal level: Muscle trauma from injury or intramuscular injection, dermatomyositis • Below-normal level: No clinical significance
Creatinine This test provides a more sensitive measure of renal damage than BUN levels because renal impairment is usually the only cause of creatinine elevation.	*Males:* 0.8 to 1.2 mg/dl *Females:* 0.6 to 0.9 mg/dl	• Above-normal level: Renal disease causing serious damage to at least half the nephrons in the kidneys • Below-normal level: Diabetes mellitus
Differential white cell count This test evaluates white blood cell (WBC) distribution and morphology, providing more information about the body's ability to resist and overcome infection than the WBC count alone. It classifies cells by	*Neutrophils:* 47.6% to 76.8%	• Above-normal level (neutrophilia): Bacterial and parasitic infections, metabolic disturbances (gout, diabetic or uremic coma) • Above-normal level of mature cells: Hemolysis, use of certain drugs (mercurial diuretics, sulfonamides), tissue breakdown (burns, MI, tumors, or hemolytic transfusion reaction)

continued

Common Laboratory Studies continued

TEST AND SIGNIFICANCE	NORMAL VALUES OR FINDINGS	ABNORMAL FINDINGS AND POSSIBLE CAUSES
Blood tests continued		
Differential white cell count continued type and subtype into granulocytes (neutrophils, eosinophils, and basophils) and agranulocytes (monocytes and lymphocytes). The test also determines the percentage of each blood cell type. To determine the absolute number for each type, multiply the percentage by the total WBC number.	*Neutrophils:* continued	• Below-normal level (neutropenia): Acute viral infections, blood diseases, toxic agents, hormonal diseases
	Eosinophils: 0.3% to 7%	• Above-normal level (eosinophilia): Hyperimmune, allergic, and degenerative reactions; antigen-antibody reactions in allergies, parasitic disease, Addison's disease, cancer, chronic skin infections • Below-normal level (eosinopenia): Increased adrenal steroid production from stress, hypersplenism; aplastic and pernicious anemias; infections (with neutrophilia)
	Basophils: 0.3% to 2%	• Above-normal level (basophilia): Granulocytic and basophilic leukemia and myeloid metaplasia (usually), chronic inflammation, polycythemia vera • Below-normal level: Acute allergic reactions, hyperthyroidism, stress reactions, prolonged steroid therapy
	Monocytes: 0.6% to 9.6%	• Above-normal level: Viral infections, bacterial and parasitic infestations, collagen diseases, hematologic disorders • Below-normal level: Prednisone treatment, hairy cell leukemia, rheumatoid arthritis, human immunodeficiency virus infection
	Lymphocytes: 16.2% to 43%	• Above-normal level: Infections, such as tuberculosis, hepatitis, infectious mononucleosis, mumps, rubella, and cytomegalovirus; immune diseases; lymphocytic leukemia

Common Laboratory Studies continued

TEST AND SIGNIFICANCE	NORMAL VALUES OR FINDINGS	ABNORMAL FINDINGS AND POSSIBLE CAUSES
Blood tests continued		
Differential white cell count continued	*Lymphocytes:* 16.2% to 43% continued	• Below-normal level: Severe debilitating illness, such as CHF, defective lymphatic circulation; high levels of adrenal corticosteroid
Electrolytes These tests provide a quantitative analysis of major extracellular electrolytes (sodium, calcium, chloride, and bicarbonate) and major intracellular electrolytes (potassium, magnesium, and phosphate).	*Bicarbonate:* 22 to 26 mEq/liter	• Above-normal level: Metabolic alkalosis caused by massive loss of gastric acids from vomiting or gastric drainage • Below-normal level: Metabolic acidosis caused by persistent diarrhea
	Calcium: 4.5 to 5.5 mEq/liter or 8.9 to 10.1 mg/dl	• Above-normal level: Metabolic alkalosis, renal disease, parathyroid disorder, cancer with bone metastasis, hyperthyroidism, excess vitamin D, immobilization, Paget's disease of bone, multiple fractures • Below-normal level: Malabsorption diarrhea, renal failure, activated vitamin D insufficiency, parathyroid disorder, acute pancreatitis, rickets
	Chloride: 100 to 108 mEq/liter	• Above-normal level: Severe dehydration, acute tubular necrosis, renal failure, primary aldosteronism, metabolic acidosis • Below-normal level: Vomiting, diarrhea, intestinal obstruction, chronic renal failure
	Magnesium: 1.5 to 2.5 mEq/liter	• Above-normal level: Renal failure, adrenal insufficiency, excess magnesium • Below-normal level: Chronic diarrhea, primary aldosteronism, diuretic therapy, malnutrition, malabsorption syndrome, impaired renal conservation
	Phosphate: 1.8 to 2.6 mEq/liter	• Above-normal level: High intestinal obstruction, decreased tubular secretion • Below-normal level: Malnutrition, malabsorption syndromes

continued

Common Laboratory Studies continued

TEST AND SIGNIFICANCE	NORMAL VALUES OR FINDINGS	ABNORMAL FINDINGS AND POSSIBLE CAUSES
Blood tests continued		
Electrolytes continued	*Potassium:* 3.8 to 5.5 mEq/liter	• Above-normal level: Crush injury, reduced sodium excretion (possibly from renal failure), metabolic acidosis, severe burns • Below-normal level: Loss of body fluids, aldosteronism, polyuria, diuretic therapy
	Sodium: 135 to 145 mEq/liter	• Above-normal level: Dehydration as in massive diarrhea, inadequate water intake, water loss exceeding sodium loss (as in diabetes insipidus), sodium retention (as in aldosteronism), excess sodium intake • Below-normal level: Syndrome of inappropriate antidiuretic hormone secretion, water intoxication
Erythrocyte sedimentation rate (ESR) This test measures the time required for RBCs in a whole blood sample to settle to the bottom of a vertical tube, displacing the plasma upward, which retards settling of other blood elements. The ESR is an early indicator of occult inflammatory or malignant diseases.	0 to 20 mm/hr Rates gradually increase with age.	• Above-normal level: Pregnancy, acute or chronic inflammation, tuberculosis, paraproteinemias, rheumatic fever, rheumatoid arthritis, some cancers, anemias • Below-normal level: Polycythemia, sickle cell anemia, hyperviscosity, low plasma protein levels
Fibrin split products (fibrinogen degradation products [FDP]) This test detects the breakdown products of fibrin and fibrinogen that occur in response to the activity of plasmin, the fibrin-dissolving enzyme that prevents excessive clotting. Fibrin split products have anticoagulant activity, so excessive levels inhibit clot formation.	*Screening assay:* < 10 mcg/ml *Quantitative assay:* < 3 mcg/ml	• Above-normal level: Primary and secondary fibrinolytic states, alcoholic cirrhosis, postcesarean birth, preeclampsia, abruptio placentae, congenital heart disease, sunstroke, burns, intrauterine death, pulmonary embolus, deep-vein thrombosis, MI, portacaval shunt, acute leukemia, incompatible blood transfusions, hypoxia, after thoracic or cardiac surgery and renal transplantation, DIC, streptokinase, urokinase • Below-normal level: No clinical significance

Common Laboratory Studies continued

TEST AND SIGNIFICANCE	NORMAL VALUES OR FINDINGS	ABNORMAL FINDINGS AND POSSIBLE CAUSES
Blood tests continued		
Gamma glutamyl trans-peptidase (GGT) This test detects increased activity of GGT, which reflects liver function.	*Males:* 6 to 47 units/liter *Females under 45 years:* 5 to 27 units/liter *Females over 45 years:* 6 to 37 units/liter	● Above-normal level: Liver disease, alcoholism, acute pancreatitis, MI (5 to 10 days after), cancer ● Below-normal level: Clofibrate, oral contraceptives
Glycosylated hemoglobin (GHB, glycohemoglobin) This test monitors the degree of glucose control in diabetes mellitus over 3 months.	5.5% to 9% of total hemoglobin	● Above-normal level: Uncontrolled diabetes mellitus ● Below-normal level: Hemolytic state resulting in loss of hemoglobin, hemoglobinopathies
Gonadotropins (follicle-stimulating hormone [FSH], luteinizing hormone [LH]) This test distinguishes a primary gonadal problem from pituitary insufficiency.	*Females FSH:* follicular phase 5 to 20 mIU/ml; mid-cycle peak 15 to 30 mIU/ml; luteal phase 5 to 15 mIU/ml; post-menopausal 50 to 100 mIU/ml *LH:* follicular phase 5 to 25 mIU/ml; mid-cycle peak 30 to 60 mIU/ml; luteal phase 5 to 15 mIU/ml; post-menopausal > 50 mIU/ml *Males FSH:* 5 to 20 mIU/ml *LH:* 5 to 20 mIU/ml	● Above-normal level: Primary gonadal failure ● Below-normal level: Pituitary insufficiency
Hematocrit A commonly performed test, HCT measures the percentage of RBCs in total blood volume.	Concentration varies with the client's age and sex *Males:* 42% to 54% *Females:* 38% to 46% *Children:* 36% to 40%	● Above-normal level: Polycythemia, dehydration, hemoconcentration from blood loss ● Below-normal level: Massive or prolonged blood loss, hemolysis, hemodilution
Hemoglobin, total This test measures the grams of hemoglobin found in a deciliter of whole blood. Hemoglobin enables RBCs to carry oxygen from the lungs and carbon dioxide from the tissues.	*Males:* 14 to 18 g/dl *Females:* 12 to 16 g/dl *Children:* 11 to 13 g/dl *Newborns:* 17 to 22 g/dl	● Increased hemoglobin: Polycythemia, dehydration, chronic obstructive pulmonary disease, living in high altitudes ● Decreased hemoglobin: Anemia, hemorrhage, hemolytic reactions to blood or blood products, increased RBC destruction

continued

Common Laboratory Studies continued

TEST AND SIGNIFICANCE	NORMAL VALUES OR FINDINGS	ABNORMAL FINDINGS AND POSSIBLE CAUSES
Blood tests continued		
Human growth hormone (hGH) This test evaluates growth hormone oversecretion.	*Males:* < 5 ng/ml *Females:* < 10 ng/ml	• Above-normal level: Acromegaly, gigantism • Below-normal level: Dwarfism
Immunoelectrophoresis This test identifies immunoglobulins IgG, IgA, and IgM in a serum sample by nephelometry. It assesses the effectiveness of chemotherapy or radiation therapy, detects hypogammaglobulinemias and hypergammaglobulinemias, and diagnoses paraproteinemias.	*IgG:* 6.4 to 14.3 mg/ml *IgA:* 0.3 to 3 mg/ml *IgM:* 0.2 to 1.4 mg/ml	• Above-normal levels of all three: Hepatic disorders such as hepatitis; other disorders such as rheumatoid arthritis and systemic lupus erythematosus • Below-normal levels of all three: Immunoglobulin disorders such as lymphoid aplasia, myelomas, and leukemias • Combinations of normal, above-normal, and below-normal levels of all three: Immunoglobulin disorders, myelomas, leukemias, hepatic disorders
Iron, serum Commonly used to confirm iron deficiency, this test measures the amount of iron bound to transferrin.	*Males:* 70 to 150 μg/dl *Females:* 80 to 150 μg/dl Level normally peaks in the morning and drops at night	• Above-normal level: Liver damage, hemochromatosis, hemolytic anemias, excessive iron intake, thalassemia • Below-normal level: Iron deficiency, chronic inflammation, chronic blood loss, pregnancy
Iron-binding capacity, total (TIBC) This test helps estimate total iron storage and evaluate nutritional status.	*Males:* 300 to 400 μg/dl *Females:* 300 to 450 μg/dl	• Above-normal level: Iron deficiency anemia, oral contraceptives • Below-normal level: Cancer, pernicious anemia, renal disease, infection
Lactic dehydrogenase (LDH) This enzyme reflects cellular damage. Two of its five isoenzymes are specific to cardiac tissue: LDH_1 and LDH_2.	*Total LDH:* 48 to 115 IU/liter *LDH_1:* 18% to 29% of total LDH *LDH_2:* 29.4% to 37.5% of total LDH	• Above-normal level: MI, rheumatic carditis, myocarditis
Leukocyte (WBC) count This test, along with the differential white cell count, establishes the quantity and maturity of WBCs in the blood.	4,100 to 10,900/mm³	• Above-normal level (leukocytosis): Infection (usually); leukemia; tissue necrosis from burns, MI, or gangrene • Below-normal level (leukopenia): Bone marrow depression related to viral infections, toxic reactions, radiation

Common Laboratory Studies continued

TEST AND SIGNIFICANCE	NORMAL VALUES OR FINDINGS	ABNORMAL FINDINGS AND POSSIBLE CAUSES
Blood tests continued		
Lipoprotein cholesterol fractionation This test measures high-density lipoproteins (HDLs) and low-density lipoproteins (LDLs).	*HDL:* greater than 50 mg/100 ml	• Above-normal level: Decreased risk of coronary artery disease • Below-normal level: Increased risk of coronary artery disease, familial alpha-lipoproteinemia, hyperthyroidsim, end-stage liver disease, diabetes, obesity, hypertriglyceridemia
	LDL: less than 130 mg/100 ml	• Above-normal level: Increased risk of coronary artery disease • Below-normal level: No clinical significance
Lymphocyte count, total (TLC) Besides helping to diagnose nutritional status, this test may suggest impaired immunocompetence.	1,500 to 3,000 mm³ (TLC value stems from differential white cell count)	• Above-normal level: Viral infection (infection may mask malnutrition, which normally depresses TLC) • Below-normal level: Protein-calorie malnutrition, possibly reflecting an impaired immune response; moderate malnutrition (900 to 1,400 mm³), severe malnutrition (below 900 mm³)
Oral glucose tolerance test This test detects diabetes mellitus and hypoglycemia.	160 to 150 mg/dl 30 to 60 min after oral glucose dose; fasting levels or lower in 2 to 3 hr	• Above-normal level: Diabetes mellitus • Below-normal level: Hypoglycemia
Osmolality Intracellular and extracellular osmolality are normally equal and reflect overall hydration and body fluid concentration.	280 to 295 mOsm/kg of water	• Above-normal level: Dehydration, kidney dysfunction • Below-normal level: Kidney dysfunction
Parathyroid hormone (PTH) This test evaluates parathyroid function.	210 to 310 pg/ml	• Above-normal level: Hyperparathyroidism • Below-normal level: Hypoparathyroidism
pH (hydrogen ion concentration) This test reflects the acid-base balance of the blood.	7.35 to 7.42	• Above-normal level: Metabolic alkalosis from vomiting, gastric drainage, or other GI fluid losses • Below-normal level: Metabolic acidosis from persistent diarrhea

continued

Common Laboratory Studies continued

TEST AND SIGNIFICANCE	NORMAL VALUES OR FINDINGS	ABNORMAL FINDINGS AND POSSIBLE CAUSES
Blood tests continued		
Phosphorus Blood concentration of phosphorus is affected by the action of vitamin D and intestinal absorption of calcium.	2.5 to 4.5 mg/dl	• Above-normal level: Hypoparathyroidism, renal failure • Below-normal level: Malabsorption, cirrhosis, starvation, antacid overdose, hyperparathyroidism
Plasma fibrinogen (Factor I) This test measures the level of plasma protein fibrinogen available for coagulation. In this test, a clot is formed and is then dissolved, and its proteins are assayed.	195 to 365 mg/dl	• Above-normal level: Hemostatic stress; nonspecific stresses such as inflammation, pregnancy, or autoimmune disorders; cancer • Below-normal level: Congenital afibrinogenemia; hypofibrinogenemia; dysfibrinogenemia; DIC; fibrinolysis; severe hepatic disease; cancer; acute illness
Plasma thrombin time (thrombin clotting time) This test estimates plasma fibrinogen levels by measuring how quickly a clot forms when thrombin is added to plasma samples from the client and a normal control.	10 to 15 seconds	• Prolonged time (> 1.3 times the control time): Effective heparin therapy, hepatic disease, DIC, hypofibrinogenemia, macroglobulinemia, multiple myeloma • Shortened time: No clinical significance
Platelet (thrombocyte) count This test assesses the number of platelets in a blood sample. It evaluates production of platelets, which are vital to coagulation; assesses the effects of chemotherapy and radiation on platelet production; and aids diagnosis of platelet disorders.	130,000 to 370,000/mm^3	• Above-normal level (thrombocytosis): Primary thrombocytosis, polycythemia vera, chronic myelogenous leukemia, hemorrhage, infectious disorders, carcinomas, iron-deficiency anemia, recent surgery • Below-normal level (thrombocytopenia): Aplastic or hypoplastic bone marrow; infiltrative bone marrow disease (such as carcinoma or leukemia); megakaryocytic hypoplasia; folic acid or vitamin B_{12} deficiency; DIC
Protein, total By measuring the sum of albumin and globulin fractions—a plasma nutrition source for body tissues—this test helps determine nutritional status and indicates hyperproteinemia or hypoproteinemia.	6.6 to 7.9 g/dl	• Above-normal level: Liver disease, dehydration, vomiting, diarrhea, diabetic acidosis • Below-normal level: Malnutrition, protein-losing condition, chronic hepatic insufficiency, nephrosis

Common Laboratory Studies continued

TEST AND SIGNIFICANCE	NORMAL VALUES OR FINDINGS	ABNORMAL FINDINGS AND POSSIBLE CAUSES
Blood tests continued		
Prothrombin time (PT) Although less sensitive than the APTT, this test aids in evaluating thrombin generation (extrinsic clotting mechanism). It indirectly measures prothrombin by measuring the time required for a fibrin clot to form in a citrated plasma sample after the addition of calcium and tissue thromboplastin.	*Males:* 9.6 to 11.8 seconds *Females:* 9.5 to 11.3 seconds	• Prolonged time: Deficiencies in fibrinogen, prothrombin, Factors V, VII, or X, or vitamin K; hepatic disease; oral anticoagulant therapy • Time exceeding 2½ times normal: Abnormal bleeding related to causes above
Red blood cell count This test reports the number of RBCs found in a microliter of whole blood. The main function of the RBC is to maintain a high concentration of circulating hemoglobin.	*Males:* 4.5 to 6.2 million/µl venous blood *Females:* 4.2 to 5.4 million/µl venous blood *Children:* 4.6 to 4.8 million/µl venous blood *Newborns:* 4.4 to 5.8 million/µl capillary blood	• Increased RBCs: Polycythemia, severe diarrhea, dehydration • Decreased RBCs: Anemia, hemorrhage
Red blood cell indices This blood test provides information about the size, hemoglobin concentration, and hemoglobin weight of an average RBC.	*Mean corpuscular volume (MCV):* 84 to 99 µ³/red cell	• Above-normal level: Macrocytic anemia, sprue, alcoholism, vitamin B and folate deficiencies, malabsorption syndromes • Below-normal level: Dehydration or chronic blood loss, microcytic or hypochromic anemia, thalassemia
	Mean corpuscular hemoglobin (MCH): 26 to 32 pg/red cell	• Above-normal level: Macrocytic anemia • Below-normal level: Microcytic anemia, thalassemia
	Mean corpuscular hemoglobin concentration (MCHC): 30% to 36%	• Above-normal level: Dehydration • Below-normal level: Microcytic or hypochromic anemia
Rheumatoid factor (RF) This test is an immunologic study specific for rheumatoid arthritis.	Nonreactive test with titer value less than 1:20	• Reactive test (with titer value greater than 1:20): Positive titer values above 1:80 are diagnostic for rheumatoid arthritis

continued

Common Laboratory Studies continued

TEST AND SIGNIFICANCE	NORMAL VALUES OR FINDINGS	ABNORMAL FINDINGS AND POSSIBLE CAUSES
Blood tests continued		
Serum glutamic-oxalo-acetic transaminase (SGOT) Also known as aspartate aminotransferase (AST), this enzyme also reflects cellular damage but is less specific than LDH.	*Adults:* 8 to 20 units/ liter *Infants:* four times adult values	• Above-normal level: MI, hepato-cellular damage, pancreatic in-flammation, primary muscle disease (such as muscular dys-trophy or muscle trauma)
Serum glutamic-pyruvic transaminase (SGPT) Also called alanine amino-transferase (ALT), this test reflects muscle tissue damage when the en-zyme, found in skeletal muscle, exceeds normal levels.	*Males:* 10 to 32 units/ liter *Females:* 9 to 24 units/liter *Infants:* twice the adult values	• Above-normal level: Hepatocel-lular damage, skeletal muscle damage, cirrhosis, hepatitis, he-patic congestion caused by heart failure, MI, infectious mononucle-osis • Below-normal level: No clinical significance
T₄ radioimmunoassay (RIA) This test evaluates thyroid function and monitors io-dine or antithyroid therapy.	5 to 13.5 mcg/dl	• Above-normal level: Hyperthy-roidism • Below-normal level: Hypothy-roidsim
T₃ RIA This test detects hyper-thyroidism if T₄ levels are normal.	90 to 230 ng/dl	• Above-normal level: Hyperthy-roidism • Below-normal level: Hypothy-roidism, nephrosis
Thyroid-stimulating hor-mone (TSH) This test detects primary hypothyroidism.	< 15 μIU/ml	• Above-normal level: Primary hypothyroidism • Below-normal level: Secondary hypothyroidism
Transferrin, serum (siderophilin) By determining the iron-transporting capacity of the blood, this test evalu-ates iron metabolism in iron-deficiency anemia.	250 to 390 μg/dl (65 to 170 μg usually bound to iron)	• Above-normal level: Severe iron deficiency; elevations occur nor-mally in children between ages 2½ and 10 and during the third trimester of pregnancy • Below-normal level: Visceral protein depletion
Triglycerides This test provides a quan-titative analysis of stored lipids.	Below 200 mg/dl	• Above-normal level: Increased risk of coronary artery disease
Uric acid A purine metabolite, uric acid clears the body via glomerular filtration and tubular secretion.	*Males:* 4.3 to 8 mg/dl *Females:* 2.3 to 6 mg/dl	• Above-normal level: Gout, im-paired renal function • Below-normal level: Defective tubular absorption

Common Laboratory Studies continued

TEST AND SIGNIFICANCE	NORMAL VALUES OR FINDINGS	ABNORMAL FINDINGS AND POSSIBLE CAUSES
Cerebrospinal fluid tests		
Cerebrospinal fluid (CSF) analysis CSF analysis aids in diagnosis of acute or chronic bacterial or viral CNS infections, hemorrhages, tumors, or brain abscesses.	*Color:* Clear, colorless	• Cloudy (caused by increased leukocytes and proteins) or xanthochromic (bloody): Infection, such as meningitis; subarachnoid, intracerebral, or intraventricular hemorrhage; spinal cord obstruction; traumatic spinal tap (usually noted only in initial specimen)
	Glucose: 50 to 80 mg/dl (or ⅔ of blood glucose)	• Above-normal level: Systemic hyperglycemia • Below-normal level: Bacterial, tuberculosis (TB), or fungal meningitis; some CNS viral infections (herpes, mumps); meningeal neoplasm; meningeal sarcoidosis; post-subarachnoid hemorrhage; brain abscess; degenerative disease
	Protein: 15 to 45 mg/dl	• Above-normal level (greater than 60 mcg/dl): Peripheral neuropathy involving nerve roots, brain tumor, encapsulated brain abscess, bacterial meningitis, viral CNS infections, degenerative CNS diseases (multiple sclerosis, neurosyphilis), Guillain-Barré syndrome, subarachnoid hemorrhage, blood in CSF from traumatic tap • Below-normal level: Rapid CSF production
	Gamma globulin: 3% to 12% of total protein	• Above-normal level: Herpes encephalitis, Guillain-Barré syndrome, neurosyphilis, multiple sclerosis • Below-normal level: No clinical significance
	Cell count: No RBCs	• Presence: Hemorrhage (subarachnoid, intracerebral), bleeding into ventricular system, CNS trauma, traumatic tap
	0 to 5 WBCs	• Increase (greater than 10): Meningitis, CNS infections, infectious mononucleosis, subarachnoid hemorrhage, thrombosis

continued

Common Laboratory Studies continued

TEST AND SIGNIFICANCE	NORMAL VALUES OR FINDINGS	ABNORMAL FINDINGS AND POSSIBLE CAUSES
Fecal tests		
Fecal occult blood test This test measures occult (concealed) blood in stool samples.	2 to 2.5 ml/day	• Above-normal level: GI bleeding, colorectal cancer • Below-normal level: No clinical significance
Stool culture This bacteriologic examination of stool sample detects pathogenic organisms causing GI disease.	No pathogens	• Presence of pathogens: Bacterial, viral, or fungal GI infection
Stool examination for ova and parasites This test confirms or rules out intestinal parasitic infestation and disease.	No parasites or ova in stool	• Presence of parasites or ova; Parasitic infestation and possible infection
Semen test		
Semen analysis This test quantifies the number of sperm in a semen sample to evaluate fertility.	60 to 150 million/ml	• Above-normal level: No clinical significance • Below-normal level: Male infertility
Sputum test		
Sputum culture and sensitivity This test is used to detect pathogens in sputum and to plan treatment for pathogens detected.	Normal throat flora, such as alpha-hemolytic streptococci or diphtheroids	• Pathogenic organisms, such as *Streptococcus pneumoniae, Mycobacterium tuberculosis,* and *Legionella pneumophila:* Pneumonia, Legionnaires' disease, TB
Urine tests		
Bilirubin This test detects bile pigments in urine.	No bilirubin	• Presence of bilirubin: Biliary obstruction
Creatinine clearance An excellent diagnostic index of renal function, this test determines how efficiently the kidneys clear creatinine from the blood. The test is performed from urine specimens collected at 2, 6, 12, or 24 hours and a blood sample obtained any time during the urine collection period.	*Males:* 90 mg/min/ 1.73 m² of body surface *Females:* 84 ml/min/ 1.73 m² of body surface *Elderly clients:* Concentrations normally decrease by 6 ml/min/ decade	• Above-normal creatinine clearance: Little diagnostic significance • Below-normal creatinine clearance: Reduced renal blood flow (associated with shock or renal artery obstruction), acute tubular necrosis, acute or chronic glomerulonephritis, advanced bilateral renal lesions (as in polycystic kidney disease, renal TB, and cancer), nephrosclerosis, CHF, severe dehydration

Common Laboratory Studies continued

TEST AND SIGNIFICANCE	NORMAL VALUES OR FINDINGS	ABNORMAL FINDINGS AND POSSIBLE CAUSES
Urine tests continued		
Culture and sensitivity Using a common culture medium, this test detects infectious microorganisms in exudate, urine, or lesions.	Absence of infectious microorganisms	• Presence of infectious microorganisms: Infection of kidney, bladder, or urethra
Divided urine test This test detects bacteria in prostatic fluid or a urine sample.	Absence of bacteria	• Presence of bacteria: Prostatitis
17-Hydroxycorticosteroids (17-OHCS) This test evaluates adrenal function.	*Males:* 4.54 to 12 mg/24 hr *Females:* 2.5 to 10 mg/24 hr	• Above-normal level: Hyperadrenalism • Below-normal level: Hypopituitarism, adrenal disease
17-Ketosteroids (17-KS) This test evaluates adrenocortical and gonadal function.	*Males:* 6 to 21 mg/24 hr *Females:* 4 to 17 mg/24 hr	• Above-normal level: Congenital adrenal hyperplasia • Below-normal level: Adrenal insufficiency
Uric acid This test reflects excretion of uric acid.	250 to 750 mg/24 hr	• Above-normal level: Multiple myeloma • Below-normal level: Gout
Urinalysis This common screening test can indicate urinary or systemic disorders. Performed on a urine specimen of at least 5 ml, it may suggest absence of major disease (normal findings) or possible disease warranting further investigation (abnormal findings).	Straw color	• Clear to black: Dietary changes; use of certain drugs; metabolic, inflammatory, or infectious disease
	Slightly aromatic odor	• Fruity odor: Diabetes mellitus, starvation, dehydration
	Clear appearance	• Turbid appearance: Renal infection
	Specific gravity between 1.005 and 1.020, with slight variations from one specimen to the next	• Above-normal specific gravity: Dehydration, nephrosis • Below-normal specific gravity: Diabetes insipidus, glomerulonephritis, pyelonephritis, acute renal failure, alkalosis • Fixed specific gravity: Severe renal damage
	pH between 4.5 and 8.0	• Alkaline pH (above 8.0): Fanconi's syndrome (chronic renal disease), urinary tract infection, metabolic or respiratory alkalosis • Acidic pH (below 4.5): Renal TB, phenylketonuria, acidosis

continued

Common Laboratory Studies continued

TEST AND SIGNIFICANCE	NORMAL VALUES OR FINDINGS	ABNORMAL FINDINGS AND POSSIBLE CAUSES
Urine tests continued		
Urinalysis continued	No protein	• Presence of protein: Renal disease (such as glomerulosclerosis, acute or chronic glomerulonephritis, nephrolithiasis, polycystic kidney disease, acute or chronic renal failure)
	No ketones	• Presence of ketones: Diabetes mellitus, starvation, conditions causing acutely increased metabolic demands and decreased food intake (such as vomiting and diarrhea)
	No sugars	• Glycosuria: Diabetes mellitus • Fructosuria: Rare hereditary metabolic disorder, excess fructose ingestion • Galactosuria: Rare hereditary metabolic disorder • Pentosuria: Rare hereditary metabolic disorder, excess pentose ingestion
	0 to 3 RBCs/high-power field	• Numerous RBCs: Urinary infection, obstruction, inflammation, trauma, or tumor; glomerulonephritis; renal hypertension; lupus nephritis; renal TB; renal vein thrombosis; hydronephrosis; pyelonephritis; parasitic bladder infection; polyarteritis nodosa; hemorrhagic disorder
	0 to 4 WBCs/high-power field	• Numerous WBCs: Urinary tract inflammation, especially cystitis or pyelonephritis • Numerous WBCs and WBC casts: Renal infection (such as acute pyelonephritis and glomerulonephritis, nephrotic syndrome, pyogenic infection, and lupus nephritis)
	Few epithelial cells	• Excessive epithelial cells: Renal tubular degeneration

Common Laboratory Studies continued

TEST AND SIGNIFICANCE	NORMAL VALUES OR FINDINGS	ABNORMAL FINDINGS AND POSSIBLE CAUSES
Urine tests continued		
Urinalysis continued	No casts (except occasional hyaline casts)	● Excessive casts: Renal disease ● Excessive hyaline casts: Renal parenchymal disease, inflammation, glomerular capillary membrane trauma ● Epithelial casts: Renal tubular damage, nephrosis, eclampsia, chronic lead intoxication ● Fatty, waxy casts: Nephrotic syndrome, chronic renal disease, diabetes mellitus ● RBC casts: Renal parenchymal disease (especially glomerulonephritis), renal infarction, subacute bacterial endocarditis, vascular disorders, sickle cell anemia, scurvy, blood dyscrasias, malignant hypertension, collagen disease, acute inflammation
	Some crystals	● Numerous calcium oxalate crystals: Hypercalcemia ● Cystine crystals (cystinuria): Inborn metabolic error
	No yeast cells	● Yeast cells in sediment: Genitourinary tract infection, external genitalia contamination, vaginitis, urethritis, prostatovesiculitis
	No parasites	● Parasites in sediment: Genitourinary tract infection, external genitalia contamination
Urobilinogen This test detects impaired liver function.	*Males:* 0.3 to 2.1 Ehrlich units/2 hr *Females:* 0.1 to 1.1 Ehrlich units/2 hr	● Above-normal level: Impaired liver function ● Below-normal level: Total biliary obstruction

Master glossary

Abdominal distention: visible enlargement of the abdominal cavity commonly caused by liquid, gas, or a tumor.

Abduction: limb movement away from the body's midline.

Abortion: spontaneous or induced termination of pregnancy before the fetus becomes viable (about 20 weeks).

Accessory muscles: muscles used for forced inspiration and active expiration, including the internal intercostal, pectoral, scalenus, sternocleidomastoid, trapezius, and abdominal rectus muscles.

Accommodation reflex: adjustment of the eyes for near vision, consisting of pupillary constriction, eye convergence, and increased lens convexity.

Acid-base balance: condition existing when the net rate at which the body produces acids or bases equals the net rate at which acids or bases are excreted. The result of acid-base balance is a stable concentration of hydrogen ions in body fluids.

Acromegaly: endocrine condition characterized by gradual, marked enlargement and elongation of the bones of the face, jaw, hands, and feet, caused by excess production of growth hormone in adults.

Addison's disease: endocrine disorder of the adrenal cortex, caused by decreased cortisol and aldosterone secretion, characterized by bronze skin and life-threatening crises.

Adduction: limb movement toward the body's midline.

Affect: outward manifestation of a person's feelings or emotions.

Agranulocyte: a nongranular leukocyte having a nucleus without lobes. Agranulocytes include monocytes and lymphocytes.

Aldosterone: mineralocorticoid produced by the adrenal cortex that regulates the sodium and potassium balance in the blood.

Alopecia: partial or complete hair loss caused by normal aging, endocrine disorders, drug reactions, chemotherapeutic agents, or skin disorders.

Amplitude: width or breadth of range or extent, especially of pulses.

Androgens: male sex hormones, primarily testosterone.

Anemia: abnormal decrease in red blood cells (RBCs) per cubic millimeter (mm^3) of blood, hemoglobin quantity, or volume of packed RBCs per deciliter of blood.

Angina: chest pain characterized as a squeezing or crushing sensation or a feeling of heaviness or tightness; caused by an inadequate oxygen supply to the myocardium when the work load of the heart is increased.

Annular: ring shaped; characteristic of a skin lesion surrounding a clear, normal skin area.

Anorexia nervosa: eating disorder involving severe self-limitation of food intake; usually seen in teenage and young adult females.

Anosmia: loss of sense of smell, indicating malfunction of cranial nerve I (olfactory).

Anovulation: lack of ovulation.

Anteflexed uterus: normal position of the uterus in which its corpus flexes forward at an acute angle.

Anteverted uterus: normal position in which the uterine corpus flexes forward, but less acutely than if anteflexed.

Anthropometric measurements: measurements of the human body, including height, weight, body frame size, skin-fold evaluation, and (in infants and young children) head and chest circumference.

Antidiuretic hormone (ADH): hormone secreted by the hypothalamus and stored in the pituitary gland; reduces urine production by increasing the water reabsorption in the renal tubules.

Antigen: any substance capable of eliciting an immune response; a foreign substance that stimulates the body to secrete specific antibodies or to proliferate activated T cells specific to the introduced antigen.

Aphasia: inability to understand or use language (or both) secondary to damage to the language control centers in the frontal and temporal brain lobes.

Master glossary continued

Aqueous humor: watery, clear fluid circulating in the anterior and posterior chambers of the eye.

Arciform: arc shaped; characteristic of a lesion forming an arc or curve.

Areola: pigmented circular area surrounding the nipple of each breast.

Ascites: collection of fluid in the abdominal cavity.

Assessment: first step in the nursing process; collection and organization of data from such sources as the client, the client's family, medical records, and laboratory and diagnostic tests.

Assimilation: loss of cultural identity when an individual becomes part of a different, dominant culture.

Astigmatism: abnormal eye condition in which light does not focus clearly on the retina, but rather spreads over a diffuse area. It occurs when the curve of the cornea or lens is not even in all parts and causes blurred vision and discomfort during close eye work.

Ataxia: impaired ability to coordinate movement, such as unsteady gait characterized by a wide base of support and staggering.

Atherosclerosis: disorder characterized by accumulation of lipids, calcium, and blood clotting products in the inner layer of arterial walls. As the debris accumulates, the vessel lumen narrows, causing ischemia in the organs the vessel supplies. In the coronary arteries, ischemia occurs when the vessels are narrowed by 70% or more.

Auscultation: physical assessment technique in which the examiner listens for body sounds to evaluate the condition of the heart, lungs, and other organs or to detect fetal heart sounds. The examiner usually uses a stethoscope to auscultate the sounds' frequency, intensity, quality, and duration.

Autoimmune disorder: abnormal response of the body to its own tissue, possibly from an inability to differentiate resident self antigens from foreign antigens.

Ballottement: palpation technique used to evaluate a floating structure by bouncing it gently and feeling it rebound. It may be used, for example, to check fetal position.

Basophil: least common granulocyte, having cytoplasmic granules containing serotonin and histamine and irregularly shaped, two-lobed, segmented nucleus.

B cell or **B lymphocyte:** white blood cell (WBC), originating in the bone marrow, that produces antibodies; responsible for humoral immunity.

Blood pressure: pressure exerted by the circulating blood volume on arterial walls. Blood pressure depends on myocardial contractile force, blood volume, size and patency of the arterial lumen, and arterial wall elasticity.

Blunt percussion: percussion performed by striking a body surface directly with the fist to elicit tenderness, *not* to create a sound.

Bronchophony: increased referred voice sounds auscultated in the periphery of the lungs. In bronchophony, the word "ninety-nine" reverberates clearly over areas of consolidation and sounds muffled over other areas.

Bruit: abnormal, murmurlike heart sound auscultated over a major vessel with turbulent blood flow.

Bruxism: grinding of the teeth, especially during sleep.

Bulbar: pertaining to the cranial nerves, which exit from the brain stem. Difficulty swallowing, slurred or nasal speech, and an impaired gag reflex are bulbar symptoms.

Bulimia: eating disorder involving alternating periods of starvation and excessive food intake with self-induced vomiting and purging; usually seen in teenage and young adult females.

Calculus: pathologic stone, formed of mineral salts, usually found in a hollow organ or duct, such as the ureter. A calculus may cause inflammation or obstruction.

Calorie: standard unit of heat; the amount of energy it takes to raise the temperature of one gram of water one degree centigrade at atmospheric pressure.

Cardiac cycle: period from the beginning of one heartbeat to the beginning of the next.

continued

Master glossary continued

Cataract: abnormal, progressive loss of lens transparency in the eye. Most cataracts result from degenerative changes that occur after age 50.

Catecholamines: epinephrine and norepinephrine – the functioning units of the autonomic nervous system.

Chloasma: brownish pigmentation of facial skin in some pregnant women. Also known as the mask of pregnancy.

Chronic obstructive pulmonary disease (COPD): disease involving airway obstruction, such as asthma, chronic bronchitis, or emphysema.

Click: high-pitched abnormal heart sound auscultated at the apex during mid- to late systole; it usually precedes a late systolic murmur.

Climacteric: period from onset to end of hormonal and related changes that cease reproductive function.

Clubbing: abnormal enlargement of the distal phalanges associated with peripheral tissue hypoxia, characterized by the loss of the angle between the skin and nail base.

Cognitive: higher skills of the cerebral cortex, such as judgment, reasoning, abstraction, and intellect.

Colostrum: fluid secreted by the breast during pregnancy and the first few days postpartum, before lactation begins. It is a thin, yellowish, serous fluid consisting of immunologically active substances, white blood cells, water, protein, fat, and carbohydrates.

Conductive hearing loss: hearing loss caused by blockage of sound waves from the external to the inner ear. It may result from a cerumen obstruction, middle ear inflammation, or sclerosis of the ear bones.

Confluent: fused or blended; characteristic of merging skin lesions.

Consensual reaction: reflex stimulation of one body side or part resulting from stimulation of the opposite side or another body part. For example, a consensual reaction to light occurs when the client's right pupil constricts as the left pupil is illuminated.

Consolidation: solidification of part of the lung into a dense mass from fluid or infection. In consolidation, percussion over the lung produces dull sounds.

Constipation: retention of feces associated with bowel hypoactivity.

Corrigan's pulse: bounding pulse in which a great surge precedes a sudden absence of force or fullness; also called a water-hammer pulse.

Costal angle: area between the two lower borders of the rib cage near the xiphoid process.

Crackles: short, moist, explosive sounds produced by air passing through liquid in the airways. Also called rales.

Crepitus: abnormal crackling or grating sound or sensation produced in the musculoskeletal system when irregular bone edges rub together.

Culture: integrated system of learned behavior patterns that are characteristic of the members of the society and are not biologically inherited. Culture affects beliefs, values, attitudes, and customs.

Cushing's syndrome: endocrine disorder, caused by excess corticosteroid production, characterized by hirsutism, trunk and abdomen obesity, and thin extremities.

Cyanosis: bluish or purplish color of the skin and mucous membranes caused by reduced oxygen in arterial blood.

Dermatome: skin area supplied with sensory nerve fibers from a single spinal nerve root.

Diabetes insipidus: endocrine disorder of the posterior lobe of the pituitary gland, caused by ineffective or decreased vasopressin secretion.

Diabetes mellitus: endocrine disorder of the pancreas involving chronically elevated blood glucose levels resulting from insufficient or ineffective insulin production, decreased insulin receptors, or post-receptor defects.

Diaphragmatic excursion: percussion technique used to determine the depth of diaphragm movement between inspiration and expiration.

Diarrhea: frequent elimination of loose stool.

Master glossary continued

Diastole: period of ventricular relaxation when blood crosses the open mitral and tricuspid valves and fills the ventricular chambers.

Diffuse: generalized or widespread, in contrast to localized or regionalized.

Digestion: breakdown of food and fluid into simple chemicals that can be absorbed into the bloodstream and transported throughout the body.

Dimpling: breast skin puckering or depression possibly caused by an underlying growth; also called retraction.

Diopter: refractive power of a lens with a 1-meter focal distance; for example, an ophthalmoscope has a lens with diopter values from − 25 to + 40.

Diplopia: double vision caused by defective extraocular muscle function or a disorder of the nerves that innervate the muscles.

Direct (immediate) percussion: percussion performed by striking the fingers directly on the body surface.

Discrete: separate and distinct; characteristic of individual, well-demarcated lesions.

Disorders of excessive daytime sleepiness: sleep disorders characterized by difficulty remaining awake during the day.

Disorders of initiating and maintaining sleep: sleep disorders characterized by changes in sleep onset, or interrupted sleep. Also called insomnia.

Disorders of sleep-wake cycle: transient or chronic sleep disorders characterized by altered or disorganized circadian rhythms caused by shift rotation, jet lag, or other interruptions in the normal sleep cycle.

Disorientation: inability to identify self, surroundings, or time correctly.

Dorsiflexion: backward bending of a joint.

Dream: vivid, internally generated sensations and perceptions.

Dysmenorrhea: menstrual discomfort or pain.

Dyspepsia: indigestion.

Dysphagia: difficulty swallowing.

Dyspnea: shortness of breath; a common symptom of cardiovascular disease.

Ecchymosis: flat, purple-blue, hemorrhagic bruise on the skin or mucous membranes caused by blood escaping into tissue from a blood vessel.

Edema: fluid accumulation in interstitial tissues that causes swelling; a common sign of cardiovascular disease.

Egophony: increased referred voice-sounds auscultated in the periphery of the lung. In egophony, the sound "e" will sound like "a" and have a nasal, bleating quality.

Ejaculation: forceful emission of semen from the urethral meatus at sexual climax.

Endocrine glands: glands that release hormones directly into the blood.

Enuresis: involuntary urination during sleep; bed-wetting.

Eosinophil: granulocyte with two lobes that responds phagocytically to allergens and parasites.

Epispadias: congenital opening of the urethral meatus on the dorsal surface of the penis.

Erection: state of penile swelling and rigidity usually associated with sexual arousal.

Erythrocyte or red blood cell (RBC): rounded, biconcave disk-shaped nonnuclear cell that contains hemoglobin and transports oxygen and carbon dioxide throughout the body.

Ethnic group: societal group within a cultural system. Ethnic groups contain racial, religious, linguistic, and ancestral traits.

Evaluation: fifth and final step in the nursing process; refers to the client's status relevant to goals described in the nursing care plan.

Exanthem: lesion that characterizes an eruptive disease, such as rubeola or varicella.

Exophthalmos: abnormal eyeball protrusion caused by trauma, intracranial lesions, intraorbital disorders, or systemic disease such as hyperthyroidism.

Extension: movement that increases the angle between two articulating bones.

Fasciculus: bundle of skeletal muscle fibers.

continued

Master glossary continued

Flaccid: weak, soft, and flabby; used to describe muscles that lack tone.

Flatus: intestinal air or gas passed through the rectum.

Flexion: movement that decreases the angle between two articulating bones.

Focal: in a limited area, as in focal skin lesions.

Fontanels: membrane-covered spaces between the bones of an infant's cranium.

Frenulum: restraining band of tissue, such as that attaching the posterior tongue to the floor of the mouth.

Gallop: abnormal heart rhythm characterized by a low-pitched extra sound during diastole; a general term for the extra heart sounds, S_3 and S_4.

Gingivae: gums.

Glands: specialized cell clusters that synthesize and release chemical substances that regulate body processes.

Glaucoma: abnormal condition of elevated intraocular pressure caused by obstruction of the outflow of aqueous humor; may be acute (closed-angle) or chronic (open-angle).

Goniometer: instrument used to measure joint range of motion.

Granulocyte: white blood cell characterized by prominent cytoplasmic granules and a single multilobed nucleus. According to the staining characteristics of their specific granules, granulocytes are known individually as neutrophils, eosinophils, or basophils and collectively as polymorphonuclear leukocytes.

Gynecomastia: enlargement of one or both male breasts, usually secondary to hormonal changes during puberty.

Health: optimal physical, social, and emotional functioning of an individual. In health, the individual tries to achieve the maximum potential for a sense of well-being by continually adapting to internal and external stressors.

Health history: collection of information obtained from a client and other sources that includes psychosocial and cultural concerns as well as physical data. It provides a significant part of the nurse's assessment data base.

Health problem or concern: anything that impairs or threatens an individual's physical, social, or emotional functioning and that causes or may cause illness or disease.

Health promotion: actions taken to develop resources that improve or maintain well-being and self-actualization, or actions taken to protect against health problems.

Heave: strong outward thrust palpated over the chest during systole; also called a lift.

Hematemesis: vomiting of bright red blood commonly caused by a bleeding ulcer or esophageal bleeding.

Hematocrit (HCT): concentration of red blood cells in total blood volume, expressed as a percentage.

Hematopoiesis: formation and development of blood cells from precursors.

Hemoglobin (Hb): oxygen-carrying pigment in red blood cells; formed by the developing erythrocyte in bone marrow. A conjugated protein, hemoglobin can carry and release oxygen. It is expressed as grams of hemoglobin per deciliter of blood.

Hernia, inguinal: protrusion of the bowel through the abdominal wall into the inguinal canal.

Herpetiform: patterned along the course of cutaneous nerves; characteristic of clusters of vesicles that appear with some herpesviruses.

High-density lipoproteins (HDLs): cholesterol carried by alpha-lipoproteins. HDLs are believed to serve as carriers that remove cholesterol from peripheral tissues and return it to the liver for catabolism and excretion; HDLs are also thought to inhibit cellular uptake of low-density lipoproteins. HDL values are inversely related to the risk of coronary atherosclerosis.

Hirsutism: excessive body hair, especially a masculine distribution in women caused by heredity, hormonal dysfunction, porphyria, or medication.

Holistic health care: system of health care that considers all facets of an individual: physical, psychological, social, and spiritual.

Master glossary continued

Holistic health-oriented approach: comprehensive health care approach that considers the client's physical, emotional, social, economic, and spiritual needs; the client's response to illness; and the impact of illness on the client's self-care capacity.

Hordeolum: purulent infection of the meibomian (sebaceous) glands of the eyelid, often caused by a staphylococcal infection. Also called a stye.

Hormone: chemical substance produced by an endocrine gland that exerts a specific regulatory effect on the activity of a certain organ or organs.

Human response: individual's reaction to a health problem.

Hyperglycemia: excessive blood glucose levels.

Hyperlipidemia: excess lipids in plasma.

Hyperparathyroidism: endocrine disorder of the parathyroid glands, caused by excess parathyroid hormone secretion and characterized by back pain and fractures.

Hypertension: elevated blood pressure that consistently exceeds 140/90 mm Hg in an adult.

Hyperthyroidism: endocrine disorder of the thyroid gland, caused by excess thyroid hormone secretion and characterized by heat intolerance, anxiety, and weight loss.

Hypoglycemia: insufficient blood glucose levels.

Hypoparathyroidism: endocrine disorder of the parathyroid glands, caused by decreased or ineffective use of parathyroid hormone and characterized by neuromuscular irritability and increased deep tendon reflexes.

Hypospadias: congenital opening of the urethral meatus on the ventral surface of the penis.

Hypothyroidism: endocrine disorder of the thyroid gland, caused by deficient or ineffective thyroid hormone levels and characterized by fatigue, dry skin, and facial puffiness.

Hypoxia: oxygen deficiency caused by a reduced oxygen-carrying capacity of the blood (as seen in anemia), insufficient oxygen in inspired air (as at high altitudes or in heavily polluted areas), impaired tissue use of oxygen (as in edema in an arm or leg), or a blood flow inadequate to transport oxygen (as in shock).

Illness: impairment of an individual's ability to adapt to internal and external environmental stressors. Stressors can be biological, such as bacterial infection; psychological, such as anxiety; or social, such as family problems.

Immunity: ability to resist or overcome disease-carrying microorganisms or the toxic effects of other antigens.

Immunodeficiency disease: disorder reflecting impairment of one or more immunity mechanisms.

Immunoglobulin: antibody, one of a class of proteins that interacts specifically with antigens, usually at the cell surface.

Immunoproliferative disease: disorder characterized by abnormal proliferation of cells that normally provide immunity, such as leukocytes and lymphocytes.

Immunosuppression: induced suppression of the immune response by such agents as radiation or drugs.

Implementation: fourth step in the nursing process; nursing actions that carry out interventions described in the nursing care plan.

Incontinence: inability to control urination or defecation. Urinary incontinence may result from infection, a spinal cord lesion, or a sphincter injury. Coughing, sneezing, or heavy lifting may trigger stress incontinence.

Indirect (mediate) percussion: percussion performed by striking a finger of one hand against a finger of the other hand, which is placed over an organ.

Insomnia: disorder of initiating and maintaining sleep, which may be transient (if less than 3 weeks in duration) or chronic (if longer).

Inspection: physical assessment technique in which the examiner uses sight, hearing, and smell to make informed observations.

continued

Master glossary continued

Intertrigo: erythematous irritation involving the skin folds, such as the axillae, the folds underneath the breasts, or the inner thighs.

Interventions: actions that the nurse uses to implement the care plan; may be independent (those the nurse can carry out alone, using acquired knowledge and skills), interdependent (those that the nurse performs in collaboration with other professionals), or dependent (those requiring a physician's order).

Involution: gradual reduction in size of the uterus after delivery.

Iris (target lesions): bull's-eye pattern; characteristic of some round, raised bullae.

Ischemia: decreased blood supply to a body organ or tissue, which interferes with normal organ or tissue function.

Kilocalorie: standard unit of heat used in metabolic studies and used to express the energy value of food. One kilocalorie is the amount of heat it takes to raise the temperature of one kilogram of water one degree centigrade at atmospheric pressure. Also called a large calorie.

Kyphosis: exaggerated dorsal convexity of the thoracic spine.

Lactation: process of synthesis and secretion of breast milk during nourishment of an infant or child.

Lanugo: fine, downy body hair on the neonate, predominantly covering the face, shoulders, and back.

Leukocyte or white blood cell (WBC): cell that constitutes an important part of the body's defense and immune system. Leukocytes may be subdivided into two groups, granulocytes and agranulocytes, or into five cell types: neutrophils, eosinophils, basophils, monocytes, and lymphocytes.

Level of consciousness: degree of wakefulness and orientation. Wakefulness represents subcortical reticular system activity; orientation represents cerebral cortex activity.

Linea nigra: black line or discoloration of the abdomen running from the umbilicus to the pubis, typically developing in the third trimester of pregnancy.

Linear: in a straight line, as in linear skin lesions.

Localized: in one area only, as in localized skin lesions.

Lochia alba: yellow-white uterine discharge consisting mainly of plasma and white blood cells that appears after delivery, after the lochia serosa and continuing for about a week.

Lochia rubra: uterine discharge of blood, mucus, and tissue that occurs during the first 6 days after delivery.

Lochia serosa: brownish uterine discharge that appears after delivery, after the lochia rubra and continuing for 3 to 4 days.

Locus of control: person's perception of who or what controls life events. An individual with an internal locus of control believes that each person has the power to control events; an individual with an external locus of control believes that events occur through the power of others or by chance.

Low-density lipoproteins (LDLs): beta-lipoproteins derived from very low-density lipoproteins (VLDL), approximately 50% cholesterol by weight. LDL values correlate closely with the risk of coronary atherosclerosis.

Lymphadenopathy: lymph node condition characterized by hypertrophy or proliferation of lymphoid tissue.

Lymphocyte: mononuclear leukocyte produced chiefly by lymphoid tissue. The smallest of the white blood cells, lymphocytes give rise to T cells and B cells, which are instrumental in cell-mediated and humoral immunity, respectively.

Malocclusion: abnormal positioning of the upper and lower teeth that prevents correct jaw alignment and chewing.

Mammogram: breast X-ray.

Meconium: first feces of a neonate, greenish black to dark brown and of tarry consistency, normally passed within 24 to 48 hours after birth.

Megakaryocyte: large, multilobed bone marrow cell that releases thrombocytes (platelets).

Master glossary continued

Memory, recent: ability to store and retrieve information acquired minutes, hours, or days earlier.

Memory, remote: ability to store information and retrieve it months or years later.

Menarche: onset of menstrual periods, usually between ages 9 and 17.

Menopause: cessation of menstrual periods with the decline of cyclic hormonal production and function usually between ages 45 and 60 but may stop earlier in life, for example, as a result of illness or the surgical removal of the uterus or both ovaries.

Metabolism: complex process of chemical changes that determines the body's use of nutrients.

Milia: tiny white papules commonly occurring on a neonate's nose, cheeks, and chin, caused by unopened sebaceous glands.

Monocyte: mononuclear phagocytic leukocyte, the largest of the white blood cells. When monocytes enter peripheral tissues, they swell and transform into fixed cells called tissue macrophages.

Multiparity: condition of having two or more pregnancies that resulted in viable fetuses.

Murmur: vibrating, blowing, or rumbling noise that is longer than a heart sound and may be heard over any cardiac auscultatory site. It results from turbulent blood flow through the heart and may be pathologic or nonpathologic.

Myocardial infarction (MI): interruption of the local blood supply to part of the heart muscle that causes necrosis (death) of muscle tissue.

Myopia: refractive error resulting from eyeball elongation, which causes light rays entering the eye parallel to the optic axis to focus in front of the retina. Also called nearsightedness.

Narcolepsy: sleep disorder characterized by abnormal sleep tendencies and pathologic manifestations of rapid-eye-movement sleep.

Neuro check: brief assessment of several key indicators of nervous system functioning, including level of consciousness, pupil size and response, verbal responsiveness, extremity strength and movement, and vital signs; used for rapid, repeated observations to detect subtle changes in nervous system status.

Neurologic screening assessment: short examination of key nervous system functions, including level of consciousness, verbal responsiveness, brief mental status screening, motor system screening, and sensory system screening; used to gather baseline data and identify nervous system dysfunctions that need more detailed assessment.

Neuropathy: disease or disorder of a nerve.

Neutrophil: granulocyte with single, multilobed nucleus. Neutrophils account for 50% to 70% of circulating white blood cells and migrate to infection sites by diapedesis. They are phagocytic.

Nightmare: bad dream that does not cause arousal.

Night terrors: sudden, fearful partial arousal in Stage 3 or 4 sleep that the client cannot recall after awakening.

Nipple: pigmented spherical protuberant nub of erectile tissue surrounded by the areola on each breast. The lactiferous ducts (channels carrying milk from the breast lobes) open into the nipple.

Nipple inversion: in turning or depression of the central portion of the nipple.

Nocturia: excessive urine excretion at night; may stem from renal disease or excessive fluid consumption shortly before bedtime.

Nulliparity: condition of never having delivered a viable infant.

Nursing diagnosis: second step in the nursing process; the identification of actual or potential client health problems that nursing intervention can help resolve, diminish, or change.

continued

Master glossary continued

Nursing process: systematic problem-solving method organized into five consecutive steps—assessment, nursing diagnosis, planning, implementation, and evaluation.

Objective data: factual data, related to the client's problem, obtained by inspection, palpation, percussion, auscultation, and diagnostic tests.

Olfactory: pertaining to the sense of smell, a function of cranial nerve I.

Ophthalmia neonatorum: severe purulent conjunctivitis in the neonate.

Osmolality: osmotic pressure of a solution; expressed in milliosmols (mOsm), a unit of measure representing the concentration of particles in a solution per kilogram of water. Osmolality of body fluids ranges from 280 to 294 mOsm/kg.

Osteoporosis: bone condition resulting in loss of bone mass, although the mineral-to-matrix ratio remains normal; occurs most commonly in menopausal women.

Palpation: physical assessment technique in which the examiner uses the sense of touch to feel pulsations and vibrations or to locate body structures and assess their texture, size, consistency, mobility, and tenderness.

Palpebral fissures: openings between the eyelids.

Palpitations: sensation of pounding, racing, or skipped heartbeats; a common symptom of cardiovascular disease.

Panhypopituitarism: endocrine disorder of the pituitary gland, caused by decreased pituitary hormone secretion; characterized in children by retarded growth and in adults by decreased libido, extreme fatigue, and apathy.

Papanicolaou test (or smear): cytologic study of a cervical tissue sample, usually performed to detect cervical cancer.

Paralysis: loss of ability to move. Hemiplegia is paralysis of one side of the body and characteristically results from a brain injury, such as cerebrovascular accident (stroke). Paraplegia is paralysis of the lower extremities, and quadriplegia is paralysis of all four extremities. Both result from spinal cord damage, but at different levels.

Paraphimosis: abnormal condition in which a retracted prepuce cannot move back over the glans penis.

Paresis: weakness. Hemiparesis (weakness of one side of the body) usually results from a cerebrovascular accident.

Paresthesia: disturbance of sensation characterized by tingling, prickling, or numbness.

Pedunculated: on a stalk or stem, as in the cutaneous skin tags found in elderly clients.

Percussion: physical assessment technique in which the examiner taps on the skin surface with the fingers to assess the size, borders, and consistency of certain internal organs, and to detect and evaluate the amount of fluid in a body cavity.

Perfusion: passage of blood through vessels. Perfusion of the pulmonary circulation, for instance, allows for gas diffusion in the alveoli and capillaries.

Pericardial friction rub: a harsh, scratching, scraping, or creaking sound auscultated at the third left intercostal space that may occur throughout systole or diastole or both.

Peristalsis: contractions that move GI contents distally toward the large intestine.

Petechia: tiny, flat, round, red or purple spot on skin caused by minute submucosal or intradermal hemorrhage.

pH: hydrogen ion concentration, reflecting a solution's acidity or alkalinity on a scale of 1 to 14. Normal urine pH, for example, ranges from 4.5 to 8.0.

Phagocytic: pertaining to the process by which a cell engulfs and destroys foreign material; involves recognizing the material as foreign, engulfing it, and digesting it.

Pheochromocytoma: rare adrenal tumor that secretes excessive catecholamines at inappropriate times.

Phimosis: abnormal tightness of the prepuce preventing its retraction from the glans penis.

Pica: craving for and ingestion of substances not normally considered food, such as starch, dirt, clay, cornstarch, ashes, and plaster. Condition may be associated with pregnancy.

Master glossary continued

Planning: third step in the nursing process in which the nurse develops goals that focus on desired client outcomes; goals are documented on the care plan and continuously modified.

Plexor: device (such as a finger) used to tap a mediating device (pleximeter) or to tap the body directly during percussion.

Polydipsia: excessive thirst, characteristically accompanying diabetes mellitus.

Polyuria: excretion of an abnormally large urine volume; may result from diuretics, diabetes mellitus, diabetes insipidus, alcohol intake, or excessive fluid intake.

Premenstrual syndrome (PMS): a cyclic cluster of signs and symptoms, such as breast tenderness, fluid retention, and mood swings, usually occurring after ovulation and before or during menses; characterized by at least 7 symptom-free days, usually in the first half of the menstrual cycle.

Projectile vomiting: forceful vomiting that is propelled away from the body.

Proprioception: sense of position; the ability to know the position of a body part without having to look at it.

Psychosocial consideration: individual's ability to process past and present information to gain a realistic perspective of oneself, one's life, and others.

Puerperium: 6-week period after childbirth, during which the uterus and vagina return to their prepregnant state.

Pulse: rhythmic beating or vibrating movement produced by left ventricular blood ejection.

Pulse pressure: difference between the systolic and diastolic blood pressures, normally 30 to 50 mm Hg.

Pulsus alternans: abnormal pulse rhythm with regular alternation of weak and strong beats.

Pulsus biferiens: abnormal pulse rhythm with a strong upstroke, downstroke, and second upstroke during systole.

Pulsus bigeminus: abnormal pulse rhythm in which premature beats alternate with sinus beats.

Pulsus paradoxus or **paradoxical pulse:** abnormal pulse rhythm with markedly decreased amplitude during inspiration.

Range of motion: amount of movement measured in degrees of a circle through which a joint can be extended or flexed.

Rectocele: herniation of the rectum through the posterior vaginal wall.

Regurgitation: backward flow of blood through the heart across a valve that does not close completely.

Religion: organized, codified behaviors, rituals, and practices that reveal a person's faith and beliefs.

Respiratory excursion: palpation technique that evaluates symmetry of chest expansion. Asymmetry could indicate pneumothorax or pleural effusion on the side with reduced excursion.

Restating: paraphrasing or rewording another's idea without altering its original meaning.

Reticulocyte: immature red blood cell (RBC) characterized by a meshlike network. Released into circulation by the bone marrow, reticulocytes mature into RBCs in about 1 day. The reticulocyte release rate about equals the rate of RBC removal by the spleen, so the reticulocyte count reflects the blood cell activity rate in the bone marrow.

Retroflexed uterus: normal position of the uterus in which its corpus flexes toward the rectum at an acute angle.

Retroverted uterus: normal position of the uterus in which its corpus flexes toward the rectum, but at a less acute angle than if retroflexed.

Rhonchi: bubbling sounds produced by air passing through fluid-filled airways. Also called gurgles.

S_1 or **first heart sound:** normal heart sound that signals the beginning of systole; the *lub* of *lub-dub*.

S_2 or **second heart sound:** normal heart sound that signals the beginning of diastole; the *dub* of *lub-dub*.

S_3 or **ventricular gallop:** low-pitched extra heart sound auscultated in the tricuspid or mitral area during early to mid-diastole; caused by left ventricular failure associated with such disorders as myocardial infarction and mitral insufficiency.

continued

Master glossary continued

S₄ or atrial gallop: low-pitched extra heart sound auscultated in the tricuspid or mitral area late in diastole just before S_1; caused by such disorders as hypertension and aortic stenosis.

Self-concept: composite of ideas, feelings, and attitudes about one's identity, self-worth, capabilities, and limitations.

Semen: viscous secretion discharged during ejaculation, containing sperm and fluids produced by the prostate, bulbourethral, and other glands.

Sensorineural hearing loss: hearing loss caused by damage to inner ear structures, such as the organ of Corti, or by damage to cranial nerve VIII (the acoustic nerve). Also called nerve deafness.

Septal defect: defect or opening in the wall separating two heart chambers.

Sign: objective finding perceived by an examiner, such as a fever or a rash. Many signs can accompany symptoms: for example, a skin rash is one sign that can accompany itching (a symptom).

Sleep apnea, central: serious disorder of excessive daytime sleepiness characterized by an absence of airflow through the nose and mouth and by an absence of inspiratory effort during sleep.

Sleep apnea, mixed: serious disorder of excessive daytime sleepiness characterized by central and obstructive sleep apnea.

Sleep apnea, obstructive: serious disorder of excessive daytime sleepiness characterized by a collapsed upper airway resulting in no airflow despite respiratory efforts during sleep.

Snap: high-pitched abnormal heart sound auscultated medial to the apex along the lower left sternal border just after S_2.

Specific gravity: relative weight of a fluid compared to the weight of an equal amount of water, determined by the amount of solids in the fluid. For example, urine with a specific gravity of 1.010 is 1.010 times heavier than water.

Sperm: spermatozoa, the mature male sex or germ cells contained in semen.

Splitting: auscultation of a single heart sound as two separate sounds. Splitting can occur with S_1 or S_2 and may be normal or abnormal.

Stress: nonspecific physical response to a demand or stressor.

Striae: lines resulting from rapid or prolonged skin stretching.

Striae gravidarum: stretch marks; these pinkish white or red lines commonly appear on the breasts, abdomen, thighs, and buttocks during pregnancy.

Subjective data: data obtained from the client's description of the problem and recorded in the client's words.

Subluxation: partial or incomplete dislocation.

Symptom: indication of a disease or change in condition as perceived subjectively by the client; some may be confirmed objectively – for example, numbness of a body part may be proved by absence of response to a pinprick.

Syncope: dizziness, especially after changing positions; a common symptom of cardiovascular disease.

Syndrome of inappropriate antidiuretic hormone secretion (SIADH): endocrine disorder of the posterior lobe of the pituitary gland, caused by continued secretion of antidiuretic hormone (vasopressin) despite contrary regulatory signals.

Systole: period of ventricular contraction when the ventricles eject blood through the open aortic and pulmonic valves into the aorta and pulmonary artery.

Tactile fremitus: voice sounds palpated on the chest wall surface. Normally, the palpation of vibrations made by voice sounds decreases as the examiner's hands move from the center to the periphery of the lungs. Equal or increased tactile fremitus indicates consolidation.

T cell or T lymphocyte: thymic lymphocyte responsible for cell-mediated immunity.

Temporomandibular joint (TMJ): connecting point between the mandible and the temporal bone.

Master glossary continued

Thrombocyte or **platelet:** disk-shaped blood cell essential for coagulation. Formed in a megakaryocyte, thrombocytes are released in clumps into the blood, where they promote hemostasis.

Tinnitus: ringing or tinkling sound in one or both ears. Tinnitus may be caused by trauma, inner ear disease, ossification of the bones of the inner ear, aging, or cerumen pressing on the tympanic membrane or occluding the external auditory canal.

Transairway pressure: pressure gradient between the mouth and the alveolar spaces.

Turbinates: bony internal nasal walls.

Uremic frost: pale, frostlike deposit of white or yellow urate crystals on the skin. Sometimes accompanying renal failure and uremia, uremic frost forms when urea compounds and other metabolic waste products cannot be excreted by the kidneys into the urine and instead are excreted through small superficial capillaries to the skin.

Urinary catheter: hollow, flexible tube inserted through the urethral meatus into the bladder to drain urine.

Urinary frequency: abnormally frequent urination, or urge to urinate, without an increase in total daily urine output.

Urinary hesitancy: decrease in the force of the urine stream, commonly accompanied by difficulty starting the urine flow. It usually results from an obstruction or a stricture between the bladder and urethral meatus.

Urinary urgency: sudden powerful urge to urinate, commonly caused by urinary tract infection.

Uvula: small, cone-shaped mass that hangs from the soft palate and is composed of muscle and mucous membranes.

Vaginitis: inflammation of the vaginal mucosa.

Valvular insufficiency: inability of the heart valves to close properly, resulting in regurgitation (backward flow) of blood.

Valvular stenosis: narrowing or constriction of the heart valves that prevents them from opening properly.

Ventilation: gas movement and distribution into and out of the pulmonary airways.

Vernix caseosa: white, cheeselike, sebaceous deposit usually covering the just-born neonate.

Vertigo: sensation of movement of self or surroundings, caused by disease of the inner ear or the vestibular branch of the acoustic nerve.

Vestibular: pertaining to sense of equilibrium and balance, originating in the semicircular canals of the inner ear and mediated through cranial nerve VIII (acoustic).

Void: to eliminate waste matter from the body, as urination.

Wheezes: musical sounds of lower pitch than crackles, produced by air passing through narrowed airways.

Whispered pectoriloquy: increased voice resonance auscultated in the periphery of the lung. In whispered pectoriloquy, the words "one-two-three" sound clear over areas of consolidation but muffled over normal areas.

Index

i refers to an illustration; t refers to a table.

C

Ear assessment continued
physical examination and, 85-87
otoscopic examination
of external canal, 86i
of infant or toddler, 87i
insertion of otoscope, 86i
Economic function of family, assessment of, 13
Elderly clients, special considerations for, 26-27, 30
Endocrine disorders
laboratory studies to detect, 243-244t
nursing diagnosis categories for, 245
Endocrine system assessment, 234-246
health history and, 234-235, 238-240
physical examination and, 240-242, 244-245
SOAPIE documentation of, 245-246
Endocrine system glands, location of, 236-237i
Esophageal reflux, chest pain and, 120-121t
Esophageal spasm, chest pain and, 120-121t
Extraocular muscles, testing function of, 77-78
Eye, anatomy of, 74i
Eye assessment, 73-81
health history and, 73, 75-76
physical examination and, 76-81
conjunctivae, inspection of, 78-79i
cover-uncover test, 77i-78i
ophthalmoscopic examination, 80i
peripheral vision, testing of, 78i
SOAPIE documentation of, 87-88

F

Facial characteristics, assessment of, 28
Facial nerve
assessment of, 191t
origin of, 184i
Family, assessment of, 8, 12-13
Family responsibility activities, assessment of, 35
Fatigue, chronic, SOAPIE documentation of, 232-233
Female genitalia, anatomy of, 162i
Female reproductive system assessment, 161-173
health history and, 161, 163-166
physical examination and, 166-172
Bartholin's glands, palpation of, 166i
cervix, bimanual palpation of, 170i
cervix, inspection of, 167-168i
obtaining specimens, 168-169i, 169t
rectovaginal palpation, 172i
speculum, insertion of, 167i
urethra and Skene's glands, milking of, 166i
uterus, bimanual palpation of
assessing adnexal areas, 171i
assessing uterine position, 171i
assessing uterine size and shape, 171i
position of hands, 170i
vaginal tone, assessment of, 167i
vaginal wall, bimanual palpation of, 170i
SOAPIE documentation of, 172-173

i refers to an illustration; t refers to a table.

Murmur
auscultation of, 129-130
grading of, 130t
Muscles, assessment of, 204-205
Muscle strength
assessment of, 207-213
grading of, 206t
Musculoskeletal disorders
laboratory studies to detect, 214t
nursing diagnosis categories for, 215
Musculoskeletal system, anatomy of,
200-201i
Musculoskeletal system assessment,
199-215
health history and, 199, 202-204
physical examination and, 204-213
SOAPIE documentation of, 214-215
Myocardial infarction, chest pain and,
118-119t

N

Nails
anatomy of, 55i
assessment of, 55, 56-57, 61
NANDA taxonomy of nursing diag-
noses, 295-297
Nasal illuminator, 17
Near vision test, 77
Neck assessment. *See* Head and neck
assessment.
Neck pain, SOAPIE documentation of,
71-72
Neonatal assessment, 289-293

Neonatal reactivity, assessment findings
during periods of, 290t
Neonatal reflex assessment, 291t
Nervous system assessment, 182-198
health history and, 182, 185-187
physical examination and, 187-189,
192-197
cerebellar function, assessment of,
189, 192-193
point-to-point localization, 193i
rapid alternating movements,
193i
tandem gait walking, 192-193i
sensory system, assessment of,
194-195
extinction, 195i
number identification, 195i
proprioception, 194i
two-point discrimination, 195i
SOAPIE documentation of, 197-198
Neurologic disorders
laboratory studies to detect, 196t
nursing diagnosis categories for, 197
SOAPIE documentation of, 197-198
Nose assessment, 65, 68, 69
Nurse-client communication, 2-4
Nursing diagnosis categories
for blood disorders, 233
for breast disorders, 139
for cardiovascular disorders, 130
for ear disorders, 87
for endocrine disorders, 245
for eye disorders, 87
for gastrointestinal disorders, 150
for hair problems, 62
for head or neck disorders, 71

i refers to an illustration; t refers to a table.

i refers to an illustration; t refers to a table.